THE BIOCHEMISTRY
OF THE
REPRODUCTIVE YEARS

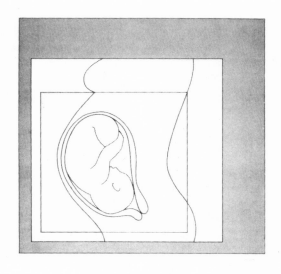

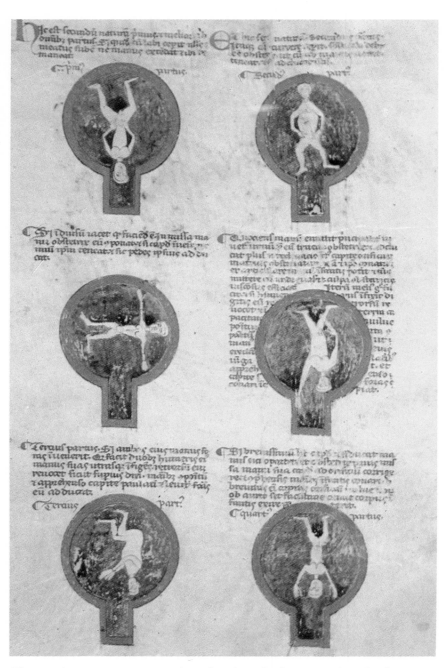

Thirteenth century representation of various fetal presentations in the uterus (ms. Lat. 161, folio 39 verso; courtesy of Bayerische Staatsbibliothek, München).

THE BIOCHEMISTRY OF THE REPRODUCTIVE YEARS

Proceedings of the Seventh Arnold O. Beckman
Conference in Clinical Chemistry

Edited by
Paige K. Besch

With a foreword by
Gerald R. Cooper

Co-Editors
Joseph W. Goldzieher
William E. Gibbons

Series Editor
Virginia S. Marcum

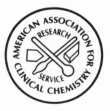

The American Association for Clinical Chemistry
1725 K Street, NW
Washington, DC 20006

Previous Proceedings of Arnold O. Beckman Conferences in Clinical
Chemistry, published by the American Association for Clinical
Chemistry:

1. Clinician and Chemist: The Relation of the Laboratory to the
   Physician
2. The Clinical Biochemistry of Cancer
3. Aging—Its Chemistry
4. Human Nutrition: Clinical and Biochemical Aspects
5. Genetic Disease: Diagnosis and Treatment
6. The Brain, Biochemistry, and Behavior

Library of Congress Cataloging in Publication Data

Arnold O. Beckman Conference in Clinical Chemistry (7th :
   1984 : Tucson, Ariz.)
   Biochemistry of the reproductive years.

   Conference held Jan. 1984 in Tucson, Ariz.
   Includes bibliographies and index.
   1. Generative organs, Female—Congresses.   2. Human
reproduction—Congresses.   3. Endocrine gynecology—
Congresses.   4. Contraception—Congresses.   5. Biological
chemistry—Congresses.   I. Besch, Paige K. (Paige Keith),
1931–   .   II. Gibbons, William E.
III. Goldzieher, Joseph W. (Joseph William), 1919–   .   IV. Title.
[DNLM: 1. Fertilization—congresses.   2. Infertility—
congresses.   3. Menopause—congresses.   4. Reproduction—
congresses. W3 AR719 7th 1948b / WQ 205 A757 1984b]

QP259.A76   1984   618   84–9171
ISBN 0–915274–24–8

Dedication

This book is dedicated to Griff T. Ross. Born July 17, 1920, in Mount Enterprise, Texas, he attended high school and college at Stephen F. Austin State University in Nacogdoches, graduate school at the University of Texas in Austin, and medical school at the Medical Branch in Galveston, Texas. After an internship at John Sealy Hospital, he returned to Mount Enterprise in 1946, where he succeeded his father in the practice of Family Medicine until called to active military duty in 1953.

After two years as a physician in the U.S. Air Force, Griff became a Fellow in Medicine of the Mayo Foundation at the Mayo Clinic in Rochester, Minnesota. Under the direction of R.C. Bahn, with advice and counsel of A. Albert, he completed requirements for a Ph.D., during which time his interest in reproductive biology and endocrinology developed.

After completing his residency in Internal Medicine, Griff was invited to join Roy Hertz and Mort Lipsett in the Endocrinology Branch of the National Cancer Institute. Research in reproductive biology at "The Branch," as it came to be called, flourished and attracted young scientists from all over the world for postgraduate training. These investigators developed radioligand-binding assays for gonadotropins and sex-steroid hormones and used these assays to determine concentrations of these hormones in biological fluids of normal persons and persons with disorders of gonadal function.

In addition to clinical studies, these scientists developed reagents for use in studying hormonal regulation of gonadal function in other mammals. Griff and his collaborators stimulated renewed interest in the role of sex-steroid hormones in regulating ovarian follicular growth, development, and differentiation in mammalian ovaries.

v

Because of these contributions to research in reproductive biology, Griff has received the Koch Medal of the Endocrine Society, the Hartmann Award of the Society for the Study of Reproduction, and honorary fellowships in the American Association of Obstetricians and Gynecologists and the American College of Obstetricians and Gynecologists. Other awards include an honorary Doctor of Science degree conferred by George Washington University, and distinguished alumnus awards from the University of Texas Medical Branch at Galveston, Stephen F. Austin State University, and the Mayo Foundation. He served as an associate editor of the *Journal of Clinical Endocrinology and Metabolism* and as a member of the Council, and subsequently as President, of the Endocrine Society.

In 1981, after 21 years at NIH, Griff retired from the Civil Service to return to Texas, where he spent several years as the associate dean of patient services at the University of Texas Medical School at Houston. Currently, he is devoting his energies as a member of the faculty to research and teaching in the Department of Obstetrics, Gynecology, and Reproductive Sciences. His return to Texas "closes the loop" on a life filled with the excitement of sharing the learning experience with students of reproductive biology and medicine, whose friendship he so greatly treasures.

Contents

Foreword: The Needs and Hopes for Scientific Facts about the Reproductive Years

Gerald R. Cooper

This conference is dedicated to the field of obstetrics and gynecology in the hope that it will enhance the well-being of women. Historically, more fantasy and emotion than scientific facts have been associated with women's problems. Many have been considered psychogenic rather than chemically based. Gradually, as research gives us a better understanding of the fundamental chemical reactions that occur in women during the reproductive years, we are recognizing that chemical deviations from the norm are the basis for many pathological conditions, disorders, and diseases. Chemistry offers facts and gives an understanding of sex-related medical disorders.

Scientists today are working more intensely on how to assure the well-being of women. All of us are interested in learning how to help women maintain excellent mental and physical health during their reproductive years and for the rest of their lives. Preventive measures are being considered as much as therapeutic measures, and the myth that women must suffer from menstrual problems is being expunged.

There is much we do not know about the reproductive years, but we have learned some basic scientific facts. For example, we have progressed greatly in our understanding of dysmenorrhea since the days when it was treated by fumigating the external genitalia with vapors of sweet wine, fennel seed and root, and rose oil; by burning a cone of wormwood on a slice of ginger on the abdomen; by applying suction cups to the breasts; or by removing the ovaries, either surgically or by radiation. Contemporary scientists, accepting the symptoms of dysmenorrhea as real and organic, have found that dysmenorrhea results from myometrial ischemia produced by highly intense contractions superimposed on increased basal tension of the uterus. These contractions are associated with changes in the concentrations and ratios of prostaglandins, changes in concentrations of endogenous opiates in the nervous system, and excesses or deficiencies in the concentrations and ratio of concentrations of certain hormones. Knowledge of the chemical reactions occurring with dysmenorrhea has helped us develop successful therapeutic measures for dealing with it.

Measurements of hormones in the clinical laboratory are highly useful, and are becoming more widely available because of improvements in analytical procedures. Measurements of progesterone can detect ovulation, defects of luteal phase, threatened abortion, and female infertility. Combined measurements of progesterone and estradiol can assess susceptibility to premenstrual syndrome, and measurements of progesterone and human choriogonadotropin can help diagnose ectopic pregnancies and pregnancies complicated by dysfunction of the corpus luteum. A battery of tests for progesterone, lutropin, follitropin, and estradiol will characterize the different phases of the menstrual cycle and can reflect the major steroidogenic reactions of the fetoplacental unit.

In addition, biochemical and immunological studies of normal pregnancy have contributed to our concepts about cancer. Normal pregnancy and cancer are two biological conditions that are tolerated by the intact immune system. Information about chemical changes in normal and abnormal pregnancies certainly has helped shape our thinking about sex-related cancers in women. Interestingly, both thyroid cancer, the cancer most likely to occur in women during their reproductive life, and breast cancer, the cancer most likely to occur during pregnancy, are metabolically influenced by pregnancy. Ovarian cancer is of great concern to physicians because it is difficult to detect early in nonpregnant women and is obscured during pregnancy by the enlarged uterus. Here, chemical profiles can aid ultrasonography in diagnosis.

Clinical chemists dream of the day when endocrinologic and immunologic profiles can be made available in the clinical laboratory with the analytical ease and low cost of current clinical chemistry profiles used for health evaluations. When this happens, we will have the potential to monitor the health of women during their reproductive years, detect subclinical disorders that pose harm to pregnant women, and uncover early cases of sex-related cancer. With such a battery, we could monitor during pregnancy the needs of the fetus, placental function, and maternal health.

At this conference, we hope to link clinical chemistry more closely with obstetrics and gynecology. Clinical chemistry is effective only if it serves helpfully in diagnosis and facilitates applied research for the various clinical disciplines of medicine. This conference presents an opportunity to discuss the latest physiological and clinical findings regarding the reproductive years. Scientific progress in this field is needed to continue improving the health of women, help physicians develop more effective therapy, and provide a means for controlling the world's serious overpopulation problems.

Preface

Just as the specialized endocrine laboratory developed in other areas of the hospital, so did the Ob/Gyn specialty lab surface outside of the main clinical laboratory. Indeed, it is still only with reluctance today that more assays associated with the reproductive years are slowly appearing in the main clinical laboratory. In general, practically all aspects of obstetrics and gynecology have been shrouded with misunderstanding throughout recorded history. A nineteenth-century incident illustrates the point well. Sir Simpson, a Scottish obstetrician, was violently opposed by members of the clergy when he proposed the use of ether for relief of pain during labor, for they argued from the Scripture ". . . in sorrow thou shalt bring forth children." A quick review of various cultural aspects of women's problems associated with the reproductive years should serve to introduce our conference.

As I have noted elsewhere,[1] as early as 2250 B.C., in the Code of Hammurabi, the medical profession in Babylon had advanced far enough in public esteem to be rewarded with adequate fees, carefully prescribed and regulated by law (the first example of socialized medicine). At that time, internal medicine was mainly concerned with endeavoring to cast out demons of disease. Inasmuch as women had always been considered the least important of mankind, and birth was construed as a natural process exhibited by all animals, little if any medical attention was directed toward obstetrics, although very stringent laws were written concerning women during their menstrual period, birth, and the puerperium—laws primarily concerned with isolating the women. The Babylo-

---

[1] Besch PK, Besch NF. Obstetric history, placental folklore, and neonatal models. In *The Neonate,* DS Young, JM Hicks, Eds., John Wiley & Sons, New York, NY, 1976, pp 3–26.

nians developed outstanding achievements in public hygiene, but they did little to attempt to understand personal hygiene related to birth.

Likewise, the Persians did little to advance obstetrics. In fact, they may have added to the misery of complicated childbirth by prohibiting incantations directed to the obstetrical patient. The main features of their approach were directed toward cult cleanliness, with particular ritual emphasis on the uncleanliness of menstruating women.

Closely connected with Mesopotamian medicine was the medicine of the Hebrews (600 B.C.). The ancient Hebrews were, in fact, the founders of prophylaxis and the high priests were true medical police. They had a definite code of ritual hygiene and cult cleanliness, gradually expanded from contact with different civilizations. The Book of Leviticus contains the sternest mandates about touching unclean objects, the proper food to be eaten, the purifying of women after childbirth, the hygiene of the menstrual periods, and many other sanctions relating to such matters as bestiality and other sexual perversions. During this period we find reference to professional midwives and particularly a striking reference to the obstetrical chair used in labor (Exod. 1:16), as Pharaoh commands the slaying of all Jewish infants of the male sex, "when ye do the office of a midwife to the Hebrew women, and see them upon the [labor] stools." Interestingly, the basic design, as seen in drawings and sculpture from 700 to 600 B.C., changed only slightly until the early nineteenth century A.D.

Very few other obstetrical and gynecological references are found—with the exception of cardiac shock in precipitate labor (1 Sam. 4:19), uniovular twins (Gen. 38:27), and gonorrhea and leukorrhea (Lev. 13:15). The Hebrews were aware of the existence of the cesarean section, but it is not clear whether they used it.

As the Hebrews attained the highest eminence in hygiene, so did the ancient Hindus excel all other nations of their time in operative surgery. However, in the earliest Sanskrit documents— the Rig-Veda (1500 B.C.) and the Atharva-Veda—we find the first fragmentary evidence relating to the placenta and remarks on obstetrics. The Hindus evidently connected the products of conception, the fetus and placenta, with copulation. Their documents also stated that the menstrual blood, absent during gestation, was stored in the body to form milk in the postpartum period. Included in an obstetrical chapter by the Susruta is an admirable section on infant hygiene and nutrition, unexcelled by anything before the time of Aurelius Celsus (50 B.C.–A.D. 7) or Soranus of Ephesus (A.D. 98–138). There we also find the first known reference to the retained placenta, with a warning that pressure should be externally applied; and if this is not successful in promoting its delivery, the patient is to be shaken; and if this is not successful, dropping the patient should be considered. Podalic version appears to have been practiced by the Hindus, but in a primitive manner.

As we move to the Middle Ages, again we find a lack of consideration for women's health. Only the insane were perhaps more deprived of medical attention than the woman with obstetrical or gynecological misfortune. Women's sicknesses were women's business. We have recently found a most delightful book, *Medieval Woman's Guide to Health, the First English Gynecological Handbook,* [2] by Beryl Rowland, a Professor of English at York University in Toronto, Canada. On facing pages are printed the manuscript (Sloane 2463, circa 1400 A.D.) and Professor Rowland's modern English translation. Although the identity of the original author is disputed, the work is ascribed to the legendary midwife of Salerno, Trotula, who was said to have had a two-mile line of mourners following her bier. This translation gives us a new and different perspective on the era and should be of intense interest to anyone wishing to gain an understanding of our past and perhaps a glimpse of the future. With the permission of Professor Rowland and her publisher, we have quoted from her book various statements that are closely related to the subjects considered by the speakers at this Seventh Annual Arnold O. Beckman Conference in Clinical Chemistry. As the authors and readers will concur, many of the problems discussed and described in Tucson today are the same as those discussed in the medieval era. We seem to have made only slight changes in resolving the persistent discomforts these problems cause, but no basic resolution of the causes—being either nature, God's will, or the evil deeds of man!

Only a long leap will span the distance from Trotula to Tucson

---

[2] Rowland B. *Medieval Woman's Guide to Health: The First English Gynecological Handbook.* The Kent State University Press, Kent, OH, 1981.

and the mid-twentieth century. Within the past two decades the universal acceptance of the value of the Pap smear has allowed great strides in dealing with gynecological cancer: we have seen extraordinary advances not only in the surgical skills of the gynecologist, but also in the early diagnosis of the disease and the life-giving treatment of the radiologist. These advances, coupled with some of the major breakthroughs in the areas receiving major attention at this conference, are indeed long leaps forward. We have tried to gather the major contributors to our knowledge over the past 20 years, in an attempt to present the most current and significant advances in all decades of reproductive life, so that we can extend our understanding of a woman's health problems throughout various ages of her life.

For a moment, consider the outstanding early experimental approaches to studies of the fetal-placental unit, as conducted by Professors K. Krantz and E. Diczfalusy.[3] This form of artificial placenta or extracorporeal perfusion apparatus could take over oxygenation, acid–base balance, and nutritional regulation, and provided very rewarding approaches to research, both in vivo and in vitro. Nonetheless, it never seemed to enjoy widespread acceptance by those concerned with "physiologically significant experimentation." Attitudes that came to predominate in the mid- and late 1960s led to the erosion and finally withdrawal of all support for this type of experiment, because many considered it to be another step toward the *Brave New World* of Aldous Huxley. By the beginning of the 1970s, these types of experiments completely disappeared from the medical literature. However, during this brief period of five to eight years, some very significant data were assembled.

Today we again face this same attitude with in vitro fertilization and embryo transfer. In the United States, the negative feeling toward use of fetal material, either in in vitro or even perhaps in vivo experiments, is the result of great suspicion and hostility from various groups. Allegedly our programs are four to five years behind the in vitro fertilization programs in England and Australia, as has been so often discussed in the lay press recently. In each succeeding decade some groups seem to become more obsessed with preventing support of use of any physiological material that

---

[3] Besch and Besch, *op. cit.*

relates to embryonic or fetal life. Could all of this only be a smokescreen for a much more fundamental reason? Is it that we are experiencing a return to the Dark Ages, with perhaps thoughts of experimenting with life, death, and the soul?

Paige K. Besch

Series Editor's Note: Throughout this book the names of various peptide hormones reflect the double system of nomenclature in current use. The American Association for Clinical Chemistry encourages use of the 1974 Recommendation of the IUPAC-IUB Commission on Biochemical Nomenclature, e.g., lutropin, follitropin, thyrotropin, choriogonadotropin, gonadoliberin or luliberin, folliberin, thyroliberin. The nomenclature adopted by the Endocrine Society and favored by most of the authors of the papers presented here is, respectively, human chorionic gonadotropin (hCG), luteinizing hormone (LH), follicle-stimulating hormone (FSH), thyroid-stimulating hormone (TSH), gonadotropin-releasing hormone (GnRH) or LH-releasing hormone (LHRH), FSH-releasing hormone (FSH-RH), and thyrotropin-releasing hormone (TRH).

Conference Participants

(1, speaker; 2, co-author; 3, session moderator)

Paige K. Besch, Ph.D.
Professor and Director
Reproductive Research Laboratory
Department of Obstetrics and Gynecology
Baylor College of Medicine
One Baylor Plaza
Houston, TX 77030

Veasy C. Buttram, Jr., M.D.[1]
Professor and Director
Division of Endocrinology-Fertility
Department of Obstetrics and Gynecology
Baylor College of Medicine
One Baylor Plaza
Houston, TX 77030

Robert J. Carpenter, Jr., M.D.[1]
Division of Maternal/Fetal Prenatal Diagnostic Center
Department of Obstetrics and Gynecology
Baylor College of Medicine
One Baylor Plaza
Houston, TX 77030

M. Linette Casey, Ph.D.[2]
Department of Obstetrics and Gynecology
University of Texas
Southwestern Medical School
5323 Harry Hines Blvd.
Dallas, TX 75235

Gerald R. Cooper, M.D., Ph.D.[3]
President, AACC, and
Research Medical Officer
Clinical Chemistry Division
Centers for Disease Control
Atlanta, GA 30333

Laurence M. Demers, Ph.D.[1]
Director, Clinical Chemistry
and Core Endocrine Laboratory
The Milton S. Hershey Medical Center
The Pennsylvania State University
Hershey, PA 17033

Giar Carlo DiRenzo, M.D.[2]
Department of Obstetrics and Gynecology
University of Texas
Southwestern Medical School
5323 Harry Hines Blvd.
Dallas, TX 75235

Melvin G. Dodson, M.D., Ph.D.[2]
Department of Obstetrics and Gynecology
Baylor College of Medicine
One Baylor Plaza
Houston, TX 77030

Karen Elkind-Hirsch, Ph.D.[1]
Department of Obstetrics and Gynecology
Baylor College of Medicine
One Baylor Plaza
Houston, TX 77030

Norman F. Gant, M.D.[1]
Department of Obstetrics and Gynecology
University of Texas
Southwestern Medical School
5323 Harry Hines Blvd.
Dallas, TX 75235

William E. Gibbons, M.D.[1,3]
Department of Obstetrics and Gynecology
Baylor College of Medicine
One Baylor Plaza
Houston, TX 77030

Joseph W. Goldzieher, M.D.[1,3]
Director, Endocrine and Metabolic Research
Department of Obstetrics and Gynecology
Baylor College of Medicine
One Baylor Plaza
Houston, TX 77030

James I. Heald, M.D., Ph.D.[2]
The M.S. Hershey Medical Center
The Pennsylvania State University
Hershey, PA 17033

Gary D. Hodgen, Ph.D.[1]
Scientific Director, The Jones Institute for Reproductive Medicine
Department of Obstetrics and Gynecology
Eastern Virginia Medical School
Norfolk, VA 23501
    Formerly Chief, Pregnancy Research Branch
    National Institute of Child Health and Human Development
    National Institutes of Health
    Bethesda, MD 20205

Bradley S. Hurst, M.D.[2]
Director of the Division of Reproductive Sciences
Department of Obstetrics, Gynecology, and Reproductive Sciences
University of Texas Medical School at Houston
Houston, TX 77030

John Johnston, Ph.D.[2]
Department of Obstetrics and Gynecology
University of Texas
Southwestern Medical School
5323 Harry Hines Blvd.
Dallas, TX 75235

Howard W. Jones, Jr., Ph.D.[1]
Department of Obstetrics and Gynecology
Eastern Virginia Medical College
Norfolk, VA 23507

Howard L. Judd, M.D.[1]
Department of Obstetrics and Gynecology
University of California Medical School
Center for the Health Sciences
Los Angeles, CA 90024

Daniel Kenigsberg, M.D.[2]
Pregnancy Research Branch
National Institute of Child Health and Human Development
National Institutes of Health
Bethesda, MD 20205

Rogerio A. Lobo, M.D.[1]
Department of Obstetrics and Gynecology
University of Southern California School of Medicine
Women's Hospital
1240 North Mission Road
Los Angeles, CA

Paul C. MacDonald, M.D.[2]
Department of Obstetrics and Gynecology
University of Texas
Southwestern Medical School
5323 Harry Hines Blvd.
Dallas, TX 75235

Richard P. Marrs, M.D.[1]
Department of Obstetrics and Gynecology
University of Southern California School of Medicine
Women's Hospital
Los Angeles, CA 90033

Murray D. Mitchell, Ph.D.[2]
Department of Obstetrics and Gynecology
University of Texas
Southwestern Medical School
5323 Harry Hines Blvd.
Dallas, TX 75235

William D. Odell, M.D., Ph.D.[1]
Professor & Chairman
School of Medicine
University of Utah
Salt Lake City, UT 84132

Takeshi Okazaki, Ph.D.[2]
Department of Obstetrics and Gynecology
University of Texas
Southwestern Medical School
5323 Harry Hines Blvd.
Dallas, TX 75235

Janice Okita, Ph.D.[2]
Department of Obstetrics and Gynecology
University of Texas
Southwestern Medical School
5323 Harry Hines Blvd.
Dallas, TX 75235

Griff T. Ross, M.D., Ph.D.[1]
Director, Division of Reproductive Sciences
Department of Obstetrics, Gynecology, and Reproductive Sciences
University of Texas Medical School at Houston
Houston, TX 77030

Norimasa Sagawa, M.D.[2]
Department of Obstetrics and Gynecology
University of Texas
Southwestern Medical School
5323 Harry Hines Blvd.
Dallas, TX 75235

Daniel Strickland, M.D.[2]
Department of Obstetrics and Gynecology
University of Texas
Southwestern Medical School
5323 Harry Hines Blvd.
Dallas, TX 75235

Joyce M. Vargyas, M.D.[2]
Department of Obstetrics and Gynecology
University of Southern California School of Medicine
Women's Hospital
Los Angeles, CA 90033

Attendees

John E. Adams
6701 North Charles St.
Towson, MD 21204

Nisar Ahmad
Central California Lab., Inc.
San Luis Obispo, CA 93401

Jagan Ahuja
485 Potrero Ave., B80
Sunnyvale, CA 94086

Sunil Anaokar
Dept. 90Y, Bldg. AP-8
Routes 137 & 43
North Chicago, IL 60064

Albert Anouna
173 Garfield Place
Maplewood, NJ 07040

A.A. Armstrong, Jr.
211 West 39
Scottsbluff, NE 69361

K. Owen Ash
Pathology Dept.
Univ. of Utah Med. Center
Salt Lake City. UT 84132

C. Dennis Ashby
BioScience Laboratories
Van Nuys, CA 91405

Donner F. Babcock
Oregon Health Sci. Univ.
Portland, OR 97201

Phillip R. Bach
CLMG, Inc., Clinical Lab.
Los Angeles, CA 90057–0990

Jannet Baldwin
10700 NE Sandy Blvd.
Portland, OR 97220

Edward W. Bermes, Jr.
Loyola Univ. Med. Center
Maywood, IL 60153

George Bernett
Bernett Labs.
Buena Park, CA 90620

Norma F. Besch
Dept. of Ob/Gyn
Baylor College of Med.
Houston, TX 77030

Lemuel Bowie
Evanston Hosp.
Evanston, IL 60201

John H. Brazinsky
24730 Summit Field Rd.
Carmel, CA 93923

Mary F. Burritt
Mayo Clinic
Rochester, MN 55905

James M. Byers
V.A. Medical Center
Lab. Service
Tucson, AZ 85723

Jacob A. Canick
Women & Infants Hosp.
Providence, RI 02908

Daniel W. Chan
Dept. of Lab. Med.
Johns Hopkins Hosp.
Baltimore, MD 21205

Allan G. Charles
6854 South Bennett Ave.
Chicago, IL 60649

Albert L. Chasson
Rex Hosp.
Raleigh, NC 27607

William L. Collinsworth
3800 Brookfield Ave.
Wilmington, DE 19803

George D. Comerci
Dept. of Pediatrics, Adolescent
   Med.
Arizona Health Sci. Center
Tucson, AZ 85724

Arlene J. Crowe
Hotel Dieu Hosp.
Kingston, Ontario
Canada K7L 346

Earl Damude, Editor
Canadian Clin. Lab.
McLean Hunter Bldg.
Toronto, Ontario
Canada M5W 1A7

Patrick Delaney
Natl. Family Planning &
   Reproductive Health Assoc.
Washington, DC 20005

James A. Demetriou
BioScience Labs.
Van Nuys, CA 91405

Sonya Dobberfuhl
11985 NW Oatfield Ct.
Portland, OR 97229

James C. Dohnal
Evanston Hosp.
Evanston, IL 60201

Philip G. Douglas
Amersham Corp.
Arlington Heights, IL 60005

John W. Dyminski
Paragon Diagnostics
Sunnyvale, CA 94089

Robert Earl
PathLab
El Paso, TX 79902

Ronald J. Elin
National Institutes of Health
Clin. Pathol. Dept.
Bethesda, MD 20205

Joseph R. Elliott
St. Luke's Hosp.
Kansas City, MO 64111

R.B. Fandino
408 North Sacaton
Casa Grande, AZ 85222

Victor S. Fang
Univ. of Chicago
Chicago, IL 60637

Iris Farries
415 Canterbury Place, SW
Calgary, Alberta
Canada T2W 2B6

Jeanne Feltner
Nuclear Med. Dept.
Miami Valley Hosp.
Dayton, OH 45409

Martin Fleisher
Memorial Sloan-Kettering
    Cancer Center
New York, NY 10021

Alfred H. Free
3752 E. Jackson Blvd.
Elkhart, IN 46516

Helen M. Free
3752 E. Jackson Blvd.
Elkhart, IN 46516

Donald Freeman
Sequoia Hosp. Lab.
Redwood City, CA 94062

Herbert A. Fritsche, Jr.
M.D. Anderson Hosp.
Dept. of Lab. Med.
Houston, TX 77030

Paul C. Fu
U.C.L.A. Harbor General Hosp.
Dept. of Pathol.
Torrance, CA 90509

A.K. Garg
Dept. of Pathol.
Royal Columbia Hosp.
New Westminister, BC
Canada V3L 3W7

Patricia E. Garrett
Dept. of Lab. Med.
Lahey Clinic
Burlington, MA 01805

George L. Gaunt, Jr.
Center for Reproductive Med.
Charlotte, NC 28207

Robert L. Habig
Duke Med. Center
Durham, NC 27710

Peggy Giddings
KUAT-TV
Tucson, AZ 85724

Bill H. Haden
Beckman Instruments
Carlsbad, CA 92008

Jerry B. Gin
Strategic Planning/Advance
  Systems
Palo Alto, CA 94304

C.E. Hagelberger
Riverside Hosp.
Newport News, VA 23601

C. Bradley Hager
Micromedic Systems, Inc.
Horsham, PA 19044

Janice Goldman
6767 W. Outer Drive
Detroit, MI 48235

Hans J. Hager
Hoffmann-La Roche, Inc.
Nutley, NJ 07110

Barbara M. Goldsmith
Children's Hosp. Natl. Med.
  Center
Dept. of Lab. Med.
Washington, DC 20010

Mary Hager
3303 52nd St., SE
Grand Rapids, MI 49508

Harold J. Grady
Baptist Med. Center
Kansas City, MO 64131

Ellen Hale
Gannett News Service
Washington, DC 20044

Stanley Grand
2040 Wellington Ct.
Westbury, NY 11590

Patricia W. Heisman
52 Talister Ct.
Baltimore, MD 21237

D.E. Greer
7840 East Broadway
Tucson, AZ 85710

Rozanne Heydenburg
736 36th St., SW
Wyoming, MI 49509

Jocelyn M. Hicks
Children's Hosp. Natl. Med.
  Center
Washington, DC 20010

Thomas J. Hockert
RIA Lab.
Mayo Clinic
Rochester, MN 55901

Earle W. Holmes
Loyola Univ. Med. Center
Clinical Labs.
Maywood, IL 60153

Green S. Hsueh
9346 Beckford Ave.
Northridge, CA 91324

Norman H. Huang
Dept. of Ob/Gyn
Baylor College of Med.
Houston, TX 77030

Robert D. Hume, Jr.
408 East Ute
Farmington, NM 87401

T. William Hutchens
Dept. of Ob/Gyn
Baylor College of Med.
Houston, TX 77030

V.T. Innanen
Div. of Clin. Chem.
Women's College Hosp.
Toronto, Ontario
Canada M5S 1B2

Nai-Siang Jiang
Endocrine Labs.
Mayo Clinic
Rochester, MN 55901

Jerome Johnson
Endo Lab.
Methodist Hosp.
Houston, TX 77030

Jean C. Joseph
Clinical Lab.
St. Mary Med. Center
Long Beach, CA 90813

Kimie Kagawa
Dept. of Pediatrics, Adolescent
  Med.
Arizona Health Sci. Center
Tucson, AZ 85724

Stephen E. Kahn
Loyola Univ. Med. Center
Maywood, IL 60153

John L. Kallmeyer
310 N. Wilmot
Tucson, AZ 85711

Raymond E. Karcher
32466 Chesterbrook
Farmington Hills, MI 48072

Terry Kenny
Univ. of Oregon
Health Sci. Center
Dept. of Clin. Pathol.
Portland, OR 97201

L.M. Killingsworth
Clin. Chem.
Sacred Heart Med. Center
Spokane, WA 99220

Jennifer Koehnen
Monoclonal Antibodies, Inc.
Mountain View, CA 94043

Gordon K. Korom
Dept. 93Y, Bldg. AP-8
Routes 137 & 43
North Chicago, IL 60064

Donna L. Kuzma
Gyn./Endocrinol. Lab.
Univ. of Wisconsin
Madison, WI 53704

Hans Laetz
KNST Radio
Tucson, AZ 85702–3068

Mitchell S. Laks
Clinical Labs.
Loyola Univ. Med. Center
Maywood, IL 60153

John C. Lankford
Monoclonal Antibodies, Inc.
Mountain View, CA 94043

Sharon Laska
Lab. Med.
Univ. Hosp.
Univ. of Washington
Seattle, WA 98195

V.A. Laxdal
Dept. of Pathol.
Univ. Hosp.
Saskatoon, Saskatchewan
Canada S7N 0X0

Janice LeCocq
Montgomery Securities
San Francisco, CA 94111

Daun Leffel
Clin. Pathol., AHSC
Tucson, AZ 85724

Theodore B. Leibman
27 Brayton St.
Englewood, NJ 07631

James W. Lohman
7878 E. Cloud Rd.
Tucson, AZ 85715

William J. Longley
Corning Medical
E. Walpole, MA 02032

James H. McBride
Clinical Labs.
UCLA Hosp. & Clinics
Los Angeles, CA 90024

P.A. Govinda Malya
Stuart Pharmaceuticals
Biomed. Research Dept.
Wilmington, DE 19897

Susan Maynard
1326 Carlton Ave.
Charlotte, NC 28203

Z.D. Meachum, Jr.
4603 Givens St.
Bossier City, LA 71111

John M. Meola
Clin. Chem. Dept.
Albany Med. Center Hosp.
Albany, NY 12208

Julie A. Miller
Science News
Washington, DC 20036

Diane Mohr
Boston Biomed. Consultants
Waltham, MA 02154

C. Roger Moritz
60 Wyoming St.
Dayton, OH 45409

Werner Mueller
691 N. Clinton Ave.
Lindenhurst, NY 11757

W.F. van Muyden
1207 Fairchild Center
Woodland, CA 95695

Karen L. Nickel
Diagnostic Products Corp.
Los Angeles, CA 90045

Leslie Nies
Serono Labs
Randolph, MA 02368

Carroll Oakley
4 Tricor Ave.
New Paltz, NY 12561

Richard T. O'Kell
St. Luke's Hosp.
Kansas City, MO 64111

Douglas R. Olson
Micromedic Systems, Inc.
Horsham, PA 19044

George Opar
Roche Diagnostic Systems
Belleville, NJ 07109

James B. Peter
Specialty Labs., Inc.
Los Angeles, CA 90025

John R. Petersen
675 McConnell Blvd.
St. Louis, MO 63134

David J. Pines
5652 Arborview Ct.
W. Bloomfield, MI 48033

John D. Praither
American Med. Labs.—RIA
Fairfax, VA 22030

Roy F. Schall, Jr.
Organon Diagnostics, Inc.
Elmonte, CA 91731

Kathleen L. Provost
Corning Medical
Medfield, MA 02052

Michael Sheehan
Lab., Good Samaritan Hosp.
Portland, OR 97210

Allen L. Pusch
906 N. Spring Ave.
LaGrange Park, IL 60525

Charlotte E. Shideler
Wesley Med. Center
Dept. of Lab. Med.
Wichita, KS 67214

Robert Rej
Clin. Chem. Section
Center for Labs. and Research
New York State Dept. of Health
Albany, NY 12201

Howard J. Sloane
Savant
Fullerton, CA 92634

Gail Rodrick-Highberg
Monoclonal Antibodies, Inc.
Mountain View, CA 94043

Mike Spiekerman
Scott and White Clinic
Temple, TX 76508

Thomas G. Rosano
Clin. Chem. Dept.
Albany Med. Center Hosp.
Albany, NY 12208

Richard L. Stouffer
Dept. of Physiol.
Univ. of Arizona Health Sci.
  Center
Tucson, AZ 85724

Jean P. Safdy
Ames Division, Miles Labs., Inc.
Elkhart, IN 46515

Gary H. Stroy
Syva Company
Palo Alto, CA 94304

Edward A. Sasse
Pathol. Dept.
Med. College of Wisconsin
Milwaukee, WI 53226

Gary D. Sullivan
115 Appian Way
Vernon Hills, IL 60061

Nancy Sullivan
115 Appian Way
Vernon Hills, IL 60061

H. Fred Voss
Hana Biologics, Inc.
Berkeley, CA 94710

Patrik Swanljung
Vertrik Bioteknik AB
Altvagen 61
S-14200 Trangsund, Sweden

Chris Walker
Dept. of Pathol.
McMaster Univ. Med. Center
Hamilton, Ontario
Canada L8S 4J9

Robert Swanson
Oregon Health Sci. Univ.
Portland, OR 97201

Robert L.A. Walker
RD #1, Box 371
Northumberland, PA 17857

Vickie Thomas
3551 S. San Joaquin Rd.
Tucson, AZ 85746

Donald L. Warkentin
P.O. Box 1269
Summit, NJ 07901

Jeffrey C. Travis
Microanalytic Research, Inc.
Laguna Hills, CA 92653

Maxine Weiselberg
Rts. 137 & 43
AP6C Dept. 94B
North Chicago, IL 60064

Richard J. Tyhach
Ames Division, Miles Labs., Inc.
Elkhart, IN 46515

David Wenke
9115 Hague Rd,
Indianapolis, IN 46250

Anne S. Vanderbilt
Abbott Laboratories
N. Chicago, IL 60064

Tom Wiggans
Serono Labs
Randolph, MA 02368

Morton A. Vodian
Beckman Instruments
Carlsbad, CA 92008

Henry A. Wilkinson
Dept. of Pathol.
Box 32861
Charlotte, NC 28232

Rodney E. Willard
Dept. of Pathol. and Lab. Med.
Loma Linda Univ.
Loma Linda, CA 92354

Thomas Woloszyn
International Clin. Labs.
Nashville, TN 37203

Leonard T. Wilson
Hoffmann-La Roche
Belleville, NJ 07109

Donald S. Young
Mayo Clinic
Rochester, MN 55905

I

NORMAL PHYSIOLOGY

Greuanunces that women haue in bering of her children comyth in two maners, that is to say kyndely & unkyndely. Whan it is kyndelich, the chyld comyth forth within a xx^{ti} throwes or withyn tho twenty, & the child comyth in fourme as it shuld: first the heued & sithen the neck & with the armes & shulders & with his other membres fourmeabely as it shuld. And also in the seconde maner, the chyld comyth forth unkyndely, & that may be in 16 maners . . .

Sicknesses that women have bearing children are of two kinds, natural and unnatural. When it is natural, the child comes out in twenty pangs or within those twenty, and the child comes the way it should: first the head, and afterward the neck, and with the arms, shoulders, and other members properly as it should. In the second way, the child comes out unnaturally, and that may be in sixteen ways. . .

—ROWLAND, *MEDIEVAL WOMAN'S GUIDE TO HEALTH*, pp 122–123

Overview of the Reproductive Years: Biochemical Markers of the Ovulatory Follicle

Griff T. Ross and Bradley S. Hurst

Introduction

From the time of their appearance during fetal life until their disappearance after the menopause, growth is initiated in groups of extant ovarian follicles. The life cycle of these growing follicles terminates in the death of the oocyte in situ and the death or de-differentiation of other cellular components of each follicle complex. This process of growth and demise is referred to as atresia, or failure to perforate (ovulate). Atresia persists during each menstrual cycle from menarche to menopause. However, one growing follicle is chosen to rupture (ovulate) and extrude an oocyte potentially capable of undergoing fertilization, cleavage, and implantation to establish a pregnancy. For the follicles that ovulate, the cells remaining after ovulation differentiate to form a corpus luteum, whose secretions are required for establishing and maintaining pregnancy.

Ovulation and corpus luteum function being essential for fertility, understanding the events that transpire during selection of the ovulatory follicle may be important for regulating fertility during the reproductive years. To characterize the process, we propose to examine the biochemical markers of the events occurring in the ovaries before, during, and after the dominant follicle is chosen.

Biochemical markers of events occurring in the life cycle of the dominant follicle may be examined in at least three sites: blood (peripheral and ovarian venous blood), antral fluid, and the cells of the follicle complexes themselves. In examining the relevant literature to describe markers at each of these loci, we

3

will attempt to identify the conditions that must be fulfilled for identifying follicles destined to ovulate.

Markers in Peripheral and Ovarian Venous Blood

During spontaneous ovulatory cycles in normal women, changes in blood concentrations of gonadotropin and sex-steroid hormones reflect either the secretory activity of the dominant follicle or the regulatory effects of these secretions on hypothalamic–pituitary function. The latter alternative requires the pulsatile secretion of a hypophysiotropic hormone variously called gonadoliberin (gonadotropin-releasing hormone, GnRH) or luliberin (luteinizing hormone-releasing hormone, LHRH), secreted by the hypothalamus and acting upon pituitary cells to stimulate gonadotropin secretion. Whether ovarian sex-steroid hormones act exclusively on the pituitary to modulate responses to invariant frequencies and amplitudes of pulses of GnRH or, alternatively, act also at hypothalamic sites to modulate frequencies and amplitudes of GnRH release remains a matter of controversy. Suffice it to say that neither positive (stimulatory) nor negative (inhibitory) effects of sex-steroid hormones on gonadotropin secretion are apparent in the absence of pulses of GnRH.

What is the evidence that cyclic changes in the concentrations of gonadotropins and sex-steroid hormones in blood reflect the secretory activity of the dominant follicle? When methods for measuring concentrations of sex steroids in specimens of peripheral blood became sufficiently specific and sensitive, it became possible to compare the concentrations of these hormones in specimens of blood collected simultaneously from ovarian veins and from a peripheral vein. Moreover, it became possible to compare the concentrations of hormones in specimens of peripheral blood collected serially at short intervals before and after ablation of either the dominant follicle or the corpus luteum. Several studies (1–3) have established that the concentrations of estrone and estradiol in venous effluent from both ovaries are greater than those in peripheral blood (collected simultaneously) throughout the menstrual cycle. However, once a difference in size identifies the pre-ovulatory follicle, one finds that concentrations of both estrone and estradiol are higher in venous effluent from the ovary bearing that follicle. The same discrepancy prevails in the luteal

4

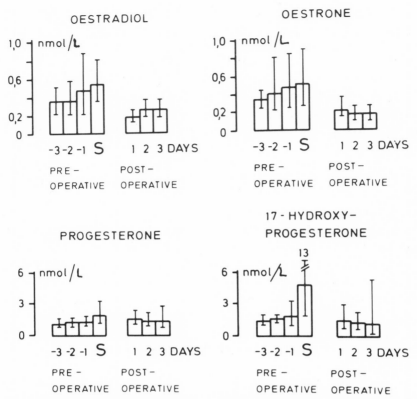

Fig. 1. Geometric means (and 95% confidence limits) of concentrations of steroids in peripheral venous blood collected from nine women on the days before (—) and after the day of surgical ablation (S) of the dominant follicle during the follicular phase of the cycle

Reproduced with permission of Aedo et al. (5)

phase, where concentrations of estrone and estradiol are higher in blood from the ovary containing the corpus luteum (3). These data are consistent with the conclusion that changing concentrations of estradiol reflect the secretory activity of the ovary containing the dominant follicle in the follicular phase and of the ovary containing the corpus luteum during the luteal phase. More recent studies, in both female rhesus monkeys and women (4–6), show that excision of the dominant follicle during the follicular phase decreases the concentrations of estradiol in peripheral blood (Figure 1), prevents the pre-ovulatory surge of lutropin (luteinizing hormone, LH), and initiates a new follicular phase that is followed by ovulation 12 to 14 days later. Similarly, excision of the corpus luteum is followed by a rapid decline in the concentrations of both progesterone and estradiol in peripheral blood and by the initiation of a new follicular phase followed by ovulation 12 to 14 days later. These data suggest not only that the dominant follicle complex and its successor, the corpus luteum, are the source of estradiol (and progesterone) but also that the dominant follicle is the "Zeitgeber" of the cycle in women and rhesus monkeys. In the context of this discussion, the concentrations of estradiol and progesterone in peripheral blood are biochemical markers of the functional status of the dominant follicle and the corpus luteum.

Serial sonographic ("ultrasound") measurements of the diameter of the dominant follicle, combined with simultaneous serial measurements of estradiol in peripheral blood, have made it possible to establish correlates of the two measurements during late follicular and peri-ovulatory periods of spontaneous cycles *(7–9)*. Results of one such study *(8)* are shown in Figure 2.

Markers in Antral Fluid

Antral fluid is a second site for examining biochemical markers of developing follicles, including the pre-ovulatory follicles. Because removing antral fluid terminates the life of a follicle, all such studies are "cross-sectional" in relation to time of sampling and size of follicle. The sources of antral fluid are follicles in ovarian tissue removed during pelvic survery for reasons unrelated to ovarian function, during surgical correction of mechanical obstruction to fallopian tubes, during elective tubal ligations for regulating fertility, and during aspiration of follicles to recover oocytes for in vitro fertilization and embryo transfer. The time in the menstrual cycle at which tissues have been harvested has been established with various degrees of precision, as based upon menstrual histories, measurements of hormone concentrations in blood, sonographic monitoring of follicle growth in spontaneous cycles, and timing studies related to use of choriogonadotropin to induce ovulation.

Given the terminal nature of this kind of study, researchers have established criteria for differentiating follicles destined to ovulate (e.g., "pre-ovulatory" or "ovulatory" or "healthy") from

6

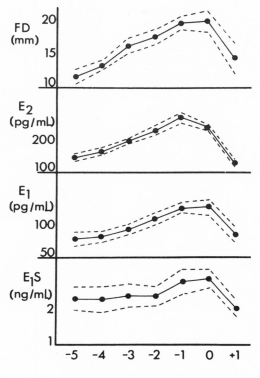

Fig. 2. Mean follicular diameter (FD) measured sonographically, and concentrations of estradiol (E_2), estrone (E_1), and estrone sulfate (E_1S) in peripheral blood on days before ($-$) and after ($+$) the surge of lutropin (LH) in 14 spontaneous ovulatory cycles in nine women

Dashed lines indicate $\pm$ SEM from the mean. Reproduced with permission from Fleming and Coutts '8)

follicles destined to undergo atresia ("pre-ovulatory healthy" or "nonovulatory" or "atretic") so that samples can be grouped for comparisons. These criteria include size (diameter), numbers of granulosa cells (10–12), pyknotic indices among granulosa cells (12), and status of the oocyte nucleus (11).

Excluding pre-ovulatory follicles harvested during the interval from the beginning of the lutropin surge until ovulation, the greatest numbers of granulosa cells in follicles 4 to 20 mm in diameter have been found in follicles in which the concentration of estradiol in antral fluid equaled or exceeded 200 ng/mL (Figure 3). More-

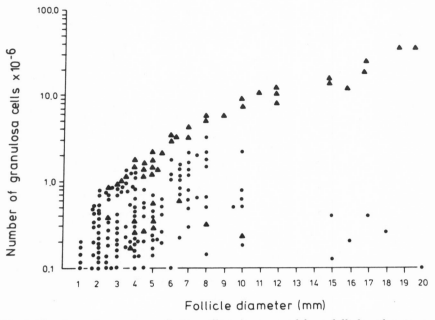

Fig. 3. Numbers of granulosa cells (in millions) recovered from follicles of various diameters

Estradiol concentrations in antral fluid were more than (▲) or less than (•) 200 ng/mL. Reproduced with permission from McNatty *(10)*

over, healthy oocytes are recovered more frequently from follicles in which the number of granulosa cells exceeded 50% of the maximal number found in follicles of a given size and in which the concentrations of estradiol were higher than average for that same consort. In follicles with maximal numbers of granulosa cells and greater estradiol content, the concentrations of progesterone tend to be higher as well.

During the interval between the onset of the lutropin surge and ovulation, the numbers of granulosa cells in pre-ovulatory follicles do not increase dramatically. In antral fluid the concentrations of estradiol decline and those of progesterone rise (Figure 4) *(12)*. It is not surprising then that high concentrations of progesterone and low concentrations of estradiol are found in antral fluid removed during aspiration of oocytes for in vitro fertilization, for which the timing of the aspiration is related to the onset of the lutropin surge in spontaneous cycles or to the administration of choriogonadotropin in induced cycles *(13)*. Given the decrease

8

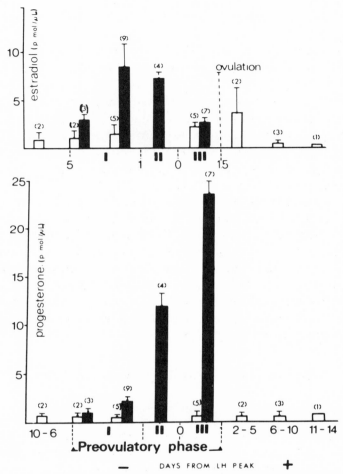

Fig. 4. Mean concentrations of estradiol and progesterone in antral fluid from ovulatory *(shaded bars)* and nonovulatory *(white bars)* follicles recovered before (−) and after (+) the day of the lutropin (LH) peak (0)

The pre-ovulatory phases are: **I,** from the beginning of the increase to the peak of the pre-ovulatory concentrations of estradiol; **II,** from the estrogen peak to the lutropin peak; and **III,** from the lutropin peak until ovulation. *Brackets* indicate the SEM; the numbers of observations are indicated in parentheses above each bar. Reproduced with permission of Bomsel-Helmreich et al. *(12)*

in the concentrations of estradiol in antral fluid during the 72 h preceding ovulation, progesterone concentrations in antral fluid may be a more reliable marker than estradiol for the quality of the oocyte.

What about the concentrations of androgens in antral fluid? The ratio of androgens to estrogens is lower in follicles having more than 50% of the maximal number of granulosa cells than in follicles having a lower percentage of granulosa cells. However, androgen concentrations do not change as dramatically as those of estrogens and progesterone during pre-ovulatory follicle growth. Indeed, during the last 72 h before ovulation, concentrations of both estrogens and androgens decline while progesterone concentrations rise (Figure 5) (14).

The data on the hormone composition of antral fluid suggest that the ability to accumulate high quantities of estradiol in antral fluid is a distinctive marker of follicles destined to ovulate. However, given that these concentrations of estradiol decline during the last 72 h before ovulation, while those of progesterone rise, one might speculate that earlier exposure to estradiol and follitropin (follicle-stimulating hormone, FSH) has programmed the luteal differentiation of granulosa cells reflected in the increase of progesterone during this period.

Markers in Cells of the Follicle Complex

Oocytes

Markers of follicular development might be expected to be predictors of oocyte maturation. In addition to completion of the first meiotic division with extrusion of an oocyte, fertilization and cleavage are markers of maturity of oocytes. These properties have been correlated with hormonal composition of antral fluid in a few studies of oocytes recovered for in vitro fertilization and embryo transfer. Carson et al. (15) found that fertilization, cleavage, and implantation correlated with high concentrations of estradiol (and progesterone) in antral fluid. More recently, Lobo et al. (16) and Fishel et al. (13) showed better correlation of these properties with progesterone concentrations in antral fluid. Considered in the light of oocyte recovery timed in relation to administration of choriogonadotropin, the concentrations of estradiol

10

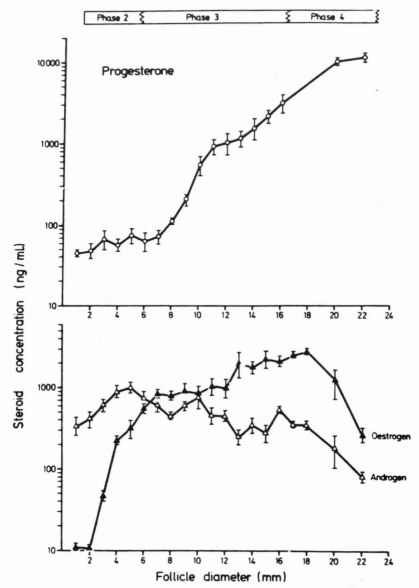

Fig. 5. Mean ± SEM concentrations of progesterone, estrogen (estradiol), and androgen (androstenedione plus testosterone) in antral fluids collected from follicles of various diameters

The pre-ovulatory phases are: *2*, for follicles enlarging from 1.0 to 5.0 mm; *3*, for follicles enlarging from 5.0 to ≥ 16 mm; and *4*, from the lutropin peak to ovulation. Reproduced with permission from McNatty *(14)*

11

might be expected to vary widely (primarily decreasing), whereas progesterone concentrations might be expected to be more uniform. Fishel et al. *(13)*, who found that fertilization occurred 90% of the time when progesterone concentrations were increased, suggested that the cause of failure should be sought elsewhere when oocytes from such an environment failed to be fertilized.

Granulosa and Theca Cells

The capacity of cells recovered from antral follicles to produce steroid hormone in vitro has been correlated with the hormonal composition of the antral fluid in the follicles from which the cells were recovered. Thus, McNatty et al. *(17)* showed that granulosa cells recovered from follicles with detectable immunoreactive follitropin, lutropin, and estradiol in the antral fluid secreted more progesterone in vitro than cells from follicles in which these hormones were below the limits of detection. Moreover, in vitro exposure of cells from these latter follicles to follitropin, lutropin, and estradiol stimulated progesterone production to quantities comparable with those of cells exposed to these hormone in vivo.

McNatty et al. *(18)* also measured the production of steroid hormones by cultured granulosa cells and theca cells recovered from healthy and atretic follicles, both <8 mm and ≥8 mm in diameter, recovered in early, middle, and late follicular phase or during the luteal phase of the cycle. Although all cells from all follicles recovered at all times were capable of de novo synthesis of progesterone, androstenedione, testosterone, dihydrotestosterone, estrone, and estradiol, differences in the relative amounts produced were related to follicle size, the time in the menstrual cycle at harvest, and the status of the follicle (healthy or atretic) from which the cells had been recovered. Granulosa cells from healthy follicles always secreted more estradiol than granulosa cells from atretic follicles; the latter consistently secreted more androstenedione than any other steroid. Theca cells also synthesized all these steroids de novo, but again, androstenedione was the major steroid secreted, irrespective of whether the theca cells were from healthy or atretic follicles.

Hillier et al. *(19)*, studying basal and follitropin-inducible estrogen synthetase (aromatase) activity in granulosa and thecal cells recovered from 11 ovaries removed during surgery for obstruction of fallopian tubes, found that these activities correlated with the concentrations of estrogen and androgen in antral fluid. As shown in Figure 6, the concentrations of estradiol and estrone in antral fluid were directly related to aromatase activity in vitro. Because the sum of the amounts of aromatizable androgen in antral fluid did not change with respect to aromatase activity, the ratio of aromatizable androgen to antral fluid estrogens (estradiol and estrone) was inversely related to the aromatase activity of the granulosa cells. This activity in granulosa cells was at least 700-fold that in theca cells from pre-ovulatory follicles. Cultures of granulosa cells from nonovulatory follicles recovered during the luteal phase had low basal aromatase activity, but this was increased seven- to 10-fold by addition of follitropin to the medium and incubation for 48 h.

Collectively, these studies suggest that acquisition of the capacity to aromatize androgens to estrogens is an early marker of the biochemical properties that distinguish the follicle destined to ovulate from its peers. Clearly, for human granulosa cells, like granulosa cells from ovaries of other species, this property depends upon sustained exposure to follitropin. Whether the granulosa cells or the theca cells, or both, contribute to the amounts of estrogen in peripheral blood remains to be determined. However, the increasing concentrations of estradiol in peripheral blood are apparently reliable indicators that one or more follicles are approaching ovulatory status in both spontaneous and induced ovulatory cycles.

In view of the apparent importance of intrafollicular estrogens in stimulating the proliferation of granulosa cells (20) and the essential role of follitropin in inducing estrogen synthesis, the mechanisms for partitioning follitropin among follicles become critical in the selection of an ovulatory follicle. Moreover, when the goal is to stimulate many follicles to mature simultaneously (e.g., in harvesting oocytes for in vitro fertilization and embryo transfer), methods for enhancing the exposure of follicles to follitropin might be useful.

An approach to therapeutic intervention requires some consideration of timing. When in their life cycle do ovulatory follicles acquire the capacity to aromatize? Alternatively, how long may this acquisition be delayed before the deficiency becomes irreversible? McNatty et al. (21), in careful studies with 12 ovaries, removed 215 follicles $\geq$ 1 mm in diameter during the luteal phase

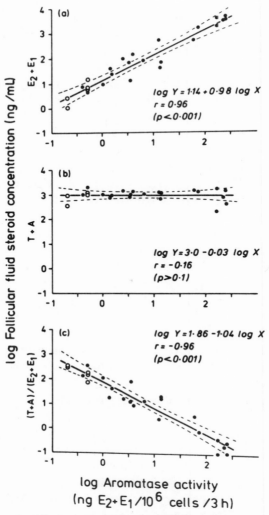

Fig. 6. Calculated best fits *(solid lines,* linear regression analysis) and 95% confidence intervals *(dashed lines)* for log concentrations of: estradiol (E_2) and estrone (E_1) *(upper panel),* testosterone (T) and androstenedione (A) *(middle panel),* and the ratio of these [(T + A)/(E_2 + E_1), *lower panel*] in antral fluid vs log aromatase activity in granulosa cells in vitro

○, values assigned to specimens in which the steroid concentrations were below the limits of detection of the assays used. Aromatase activity was measured by the production of estrone and estradiol. Reproduced with permission of Hillier et al. *(19)*

14

of the cycle. Using the criteria of numbers of granulosa cells and viability of the oocytes, they judged 202 (94%) of the follicles to be atretic. The mean number of normal follicles (<5 mm in diameter) per ovary did not vary significantly among ovaries obtained early, midway, and late in the luteal phase. Interestingly, they found no obvious differences between healthy and atretic follicles for estradiol concentrations in antral fluid. Moreover, the ratio of the total concentration of aromatizable androgens (androstenedione + testosterone) to the concentration of estradiol ranged from 74 to 384 (indicating low estradiol content) in luteal-phase follicles, in contrast to ratios of <1 in pre-ovulatory follicles sampled before the onset of the lutropin surge in the follicular phase. In terms of aromatase activity, granulosa cells from healthy follicles recovered during the luteal phase had 0.5% of the activity seen in the pre-ovulatory follicles. However, aromatase activity in granulosa cells recovered from follicles harvested during the luteal phase increased when follitropin was added to the medium. In summary, antral follicles ranging from 1.5 to 4.5 mm in diameter had low concentrations of antral fluid estradiol, and granulosa cells from these follicles had low aromatase activity in vitro. However, exposure to follitropin increased aromatase activity, which suggests that these follicles might be responsive to follitropin in vivo and thus might be potential ovulatory follicles. Apparently, exposure to follitropin in excess of the amount required for antrum formation per se, at about the time the antral follicle reaches a diameter of 5 mm, optimizes the likelihood that that follicle will be selected to ovulate. This exposure appears to occur in the late luteal or the early follicular phase of spontaneous cycles.

These observations are consistent with the demonstrated efficacy of administering clomiphene or exogenous gonadotropins, or both, beginning on the third to fifth day after onset of menses. The fact that menses is a marker of endometrial rather than ovarian events, however, probably accounts for some of the variance in numbers of mature oocytes harvested following these regimens.

Thus far, we have not considered nonsteroidal markers of follicular maturation. Various peptides that modulate the in vitro responses of follicular cells, particularly to gonadotropins, have been described (22). However, the roles of these substances under physiological conditions remain controversial.

Recently, the concentrations of some serum proteins in antral fluid have been correlated with outcomes of in vitro fertilization *(23)*. Here again, additional studies are required to validate initial observations.

Conclusions

At the outset, we proposed that understanding events transpiring during choice of the ovulatory follicle might be important for regulating fertility during the reproductive years. Superficial though it be, our understanding of hormonal regulation of follicle maturation and ovulation has already contributed to the successes of in vitro fertilization and embryo transfer.

However, pregnancies are achieved in only 20% of patients from whom oocytes are recovered. This rate is not entirely satisfactory for treatment of infertility related to tubal factors, and may well be less than might be expected if our understanding of the substances regulating oocyte maturation were better. Thus, DeCherney *(24)* noted in an epilogue to a thoughtful editorial, "How quaint that a 20% success rate was considered acceptable; that we were unaware of the repressor substances in follicular fluid which inhibited proper maturation which, once discovered, allowed for an 80% success rate." Important as the discovery of these noxious substances might be for successful pregnancies after in vitro fertilization, there are other applications that may be equally if not more important. For example, the ability to control inhibitors will indubitably be important in manipulations required for inserting information into pronuclei in the fertilized egg if the goals of gene therapy are to be realized. Furthermore, as Marrs et al. *(25)* have pointed out, information acquired during these investigations may facilitate therapies for other varieties of infertility.

Finally, investigations of the problem of fertility regulation can be extended to limiting fertility in otherwise healthy subjects throughout the world. Additional esthetically and ethically acceptable, reversible methods are needed if the problems of overpopulation are to be solved.

16

References

1. Mikhail G. Hormone secretion by the human ovaries. *Gynecol Invest* **1**, 5–20 (1970).
2. Lloyd CW, Lobotsky J, Baird DT, et al. Concentration of unconjugated estrogens, androgens and gestagens in ovarian and peripheral venous plasma of women: The normal menstrual cycle. *J Clin Endocrinol Metab* **32**, 155–166 (1971).
3. Baird DT, Fraser IS. Blood production and ovarian secretion rates of estradiol-17β and estrone in women throughout the menstrual cycle. *J Clin Endocrinol Metab* **38**, 1009–1017 (1974).
4. Goodman AL, Hodgen GD. Between-ovary interaction in the regulation of follicle growth, corpus luteum function, and gonadotropin secretion in the primate ovarian cycle. I. Effects of follicle cautery and hemiovariectomy during the follicular phase in cynomolgus monkeys. *Endocrinology* **104**, 1304–1309 (1979).
5. Aedo A-R, Pedersen SC, Diczfalusy E. Ovarian steroid secretion in normally menstruating women. I. The contribution of the developing follicle. *Acta Endocrinol (Copenhagen)* **95**, 212–221 (1980).
6. Nilsson L, Wikland M, Hamberger L. Recruitment of an ovulatory follicle in the human following follicle-ectomy and luteectomy. *Fertil Steril* **37**, 30–34 (1982).
7. Kerin JF, Edmonds DK, Warnes GM, et al. Morphological and functional relations of graafian follicle growth to ovulation in women using ultrasonic, laparoscopic and biochemical measurements. *Br J Obstet Gynaecol* **88**, 81–90 (1981).
8. Fleming R, Coutts JRT. Oestrogen levels during follicular maturation in women. In *Functional Morphology of the Human Ovary*, JRT Coutts, Ed., University Park Press, Baltimore, MD, 1981, pp 102–108.
9. Vargyas JM, Marrs RP, Kletzky OA, Mishell DR Jr. Correlation of ultrasonic measurements of ovarian size and serum estradiol levels in ovulatory patients following clomiphene citrate for in vitro fertilization. *Am J Obstet Gynecol* **144**, 569–573 (1982).
10. McNatty KP. Ovarian follicular development from the onset of luteal regression in sheep. In *Follicular Maturation and Ovulation*, R Rolland, EV van Hall, SG Hillier, KP McNatty, J Schoemaker, Eds., Excerpta Medica, Amsterdam, Holland, 1982, pp 1–18.
11. McNatty KP, Smith DM, Makris A, et al. The microenvironment of the human antral follicle: Interrelationships among the steroid levels in antral fluid, the population of granulosa cells, and the status of the oocyte in vivo and in vitro. *J Clin Endocrinol Metab* **49**, 851–860 (1979).

12. Bomsel-Helmreich O, Gougeon A, Thebault A, et al. Healthy and atretic human follicles in the preovulatory phase: Differences in evolution of follicular morphology and steroid content of follicular fluid. *J Clin Endocrinol Metab* **48,** 686–694 (1979).
13. Fishel SB, Edwards RG, Walters DE. Follicular steroids as a prognosticator of successful fertilization of human oocytes in vitro. *J Endocrinol* **99,** 335–344 (1983).
14. McNatty KP. Intraovarian aspects of follicular maturation in women. In *Biology of Relaxin and Its Role in the Human,* MK Bigazzi, FC Greenwood, F Gasparri, Eds., Excerpta Medica, Amsterdam-Oxford-Princeton, 1982, pp 247–260.
15. Carson RS, Trounson AO, Findlay JK. Successful fertilization of human oocytes in vitro: Concentration of estradiol-17β, progesterone, and androstenedione in the antral fluid of donor follicles. *J Clin Endocrinol Metab* **55,** 798–800 (1982).
16. Lobo RA, Vargyas JM, Marrs RP. Androgen levels in follicular fluid and its relationship to the maturity of the oocyte and its ability to be fertilized in vitro. *Fertil Steril* **40,** 412–413 (1983).
17. McNatty KP, Hunter WM, McNeilly AS, Sawers RS. Changes in the concentration of pituitary and steroid hormones in the follicular fluid of human graafian follicles throughout the menstrual cycle. *J Endocrinol* **64,** 555–571 (1975).
18. McNatty KP, Makris A, De Grazia C, et al. The production of progesterone, androgens, and estrogens by granulosa cells, theca tissue, and stromal tissue from human ovaries in vitro. *J Clin Endocrinol Metab* **49,** 687–699 (1979).
19. Hillier SG, Reichert LE Jr, van Hall EV. Control of the preovulatory follicular estrogen biosynthesis in the human ovary. *J Clin Endocrinol Metab* **52,** 847–856 (1981).
20. Ross GT, Lipsett MB. Hormonal correlates of normal and abnormal follicle growth after puberty in humans and other primates. *Clin Endocrinol Metab* **7,** 561–575 (1978).
21. McNatty KP, Hillier SG, van den Boogaard AM, et al. Follicular development during the luteal phase of the human menstrual cycle. *J Clin Endocrinol Metab* **56,** 1022–1031 (1983).
22. Weiss G (guest ed.). Reproductive peptides. *Semin Reprod Endocrinol* **1,** 269–365 (1983).
23. Nayudu PL, Lopata A, Leung PCS, Johnston WIH. Current problems in human in vitro fertilization and embryo implantation. *J Exp Zool* **228,** 203–213 (1983).
24. DeCherney AH. Doctored babies. *Fertil Steril* **40,** 724–727 (1983).
25. Marrs RP, Vargyas JM, Saito H, et al. Clinical applications of techniques used in human in vitro fertilization research. *Am J Obstet Gynecol* **146,** 477–481 (1983).

The Neurophysiological Role of Hypothalamic Hypophysiotropic Hormones in the Control of Reproductive Processes

Karen Elkind-Hirsch

Historical Perspective

The hypothesis that the control impulses from the hypothalamus are hormonally mediated by the anterior pituitary gland was launched 4½ decades ago. Early studies of the vasculature of the hypothalamic–hypophyseal portal system in birds and mammals included descriptions of a portal system in close contact with neurosecretory cells of the median eminence of the hypothalamus and draining to the anterior pituitary (1). However, it remained for the anatomist Geoffrey Harris to provide the necessary anatomical evidence on the vascular linkage of the hypothalamus to the pituitary that enabled him to postulate the "portal vessel–chemotransmitter hypothesis" (2). In a series of classic experiments, Harris and Jacobsohn (3) demonstrated the crucial role of the blood vessels of the pituitary stalk in adenohypophyseal regulation. According to the neurovascular concept formulated by Green and Harris (4), humoral mediators—later known as releasing factors and finally as releasing hormones—are poured into the proximal capillary plexus of the hypophyseal portal system from nerve endings in the median eminence. These specific "pituitary-regulatory" substances are then transported by the portal veins to the anterior pituitary gland, where they activate or inhibit release of pituitary hormones. A major concept was added to this by the Hungarian workers (5, 6), who demonstrated that a small region of the medial hypothalamus contains substances capable of maintaining the basal anterior pituitary structure and secretory function. The term "hypophysiotropic area" was coined by Halasz et al. *(6)* and applied to this half-moon-shaped region of the medial basal hypothalamus.

The involvement of the central nervous system in the control of gonadotropin secretion by neurohumoral mechanisms has been demonstrated experimentally by several methods. The evidence that established the fundamental importance of the hypothalamus and hypothalamo–hypophyseal portal vessels came mainly from experiments involving transection of the pituitary stalk, transplantation of the pituitary gland to a site remote from the sella turcica, or electrical stimulation of the hypothalamus *(2, 7, 8)*. In a classic experiment by Marshall and Verney *(9)*, an electrical current passed through the heads of estrous rabbits could elicit ovulation and pseudopregnancy. The realization that the hypothalamus contained substances capable of affecting pituitary activity naturally led to attempts to isolate and identify these neurohormones. The first demonstration of gonadotropin-releasing factor in hypothalamic extracts was made independently in 1960 by McCann et al. *(10)* and Harris *(11)*. However, 11 more years of intensive research by others, notably Schally *(12)* and Guilleman *(13)*, elapsed before this substance was conclusively characterized as a decapeptide and its effects were demonstrated.

Despite the suggestion of Schally et al. *(14)* that these hypothalamic substances controlling pituitary function be conventionally referred to as factors (F) if the activity of simple extracts of the hypothalamus were being studied, or as hormones (H) if their structures had been elucidated, there is no clear consensus regarding the terminology for gonadotropin-releasing hormone. This peptide has been referred to as LHRH, LHRF, LH/FSH RF (H), GnRH, luliberin, and gonadoliberin. With the detection of LHRH synthesis and receptors for this substance remote from the hypothalamus, it appears LHRH is truly a hormone and not just a factor. Some investigators still believe there is a separate follitropin (FSH)-releasing hormone and prefer to reserve the term LHRH to describe its most prominent effect, lutropin (LH) release. For consistency within this paper (and until this issue is more definitively resolved) I will use the abbreviated term LHRH, as adopted by the Endocrine Society.

Hypothalamic–Hypophyseal–Gonadal Relationships

As outlined above, it has become increasingly evident that a major component of endocrine regulation is a function of the brain and in particular, of the hypothalamus. In the human, the hypothalamus accounts for about 10 g of the 1200 to 1400 g of brain mass and is located at the base of the brain just above the point where the optic nerves converge to form the optic chiasma *(15)*. The median eminence, a specialized area of the hypothalamus located beneath the inferior portion of the third ventricle, forms the final common pathway for neurohumoral control of the anterior pituitary. The adenohypophysis receives few, if any, nerve fibers but is linked to the median eminence area of the hypothalamus by a highly specialized portal vascular system, from which it receives its entire blood supply *(15, 16)*. Ramifying in the interstitial space of the median eminence are the nerve endings of the "tuberohypophyseal" or "tuberoinfundibular" neurons, i.e., neurons arising in the hypophysiotropic area of the medial basal hypothalamus, which terminate directly on the capillaries of the portal vessels *(16)*. These "peptidergic" neurons act as "neuroendocrine transducers" to modify the neural inputs from different brain areas into neurochemical commands that turn on or off the secretion of the different hormones from the anterior pituitary. The tuberohypophyseal neurons are believed to synthesize, transport, and release the regulatory factors from the hypothalamus that control hormone secretion by the anterior pituitary. The term "stalk–median eminence," now widely used in neuroendocrinology, includes the median eminence and the upper part of the neural stalk; together these make up the contact zone between the endings of the hypophysiotropic neurons and the capillaries of the hypophyseal portal circulation *(17)*. The median eminence and upper stalk have distinctive ependymal cells, capillary structures, and interstitial spaces, thus providing a functional definition in addition to the gross appearance.

The hypothalamus as well as the gonadal steroids are now well established to be of major importance in regulating the secretion of the gonadotropins, LH and FSH, from the anterior pituitary gland. The mechanism of this regulation is extremely complex. It now appears that gonadotropin secretion is controlled by the interaction of the sex steroids and a single hypothalamic hormone capable of releasing LH, FSH, or both, depending upon the circumstance (18) (Figure 1). The LH and FSH released act upon the gonads. The ovaries or testes secrete steroids, which act to block the release of LH and FSH by suppressing the endogenous secretion of hypothalamic LHRH (known as the long negative-feedback loop). There is a negative feedback of gonadal steroids to inhibit gonadotropins during most of the female cycle, but under certain circumstances, especially in small doses under physiological conditions during the estrous or the menstrual cycle, estrogen can stimulate the release of LH (and LHRH) or enhance the effect of the releasing hormone on the pituitary, thereby creating a condition of positive feedback (18, 19). The term "positive-feedback loop" is used to describe the stimulatory action of estradiol on gonadotropin secretion, largely to distinguish it from the negative feedback (inhibition) caused by the steroid. The direct action of the sex steroids on the pituitary has also been demonstrated by studies with tritiated estradiol, testosterone, and progesterone, which indicate that sensors (steroid receptor-binding sites?) sensitive to the long feedback loop of sex steroids that exist mainly in the hypothalamus also exist in the pituitary and may regulate secretion of LH and FSH (19). A short "internal" or "autofeedback" system has been described, in which the inhibitory activity is provided by LH and FSH themselves (20). In addition, electrophysiological evidence has been presented for feedback action of LHRH on arcuate neurons as well as on the short feedback loop of LH (21). Perhaps the brain contains receptors sensitive to the circulating concentrations of LHRH such that LHRH might directly regulate its own production through a so-called "ultrashort" feedback loop.

Existence of LH- and FSH-Releasing Hormone in the Hypothalamus

Isolation and Structure

Luteinizing hormone-releasing hormone (LHRH) was structurally isolated from porcine hypothalami in 1971 by Schally and his coworkers (12) in two successive purification steps (see ref. 22 and 23 for details). During purification, LHRH activity was

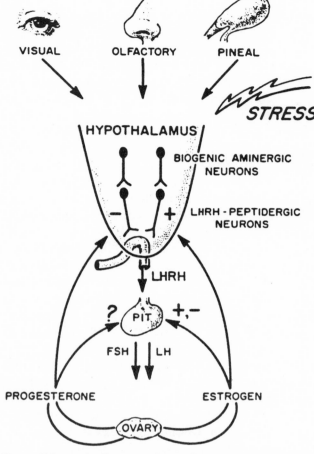

Fig. 1. Schematic diagram of gonadotropin-control systems
in women, showing the interaction of neural and hormonal
feedback

As shown, control of anterior pituitary function involves negative
as well as positive adenohypophyseal feedback circuits. Secretions
of the LHRH peptidergic neurons are in turn regulated by the bio-
genic-aminergic systems, through which a variety of nonhormonal
signals can influence reproductive function. Source: *51* (p 105), used
with permission

monitored by measuring the increase by bioassay or radioimmunoassay (RIA) of LH in plasma of ovariectomized rats pretreated
with estrogen and progesterone. FSH-releasing hormone (FSH-
RH) activity was determined in vitro by measuring by RIA the
stimulation of FSH release from isolated rat pituitaries *(18, 19)*.

The structure of LHRH was determined to be a simple linear decapeptide: (pyro) Glu-His-Trp-Ser-Tyr-Gly-Leu-Arg-Pro-Gly-NH$_2$.

Initially, two different substances (then called "releasing factors") were thought to be responsible for stimulating the secretion of LH and FSH. However, this belief came into question when highly pure porcine LHRH was shown to stimulate the release of LH and FSH in rats (14). Extensive in vivo and in vitro studies with purified LHRH showed that only one 10-amino-acid sequence needs to be present for the decapeptide to possess *both* LHRH and FSH-RH activity (14, 18, 19). Chemical and enzymic inactivation of LHRH was always accompanied by a loss of FSH-releasing activity; moreover, LHRH activity could not be separated from FSH-RH activity by the most advanced techniques of fractionation (24). In clinical studies, highly purified porcine LHRH caused the marked release of LH and FSH in men and women with normal pituitary function (18, 19). The observation that LHRH also possessed intrinsic FSH-releasing activity led Schally et al. (14) to propose that only one gonadotropin-releasing hormone exists, not two. This controversial suggestion has gained general acceptance because a separate FSH-RH has yet to be isolated, and because gonadotropin-hormone-releasing effects of hypothalamic extracts are blocked by antibody to the LHRH decapeptide. In addition, the synthetic decapeptide corresponding in molecular structure to native porcine hypothalamic LHRH possessed the same physiochemical and biological properties as the highly purified natural hormone; it released both LH and FSH in vivo and in vitro in animals, and its actions were indistinguishable from those of the natural hypothalamic LHRH (25). The synthetic decapeptide also caused a dose-related increase in circulating concentrations of LH and FSH in humans, further substantiating the view that natural LHRH and synthetic are identical. The peak values for FSH concentrations after LHRH injections are less than the peak LH values. In immature rats and humans, the peptide tends to produce greater FSH release than in adults (19, 26). The frequent discordant secretions of LH and FSH in various physiological and pathological states can be explained by variations in dose, time course, and steroid hormone interaction at the pituitary with only a single gonadotropin-releasing hormone (26). Furthermore, the pituitary-stimulating effects of LHRH are specifically restricted to changes in the secretion of gonadotropin hormones; none of the other anterior pituitary hormones are released in response to injection with this hypothalamic hormone (26).

Biological Properties of LHRH

LHRH stimulates the release of LH and FSH from the gonadotropic cells of the anterior pituitary in several animal species, including humans. Administration of synthetic LHRH to females increases release of LH and FSH, stimulates follicular maturation, and results in ovulation in many species tested (18, 19, 24, 26). In males, LHRH increases the release of LH and stimulates spermatogenesis and androgen secretion. Antisera to LHRH decrease the concentrations of LH and FSH in several species, produce gonadal atrophy in rabbits, delay vaginal opening in immature female rats, and decrease sperm production in male rats (18, 19, 24, 26).

Intravenous administration of as little as 250 to 625 pg of LHRH increases the concentration of LH in plasma of ovariectomized rats pretreated with estrogen and progesterone (25), the stimulation of FSH and LH release being related to the log dose of LHRH (within the range 1.5–13.8 ng/mL). In humans, LH release after intravenous, subcutaneous, or intramuscular administration of LHRH will peak within the first hour (18, 19, 26).

Further observations of ovariectomized rats pretreated with estrogen and progesterone indicated a lack of response to the FSH-releasing activity of synthetic LHRH administered in a rapid infusion. The FSH-releasing potency varied with the hormonal state of the animal and the frequency of LHRH injections (26). Presumably, less FSH than LH was released after administration of LHRH in vivo because of different affinities of pituitary LH- and FSH-secreting cells (gonadotrophs) to a single hypothalamic neurohormone (14, 26). The duration of exposure of pituitary gonadotrophs to LHRH appeared to be the most important factor in obtaining an increase in FSH in plasma, the rapidity of responsiveness to LHRH differing between the LH and FSH gonadotrophs.

The action of LHRH on a gonadotroph is presumably mediated by binding to highly specific receptors on the surface of the pituitary cells, with subsequent activation of cAMP (27). Apparently, pyroglutamic acid, histidine, and tryptophan (the first three amino acids of LHRH) determine the biological activity of the LHRH molecule, the second and third amino acids being critical for activating the adenylcyclase system with subsequent gonadotropin release. Pyroglutamic acid at position 1 and glycine in positions 6 and 10 are critical for maintaining conformation of the structure and its particular binding characteristics *(28)*. Pituitary responsiveness to LHRH might be altered by changes in the number of receptors for LHRH on the plasma membrane *(29)*. LHRH exerts a "self-priming effect"; that is, exposure of pituitaries to LHRH augments the response to additional exposure some 30 to 60 min later, but continuous exposure to LHRH decreases pituitary sensitivity to the peptide *(30)*. Finally, regarding the termination of LHRH action, the peptide is known to be internalized into gonadotrophs, where it is believed eventually to be degraded in the lysosomes *(29, 31)*. In addition, peptidases that degrade unbound LHRH are found in brain, pituitary, and blood; thus, the neurohormone can be degraded enzymically and subsequently excreted via the kidney *(31)*.

Apart from causing the rapid release of LH and FSH from the pituitary, some evidence indicates that the decapeptide also stimulates gonadotropin synthesis. LHRH added to cultures of anterior pituitary glands from rats increased the total content of LH and FSH in both tissues and medium, and led to increased incorporation of [^{3}H]glucosamine into the LH and FSH glucoproteins *(32)*. However, whereas the releasing hormone may control the cytological structure of the pituitary and the synthesis of tropic hormones, its most prominent effect is on their release.

Synthesis and Release of LHRH

An intimate balance between biosynthesis, degradation, and release of LHRH regulates the amount of releasing hormone secreted into the portal circulation, at least to the anterior pituitary. Changes in hypothalamic content of LHRH reflect concomitant alterations in synthesis, metabolism, or release of LHRH. The synthesis of peptides in the brain is apparently governed by the same general mechanisms as have been described for all polypeptide hormones, i.e., from post-translational proteolytic cleavage of larger precursor molecules that have little, if any, biological activity themselves *(33)*. It is highly likely that synthesis of LHRH occurs by a ribosomal mechanism. Studies by McKelvy et al. *(31)* show that not only does the incorporation of radiolabeled proline and tyrosine into LHRH take place primarily in cell fractions containing ribosomes but also this incorporation can be suppressed by puromycin and cyclohexamine, compounds known to inhibit ribosomal synthesis of protein.

Very little is known about the packaging and transport of LHRH in neurons. Perhaps it is packaged in the Golgi apparatus, with the resulting granules that contain LHRH being transported along the axon. The mechanisms for release of LHRH from nerve terminals in the median eminence have been studied in more detail. LHRH release from mediobasal hypothalamic fragments can be evoked by high concentrations of K^+ or by direct electrical stimulation. This enhanced release depends on the external concentration of Ca^{2+}, the effect of which is mediated through voltage-dependent calcium channels (34).

The activity of LHRH in the hypothalamus and pituitary can further be altered by stimuli that affect LHRH degradation. Brain peptidases not only generate bioactive LHRH in the median eminence but also, in concert with pituitary peptidases, degrade the peptide after it is secreted. Peptidases capable of degrading LHRH may also form part of the mechanisms involved in the hormonal feedback control of hypothalamic hormones. The hypothalamus and pituitary contain specific peptidases that metabolize LHRH, and their activity and (or) concentration are increased by estrogen or LH (35–37). Conversely, progesterone or gonadectomy decreases the activity of degradative enzymes (38, 39).

Now that LHRH has been synthesized, researchers have shown that nearly the complete decapeptide structure is essential for its activity. On the other hand, its activity can be increased by modifications that appear to slow the very rapid degradation of the molecule in the circulation (40). Reports of metabolic clearance rates for LHRH range from 1028 to 1640 ± 59.7 mL/min, and its half-life from 2 to 8 min (41, 42). The LH-releasing activity of the molecule is markedly enhanced by substituting for glycine in position 6 with D-leucine, D-alanine, or D-tryptophan; the L-isomers are less effective (28). One plausible explanation of the prolonged gonadotropin secretion these analogs cause is that the D-amino acid substitution increases the resistance of the peptide to enzymic degradation and thus prolongs its biologically active half-life. Other substitutions may increase its binding affinity, thus enhancing its potency above that of the natural product.

In addition to superactive LHRH agonists, various analogs that inhibit the release of LH and FSH have also been synthesized. Most of these antagonists are nonpeptides *(28)*.

Effect of Sex Steroids on LH and FSH Release

Negative- and positive-feedback effects. The influence of gonadal steroids on the release of gonadotropins may be both stimulatory and inhibitory, in part direct and exerted on the pituitary, and in part indirect and exerted by the hypothalamus. The concept of negative feedback proposes that the secretion of LH and FSH from the pituitary is inversely related to the concentrations of sex steroid (see Figure 1). Estrogen and progesterone can act on the hypothalamus and pituitary, or both, to further reduce the secretion of LH and FSH *(43)*. Very small doses of estrogen can inhibit the release of both gonadotropins, and larger or chronic administration of estrogen is even more effective. The inhibitory effects of progesterone are less spectacular than those of estrogens *(43)*. In ovariectomized rats, progesterone even in very large doses is a poor inhibitor of LH release, but given with estrogen it readily suppresses gonadotropin secretion *(43, 44)*. Pretreatment of male rats with testosterone propionate can also inhibit release of LH and FSH.

The sites of negative-feedback action remain controversial. Most workers believe that the ability to release gonadotropins in a pattern of ovulatory surge means that the hypothalamus–pituitary axis has a positive-feedback capacity; the exact site of positive-feedback receptor(s) is still under study, however. Estrogen appears to exert a negative-feedback effect on LH release, which is superseded by a positive-feedback effect when a higher concentration of estrogen is sustained for 36 h *(45)*. Nakai et al. *(46)* have demonstrated that these effects occur, at least in part, at the pituitary gland. Estradiol seems to be necessary for the increased responsiveness of the gonadotrophs to LHRH. The pituitary's response to LHRH varies throughout the estrous or menstrual cycle, being most sensitive at midcycle *(47, 48)*; however, estradiol may also exert positive- and negative-feedback effects at the hypothalamus or higher brain centers to modulate LHRH production *(43, 44)*. Most of the data from in vivo experiments suggest that progesterone acts principally at the hypothalamus, although some studies in rats and rabbits suggest that some of

28

its negative-feedback effects are exerted directly on the pituitary gland (49). Furthermore, at certain stages of the female cycle, estrogen and progesterone heighten the response of pituitary gonadotropins to LHRH. The action of progesterone depends on the previous exposure of the hypothalamic–pituitary complex to estrogen (45). The stimulatory effects of estrogen and progesterone are thought to result from direct actions of the steroid on the hypothalamus and anterior pituitary gland, although for its full effect progesterone may also require the integrity of connections of the hypothalamus with other areas of the brain (50).

Menstrual cycle. Under usual circumstances, women menstruate regularly at approximately 28-day intervals and ovulate on the 14th day of the cycle (51). The menses represent withdrawal bleeding, caused by loss of the endometrium-stimulating effects of 17β-estradiol and progesterone, the concentrations of which drop in plasma and are at their lowest level of the cycle. The characteristic pattern of hormone secretion during the cycle shows that during the first half (follicular stage) the follicle grows and matures under the predominant influence of FSH and some LH (Figure 2). Early in the follicular phase the ovarian hormonal secretion is modest, but toward the middle of the cycle a burst of estrogen (estradiol) is secreted, accompanied by an increase in 20α-progesterone (51). The spurt of estradiol appears to be crucial in triggering the neuroendocrine mechanisms that bring about ovulation (47). The pre-ovulatory discharge of LH is brought about by three mechanisms: the chronic exposure to estrogen appears, first, to sensitize the pituitary to LHRH and, second, to increase the secretion of LHRH; third, the initially released LHRH has a self-priming action (30, 45). The sum result is a massive discharge of LH, much more than needed to provoke ovulation.

At midcycle, a surge of LH secretion is responsible for ovulation. The function of the accompanying less-marked surge of FSH is not clearly defined (51). Although the pre-ovulatory secretion of estradiol is mainly responsible for triggering the release of LH, progesterone may also be needed for this response to occur. After ovulation, the developed egg leaves the ovary and the remaining follicular cells in the ovary, under the influence of LH, undergo luteinization—the conversion to a progesterone-secreting structure, the corpus luteum. The life history of the corpus luteum, which involutes after about 12 days of secretion, is largely deter-

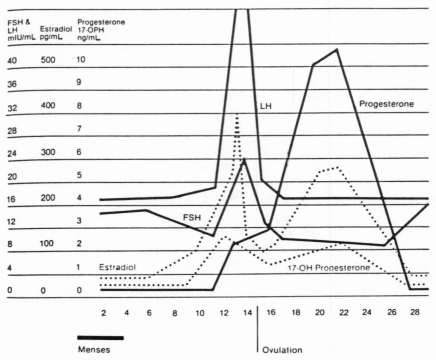

FSH & LH mIU/mL	Estradiol pg/mL	Progesterone 17-OPH ng/mL
40	500	10
36		9
32	400	8
28		7
24	300	6
20		5
16	200	4
12		3
8	100	2
4		1
0	0	0

LH

Progesterone

FSH

Estradiol

17-OH Progesterone

2 4 6 8 10 12 14 16 18 20 22 24 26 28

Menses

Ovulation

Fig. 2. Pattern of secretion of sex steroids and gonadotropins during the reproductive cycle in women

The crucial event for neuroendocrine control of ovulation is believed to be the trigger to hypothalamus and pituitary from the rising concentration of estrogen. Source: 96 (p 81), used with permission

mined genetically (51). The consequent decrease in the concentrations of estrogens and progesterone in plasma leads to withdrawal bleeding and the cycle begins again.

The crucial event for neuroendocrine control of ovulation is believed to be the trigger to the hypothalamus and pituitary from the increase in estradiol. Thus, in the normal cycle, the ovary signals its readiness to ovulate by secreting pre-ovulatory estrogen ["The clock is in the pelvis," states Knobil (52)]. Alterations in brain function that prevent normal LHRH responses at appropriate times can cause menstrual disturbance by interfering with LHRH secretion.

Localization of LHRH

Quite independently, McCann et al. *(10)* and Harris *(11)* demonstrated LH-releasing activity in extracts of the median eminence by using the ovarian ascorbic acid depletion assay of Parlow to measure LH released after injections of acid extracts of the stalk-median eminence. At the same time, similarly prepared extracts injected into the pituitary were shown to evoke ovulation. The bulk of this bioassayable activity resided in the infundibular stalk and median eminence; some was also found in the anterior basal hypothalamus and more rostrally in the regions of the pre-optic area and the suprachiasmatic nucleus. Further studies on the localization of LHRH by RIA with hypothalamic extracts have confirmed the localization data obtained by bioassay. In studies of serial sections of hypothalami in different planes, high concentrations of LHRH were localized in the retrochiasmatic, arcuate, and median eminence regions and in a prechiasmatic area that included the pre-optic and anterior hypothalamic region *(53, 54)* (Figure 3). Extracts of the medial basal hypothalamus and pre-optic area gave dose–response curves parallel to that of the synthetic peptide in the RIA, indicating that the activities of the extracts were immunologically similar to that of the decapeptide. Combining RIA and the hypothalamic nuclear "punch" techniques (in which tiny cylinders of brain tissue are punched out of frozen sections of brain and pooled for assay determinations), Palkovits et al. *(55)* and Kizer et al. *(56)* provided the first quantitative assessment of LHRH in discrete regions of the diencephalon and in several circumventricular organs of the brain, including the organum vasculosum of the lamina terminalis, a highly vascular structure at the top of the third ventricle in the pre-optic region that is also known as the supra-optic crest.

The availability of pure synthetic LHRH shed new light on this subject by enabling immunologists to produce antibodies to LHRH–protein complexes. These antisera to LHRH have been used primarily in two kinds of procedures to characterize the distribution of the decapeptide. In the first, as described above, the antisera are used in RIAs to quantify LHRH in microdissected brain regions. Immunoassays indicate that a similar compound is found in the hypothalamus, blood, and cerebrospinal fluid of

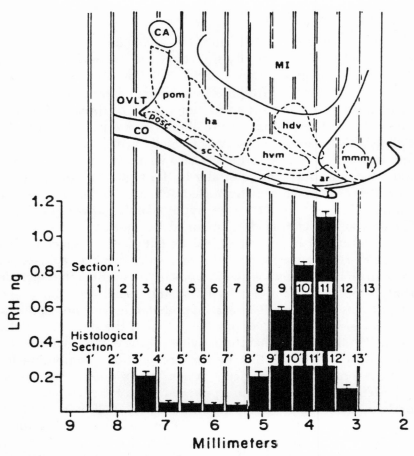

Fig. 3. A parasagittal section through the hypothalamic region of the rat; the actual content of immunoassayable LHRH contained in extracts of 400-μm-thick frontal sections is indicated on the *lower panel*

Note in particular the location of the organum vasculosum lamina terminalis (OVLT), the arcuate nucleus (ar) with overlying median eminence and pituitary stalk. Abbreviations for the remaining hypothalamic structures are as follows: ha, nucleus anterior (hypothalamus); hdv, nucleus dorsomedialis (hypothalamus); hvm, nucleus ventromedialis (hypothalamus); pom, nucleus pre-opticus medialis; posc, nucleus pre-opticus pars suprachiasmatic; mmm, nucleus mammillaris medialis pars medialis; sc, nucleus suprachiasmaticus; CA, commissura anterior; CO, chiasma opticum; MI, massa intermedia. Source: *54* (p 32), used with permission

humans; a breakdown product of LHRH is found in urine *(57)*. With the second procedure, utilizing antisera to LHRH for immunocytochemical analysis of LHRH in brain sections, one can determine the cellular profile of the intracellular compartment in which LHRH is stored—perikarya, dendrites, fibers in passage, or synaptic terminals.

The localization of LHRH by RIA has generally produced consistent results, but immunohistochemical studies to localize the perikarya responsible for the synthesis of the decapeptide are more controversial. Nonetheless, our understanding of LHRH-related neuroanatomy is directly related to steady improvements in the technology of visualizing by immunohistochemical methods the sites of LHRH localization in thin sections of brain tissue. The enormous loss of LHRH during tissue processing (e.g., by alcohol dehydration) has been minimized by the application of vibratome techniques *(58, 59)*, which do not require tissue embedding or exposure to freezing, heating, or organic solvents and have resulted in superior localization of most substrates. Recent modifications in immunocytochemical techniques such as examination of LHRH neurons in sagittal hypothalamic slices and use of well-controlled fixation time in organic solvents have increased sensitivity and improved the localization of LHRH-producing cell bodies in the brain *(58, 59)*.

Given the development of various fixatives and tissue-preparation techniques that preserve antigenicity (immunological activity), the selection of appropriate animal models, and the generation of antisera against different portions of the LHRH molecule, we can now describe the distribution of LHRH cells and their processes in several species, including humans—and a substantial number of studies have done so. Despite the variety of antisera and preparative procedures used in studying these species, there are some underlying consistencies. The distribution of LHRH-containing perikarya among species appears similar, the greatest number being present in an apparent continuum from the septal nuclei and diagonal band of Broca, through the pre-optic region, and extending into the anterior hypothalamic areas (see ref. *60* for a review). LHRH cells are present in the medial basal hypothalamus, i.e., in arcuate or infundibular nuclei, in numerous species, including humans (see ref. *60*). Perhaps the interspecies differences in the detectability of LHRH can be explained by differences in the processing of a precursor protein(s). The difficulty in localizing LHRH cells may result not only from different immunocytochemistry techniques or low concentrations of LHRH but also from the use of antisera with different antigenic properties. Moreover, if LHRH were bound within a larger protein, it might not interact with antibodies until uncovered by a local degrading enzyme. King et al. *(61)* have hypothesized that LHRH may be bound at the N or C terminus in a prohormone state in perikarya, whereas the LHRH found in fiber regions is the mature decapeptide. Alternatively, the immunoreactivity of the precursor may play a crucial role in the detection of cellular LHRH; such a protein may react with an antiserum directed against one portion of the neurohormone but not with other antisera directed against different portions. Chromatography of sheep hypothalamic extracts on Sephadex G-25 demonstrated three different molecular-mass species of immunoreactive LHRH *(62)*, additional evidence for the existence of a prohormone for LHRH that may be enzymically cleaved.

Regardless of the location within the central nervous system, LHRH neurons have now been shown to be small, generally fusiform or round (depending on the plane of section), and measuring 8 to 12 μm across the nucleus. Most of these cells have one or two dendrites; in the latter case, the dendrites extend from opposite poles of the perikaryon *(58–60)*. LHRH axons have also been made visible in cryostat or paraffin sections in numerous immunocytochemical studies. LHRH is seen as a brown precipitate in the immunoperoxidase system and as fluorescent granules in immunofluorescent preparations. High concentrations of the neurohormone have been seen repeatedly in the external zone of the median eminence, especially at its lateral angle *(60)*. Visualization of LHRH in granules within axon terminals close to the portal capillaries in the median eminence suggests that the releasing hormones are transported along the axons of the parvicellular nuclei and secreted directly into the hypophyseal portal blood vessels. The axons also project to the organum vasculosum of the lamina terminalis and more caudal structures *(58–60)*. In general, the reaction product for LHRH within the axons has a beaded appearance; whether this beading has a functional significance is not known at this time.

The LHRH activity in the rostal region overlying the optic chiasma can be related to the presence of cell bodies of LHRH neurons in this region, which has been demonstrated by immunocytochemical techniques (58–60). Localization of LHRH in the organum vasculosum of the lamina terminalis has led some to postulate that releasing hormone may be secreted from this vascular structure into the third ventricular cerebrospinal fluid and be carried to the base of the third ventricle, where it could be taken up by specialized ependymal cells known as tanycytes (16, 17). These tanycytes might transport the LHRH across the median eminence to the hypophyseal portal vessels for uptake and transport to the pituitary. However, morphological studies support only conjectures about LHRH release into the cerebrospinal fluid; the primary route is believed to be neuronal, by migration of LHRH from cell bodies, down the axons, to the median eminence, for release from axon terminals into portal vessels (60).

With the availability of pure hypothalamic hormones, immunoassays and immunohistochemical studies have been developed that demonstrate substantial amounts of different releasing hormones in hypothalamic and extrahypothalamic tissues. There are clear differences in the distribution of peptide-containing cell bodies in the brain. Some peptides, such as vasointestinal peptide, have their highest concentrations within cortical areas, whereas others, including the hypothalamic-releasing hormones (63), are present in highest concentrations in the hypothalamus. Some peptides are present in cell bodies that are restricted to one area of the central nervous system; e.g., LHRH is found, depending on the species, in the mediobasal hypothalamic or pre-optic area (or both). In contrast, some peptides appear to occur in multiple areas in cell bodies with short projection systems—e.g., substance P, thyroliberin, and somatostatin (63). Furthermore, the cellular distribution of LHRH in the brain does not appear to resemble closely the distribution of any other neuroactive substance localized so far (63).

Numerous reports (64–66) describe the concentrations of LHRH in plasma of several species. More recent studies indicate that antiserum specificity, affinity, and method of radioiodination can influence the amount of plasma LHRH detected. Attempts to reduce or eliminate nonspecific interference in plasma determinations by extracting LHRH with methanol or Florisil have had some success *(67, 68)*; however, the rapid degradation of LHRH in plasma necessitates use of a most sensitive assay.

Secretion Patterns of LHRH

In the course of validating an RIA for LH in rhesus monkeys over a decade ago, Dierschke et al. *(69)* observed abrupt pulsatile increases of LH that then declined exponentially with the half-life of this polypeptide in the monkey circulation. Shortly thereafter, a rhythmic pulsatile pattern of gonadotropin secretion was described in several other mammals, including humans *(70)*. The release of LH from the pituitaries of several species was found to be episodic, peaking at 20- to 60-min intervals *(70–72)*. This pattern was presumably induced by intermittent stimulation by the hypothalamic gonadotropin-releasing hormone (LHRH) released into the pituitary portal system in a similar intermittent pattern *(69)*, which suggested that the functioning of the hypophyseotropic control system that directs gonadotropin secretion was episodic rather than continuous. This view was strengthened by the subsequent direct observation of pulses of LHRH in the portal venous blood of rhesus monkeys, at rates that fluctuated with a frequency consonant with the circhoral mode of gonadotropin secretion *(73)*.

The physiological significance of this secretory pattern remained obscure until the recent findings of Knobil and coworkers *(46, 74, 75)*: Female monkeys with lesions of the arcuate nuclei that abolished endogenous LHRH production resumed their normal pituitary function when given an intermittent infusion of the synthetic decapeptide at a frequency of one pulse per hour, whereas continuous infusion of LHRH was incapable of re-establishing sustained secretion of gonadotropin. Furthermore, continuous infusion of LHRH inhibited the gonadotropin secretion that had been established by pulsatile administration, a situation that was reversed to the normal pattern of gonadotropin secretion when the regimen of pulsatile infusion was reinstated *(76)* (Figure 4). The influence of the pattern of hypophyseotropic stimulation is presumably related to the phenomenon of "desensitization" or "down regulation"; i.e., prolonged exposure to a high concentration of hormone in the extracellular fluid decreases the response of the target tissue. Knobil and Pohl *(74, 75)* theorized that an

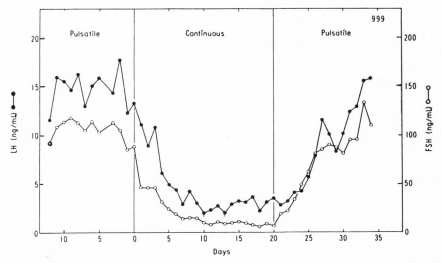

Fig. 4. Suppression of plasma LH and FSH concentrations in an ovariectomized monkey with a radiofrequency lesion in the hypothalamus after initiation on day 0 of a continuous LHRH infusion (1 μg/min)

Gonadotropin secretion had been reestablished by the intermittent (pulsatile) administration of the decapeptide (1 μg/min for 6 min once per hour). The inhibition of gonadotropin secretion was reversed after reinstitution of the intermittent mode of LHRH stimulation on day 20. Source: *76* (p 632), used with permission

intermittent presentation of hypophyseotropic hormone to the gonadotrophs permits the regeneration of receptors to LHRH, whereas the continuous mode of stimulation does not. Clinical support for the hypothesis comes from a recent study of Comite et al. *(77)*, in which the administration of a long-acting LHRH analog to girls with idiopathic precocious puberty suppressed the concentrations of gonadotropins and estradiol to values character- istic of prepubertal patterns. The daily administration of this long- acting LHRH agonist was suggested to desensitize the pituitary as the natural decapeptide did when given continuously. Subse- quent findings by Wildt et al. *(78)* in ovariectomized monkeys with arcuate nuclei lesions showed that small changes in the fre- quency of the administered LHRH pulses had profound qualita- tive and quantitative effects on the concentrations of LH and FSH in the blood and on the ratio of LH to FSH. Frequent pulses of LHRH provoked primarily release of LH; with more infrequent pulses, however, FSH appeared to predominate, perhaps in part

37

because of the longer half-life for disappearance of FSH from the circulation (Figure 5). The central importance of the neural mechanisms that generate the pulsatile release of LHRH into the pituitary portal circulation to control gonadal function in primates was demonstrated by the re-establishment of recurring ovulatory menstrual cycles of normal duration by a regimen of LHRH replacement, consisting of one pulse of the decapeptide (1 μg/min for 6 min) per hour by programmed infusion pumps for several months. In collaboration with M. Ferin and colleagues, Knobil et al. (79) obtained identical results in stalk-sectioned monkeys treated by the same LHRH-replacement regimen. Therefore, the intermittence of the neuroendocrine signal to the gonadotrophs is an essential component of the control system.

The biological importance of a particular mode of pulsatile release of LHRH for pubertal development was demonstrated by studies in which pulsatile administration of LHRH to immature female rhesus monkeys advanced the first ovulation and generated a pattern of hormone concentrations in serum that was indistinguishable from that seen during normal puberty (80). After discontinuation of the LHRH infusions, the animals reverted to their prepubertal state: the gonadotropins and ovarian hormones disappeared from plasma, and administration of estradiol failed to induce gonadotropin discharges. From this we can conclude that neither adenohypophyseal nor ovarian competence is limiting in the initiation of puberty in the rhesus monkey; rather, puberty is normally initiated by activating the hypothalamic mechanisms that control the circhoral pulsatile release of LHRH into the pituitary portal circulation.

Clinical Applications

Dynamic Testing with LHRH

The advent of solid-phase peptide synthesis of LHRH has permitted the rapid and economical synthesis of large amounts of the hypothalamic hormone for clinical use, and the availability of LHRH has led to the first direct evaluation of pituitary function. To differentiate among gonadal, pituitary, and hypothalamic causes of hypogonadism and to determine reserves of pituitary gonadotropins, 100 μg of LHRH is administered, and blood for

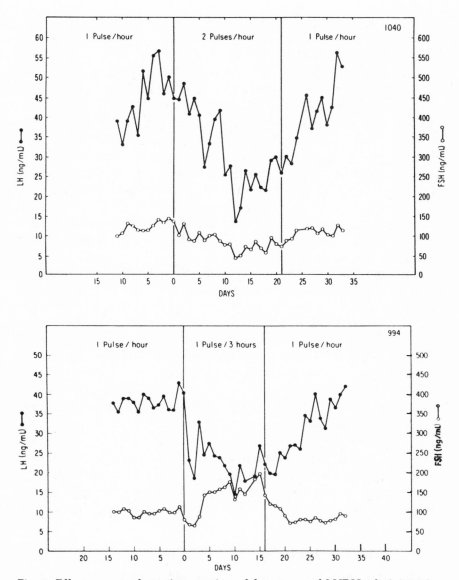

Fig. 5. Effect on gonadotropin secretion of frequency of LHRH administration

Top: LHRH pulses, 1 μg/min for 6 min, were increased from one per hour to two per hour on day 0. After reinstitution of the one pulse per hour frequency on day 21, LH and FSH concentrations gradually returned to control values. *Bottom:* reducing the frequency of pulsatile LHRH administration in a rhesus monkey with a hypothalamic lesion from one pulse per hour to one pulse every 3 h on day 0 led to a dramatic rise in FSH concentrations and a decrease in LH during the experimental period. Reinstitution of the standard frequency of one pulse per hour on day 16 reestablished the initial FSH and LH concentrations. Source: *78* [pp 379 (top) and 381 (bottom)], used with permission

determination of LH and FSH is collected 0, 30, and 60 min later. The maximal response occurs 30–60 min after injection. In a "normal" response, serum LH increases to at least 45 int. units/mL.

The value of LHRH as a diagnostic tool in clinical endocrinology is not as clear as was originally hoped. The initial studies with this test *(81)* showed that so-called "isolated gonadotropin deficiency" (in which patients show absent or partial puberty, no or low concentrations of circulating gonadotropin, no response to clomiphene, and no evidence of other pituitary hormonal deficiency) was due, in fact, to a hypothalamic defect with a LHRH deficiency rather than a defect in pituitary function, because these patients do show LH and FSH responses to LHRH. The few patients with this condition who do not respond after the first injection of LHRH do respond after repeated administration, which is additional evidence that the decapeptide can promote synthesis as well as release of LH and FSH. Further studies *(82)*, however, demonstrated that use of LHRH could not differentiate between acquired pituitary and hypothalamic dysfunction; primary gonadal failure could be differentiated, because it resulted in an exaggerated response, but LHRH increased circulating concentrations of LH or FSH in patients regardless of whether the primary cause of amenorrhea was at the pituitary or hypothalamus. About 15% of the individuals with pituitary tumors have a normal response to LHRH, whereas many of the individuals with "hypothalamic nutritional amenorrhea" have a blunted response *(83)*. Currently, the test may help corroborate other clinical and laboratory data, but it lacks adequate sensitivity and specificity for definitive diagnoses. However, the LHRH test is of considerable diagnostic value in the assessment of pituitary gonadotropin reserve in patients after transsphenoidal surgery and pituitary irradiation *(84)*.

Use of LHRH in Treatment of Infertility

The first report of stimulation of LH-release in humans by highly purified porcine LHRH was published in 1969 *(85)*. However, attempts to induce ovulation by a single intravenous injection of LHRH in women with secondary amenorrhea or in normal women on day 9 of the menstrual cycle were unsuccessful, in spite of significant increases of serum concentrations of LH and FSH *(86)*. Kastin et al. *(87)* reported the first conception after therapy with LHRH in 1971, but high-dose LHRH injections at infrequent intervals did not reliably induce ovulation. Investigators using constant infusion of LHRH failed to initiate and sustain follicular development and observed that the initial rise in LH and FSH was followed by persistently low values for serum FSH and LH. These findings in humans parallel observations with non-human primates *(88)* and other laboratory animals that continuous infusions of LHRH transiently increase circulatory concentrations of LH and FSH but decrease them as the infusion continues. Repeated injections of long-acting analogs of LHRH have also been used in attempts to induce ovulation, but with little success *(89, 90)*. The reason for these failures became clear when it was realized that *(a)* secretion of LH, FSH *(70)*, and LHRH *(73)* is pulsatile, and *(b)* for many polypeptide hormones, continuous infusion of high doses can desensitize (or down-regulate) the hormone action. Using these observations, Knobil and coworkers *(74–76)* demonstrated that in monkeys with arcuate nucleus lesions, the pulsatile administration of low doses of LHRH produced sustained increments in LH and FSH. They also demonstrated *(78)* that increasing the amplitude and (or) pulsation frequency of LHRH to supraphysiological values would decrease the circulating concentration of LH and FSH.

It is now apparent that with suitable regimens of intermittent LHRH therapy by subcutaneous injection, intranasal spray, or, preferably, by pulsatile mini-pumps to mimic the pulsatile surges of LHRH, ovulation can be induced in humans by the peptide and its analogs. Leyendecker et al. *(91)* first demonstrated the effectiveness of high-frequency pulsatile LHRH therapy in stimulating ovulation in women, and reported the successful treatment of patients having hypothalamic amenorrhea (Figure 6). Crowley and McArthur *(92)* subsequently demonstrated the potential of pulsatile LHRH therapy by the successful induction of ovulation in a patient with Kallmann's syndrome (hypothalamic hypogonadism). These findings have now been confirmed by numerous other investigators (see ref. *93* for recent review). Subsequent clinical trials have shown pulsatile LHRH therapy to be effective in inducing ovulation at pulses varying from 2.5 to 20 μg of LHRH, administered subcutaneously or intravenously, and at frequencies varying from 60 to 120 min *(93)*. The pulsatile administration of LHRH to women with hypothalamic amenorrhea has

41

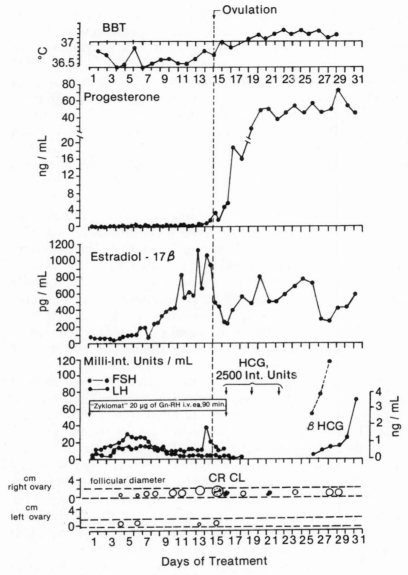

Fig. 6. Basal body temperature (BBT), follicular diameter, and serum concentrations of LH, FSH, choriogonadotropin (HCG) β-subunit, HCG-(- - -), estradiol-17β, and progesterone in patient P.S. during and after treatment with 20 μg of GHRH intravenously every 90 min over a period of 16 days by means of a portable pump (Zyklomat)

nd = not detectable; CR = corpus rubrum; CL = corpus luteum. Source: *91* (p 1215), used with permission

led to ovarian development, ovulation, and pregnancy in a significant number of cases.

In addition to inducing ovulation in anovulatory infertile women, pulsatile LHRH has also successfully induced pubertal gonadotropin changes and sexual development in men and women with delayed puberty subsequent to primary idiopathic hypogonadotropic hypogonadism *(94)*. In infertile men with Kallmann's syndrome, pulsatile LHRH therapy has effectively induced testosterone production and spermatogenesis *(95)*.

Although results of large clinical trials with pulsatile induction of ovulation and puberty have not yet been published, preliminary studies indicate that pulsatile therapy with low-dose LHRH is a promising advance in the treatment of both female and male infertility caused by gonadotropin deficiency.

References

1. Scharrer E, Scharrer B. Hormones produced by neurosecretory cells. *Recent Prog Horm Res* **10**, 183–240 (1954).
2. Harris GW. *Neural Control of the Pituitary Gland*, Edward Arnold Publishers, London, 1955, 298 pp.
3. Harris GW, Jacobsohn D. Functional grafts of anterior pituitary gland. *Proc R Soc Ser B* **139**, 263–268 (1952).
4. Green JD, Harris GW. The neurovascular link between the neurohypophysis and adenohypophysis. *J Endocrinol* **5**, 136–146 (1947).
5. Szentagothai J, Flerko B, Hess B, Halasz B. *Hypothalamic Control of the Anterior Pituitary*, 3rd rev. ed., Akademia Kiado, Budapest, 1968, 259 pp.
6. Halasz B, Pupp L, Uhlarik S. Hypophysiotropic area in the hypothalamus. *J Endocrinol* **25**, 147–154 (1967).
7. Halasz B. The endocrine effects of isolation of the hypothalamus from the rest of the brain. In *Frontiers of Neuroendocrinology*, WF Ganong, L Martini, Eds., Oxford University Press, New York, NY, 1969, pp 307–342.
8. Markee JE, Everett JW, Sawyer CH. The relationship of the nervous system to the release of gonadotropin and the regulation of the sex cycle. *Recent Prog Horm Res* **7**, 139–163 (1952).
9. Marshall FHA, Verney EG. The occurrence of ovulation and pseudopregnancy on the rabbit as a result of central nervous stimulation. *J Physiol (London)* **86**, 327–336 (1936).

10. McCann SM, Talesnik S, Freidman HM. LH releasing activity in hypothalamic extracts. *Proc Soc Exp Biol Med* **104,** 432–434 (1960).
11. Harris GW. The pituitary stalk and ovulation. In *Control of Ovulation,* C Villee, Ed., Pergamon Press, London, 1961, pp 56–74.
12. Matsuo H, Baba Y, Nair R, et al. Structure of the porcine LH and FSH releasing hormone. I. The proposed amino acid sequence. *Biochem Biophys Res Commun* **43,** 1334–1339 (1971).
13. Burgus R, Butcher M, Ling N, et al. Structure moléculair du facteur hypothalamique (LRF) d'origine ovine controlant la sécrétion de l'hormone gonadotrope hypophysaire de luteinisation (LH). *CR Acad Sci Ser D* **273,** 1611–1616 (1971).
14. Schally AV, Arimura A, Kastin AJ, et al. Gonadotropin releasing hormone: One peptide regulates secretion of luteinizing and follicle stimulating hormone. *Science* **173,** 1036–1038 (1971).
15. Knigge KM, Silverman AJ. Anatomy of the endocrine hypothalamus. In *Handbook of Physiology: Endocrinology* **4,** E Knobil, WH Sawyer, Eds., American Physiological Society, Washington, DC, 1974, pp 1–32.
16. Ezrin C, Kovacs L, Horvath E. A functional anatomy of the endocrine hypothalamus and hypophysis. *Med Clin North Am* **62,** 229–233 (1978).
17. Reichlen S. Regulation of the endocrine hypothalamus. *Med Clin North Am* **62,** 235–250 (1978).
18. Schally A, Kastin AJ, Arimura A. Hypothalamic follicle stimulating hormone (FSH) and luteinizing hormone (LH) regulating hormone: Structure, physiology and clinical studies. *Fertil Steril* **22,** 703–721 (1971).
19. Arimura A, Schally AV. Physiological and clinical studies with natural and synthetic luteinizing hormone releasing hormone. *Med J Osaka Univ* **23,** 77–100 (1972).
20. Corbin A. Pituitary and plasma LH of ovariectomized rats with median eminence implants. *Endocrinology* **78,** 893–901 (1966).
21. Kawakami M, Sakuma Y. Responses of hypothalamic neurons to the microiontophoresis of LHRH, LH and FSH under various levels of circulating ovarian hormones. *Neuroendocrinology* **15,** 290–307 (1974).
22. Baba Y, Matsuo H, Schally AV. Structure of porcine LH and FSH releasing hormone II. Confirmation of the proposed structure by conventional sequential analysis. *Biochem Biophys Res Commun* **44,** 459–463 (1971).
23. Schally AV, Nair RMG, Redding TW, Arimura A. Isolation of the luteinizing hormone and follicle stimulating hormone releasing hormone from porcine hypothalami. *J Biol Chem* **246,** 7230–7236 (1971).
24. Baba Y, Arimura A, Schally AV. Studies on the properties of hypo-

thalamic luteinizing hormone-releasing hormone. *J Biol Chem* **246,** 7581–7585 (1971).

25. Arimura A, Matsuo H, Baba Y, et al. Stimulation of release of LH by synthetic LHRH *in vivo*. I. Comparative study of natural and synthetic hormone. *Endocrinology* **90,** 163–168 (1972).

26. Schally AV, Kastin AJ, Arimura A. The hypothalamus and reproduction. *Am J Obstet Gynecol* **114,** 423–442 (1972).

27. Labrie F, Borgeat P, Drovin J, et al. Mechanism of action of hypothalamic hormones in the adenohypophysis. *Annu Rev Physiol* **41,** 55 (1979).

28. Coy DH, Schally AV. Gonadotropin releasing hormone analogues. *Ann Clin Res* **10,** 139 (1978).

29. Marshall JC, Bourne GA, Frager MS, Pieper DR. Pituitary gonadotropin releasing hormone receptors—physiological changes and control of receptor number. In *Functional Correlates of Hormone Receptors in Reproduction,* VB Mahesh, TG Muldoon, BB Saxena, WA Sadler, Eds., Elsevier-North Holland, New York, NY, 1981, pp 93–108.

30. Aiyer MS, Chiappa SA, Fink G. A priming effect of luteinizing hormone releasing factor on the anterior pituitary gland in the female rat. *J Endocrinol* **62,** 573–579 (1974).

31. McKelvy JF, Krause JE, Advis JP. Neuropeptide degradation. In *Molecular Genetic Neuroscience,* FO Schmitt, S Bird, FE Bloom, Eds., Raven Press, New York, NY, 1982, pp 189–213.

32. Redding TW, Schally AV, Arimura A, Matsuo H. Stimulation of release and synthesis of luteinizing hormone (LH) and follicle stimulating hormone (FSH) in tissue cultures of rat pituitaries in response to natural and synthetic LH and FSH releasing hormone. *Endocrinology* **90,** 764–770 (1972).

33. Millar RP, Denniss P, Tobler C, et al. Presumptive prehormonal forms of hypothalamic peptide hormones. In *Cell Biology of Hypothalamic Neurosecretion,* JD Vincent, E Kordon, Eds., National Center of Scientific Research, Paris, 1978, pp 488–510.

34. Hartter DE, Ramirez VD. The effects of metabolic inhibitors and colchicine on luteinizing hormone-releasing hormone release from superfused rat hypothalami. *Endocrinology* **107,** 375–382 (1980).

35. Koch Y, Baram T, Chobsieng P, Fridkin M. Enzymatic degradation of luteinizing hormone releasing hormone by hypothalamic tissue. *Biochem Biophys Res Commun* **61,** 95–103 (1974).

36. Griffiths EC, Hooper KC. The stimulatory influence of gonadal steroids and methallibure (ICI 33.828) on peptidase activity in the female rat hypothalamus. *Fertil Steril* **24,** 269–274 (1973).

37. Swift AD, Crighton DB. The effects of certain steroid hormones

on the activity of ovine hypothalamic luteinizing hormone releasing hormone (LHRH) degrading enzymes. *FEBS Lett* **100**, 110–112 (1979).

38. Griffiths EC, Hooper KC, Jeffcoate SL, Holland DT. The effects of gonadectomy and gonadal steroids on the activity of hypothalamic peptidases inactivating luteinizing hormone releasing hormone (LHRH). *Brain Res* **88**, 384–388 (1975).

39. Kuhl H, Taubert HD. Short-loop feedback mechanism of luteinizing hormone (LH) stimulates L-cystine arylamidase to inactivate LHRH in the rat hypothalamus. *Acta Endocrinol (Copenhagen)* **78**, 649–663 (1975).

40. McCann SM. Progress in neuroendocrinology: LH releasing (LHRH), basic and clinical aspects. *J Endocrinol Invest* **6**, 243–252 (1983).

41. Jeffcoate SL, Greenwood RH, Holland DT. Blood and urine clearance of luteinizing hormone releasing hormone in man measured by radioimmunoassay. *J Endocrinol* **60**, 305–314 (1974).

42. Arimura A, Kastin AJ, Gonzales-Barcena D, et al. Disappearance of LH-releasing hormone in man as determined by radioimmunoassay. *Clin Endocrinol* **3**, 421–425 (1974).

43. Fink G. Feedback actions of target hormones on hypothalamus and pituitary with special reference to gonadal steroids. *Annu Rev Physiol* **41**, 571 (1979).

44. Goodman RL. A quantitative analysis of the physiological role of estradiol and progesterone in the control of tonic and surge secretion of luteinizing hormone in the rat. *Endocrinology* **102**, 142–150 (1978).

45. Libertun C, Orias R, McCann SM. Biphasic effect of estrogen on the sensitivity of the pituitary to luteinizing hormone-releasing factor. *Endocrinology* **94**, 1094 (1974).

46. Nakai Y, Plant TM, Hess DL, et al. On the sites of the negative and positive feedback actions of estradiol in the control of gonadotropin secretion in the rhesus monkey. *Endocrinology* **102**, 1008–1114 (1978).

47. Yen SSC, Vandenberg G, Rebar R, Ehara Y. Variation of pituitary responsiveness to synthetic LRF during different phases of the menstrual cycle. *J Clin Endocrinol* **35**, 931–934 (1972).

48. Cooper KJ, Fawcett CP, McCann S. Variations in pituitary responsiveness to luteinizing hormone releasing factor during the rat estrous cycle. *J Endocrinol* **57**, 187 (1973).

49. Spies HG, Stevens KR, Hillard J, Sawyer CH. The pituitary as a site of progesterone and chlormadinone blockade of ovulation in the rabbit. *Endocrinology* **84**, 277–284 (1969).

50. Kalra SP, Kalra PS. Neural regulation of luteinizing hormone secretion in the rat. *Endocr Rev* **4**, 311–351 (1983).

51. Martin JB, Reichlin S, Brown GM. Neuroendocrinology of reproduc-

tion. In *Clinical Neuroendocrinology*, F.A. Davis Co., Philadelphia, PA, 1977, pp 93–128.

52. Knobil E. On the control of gonadotropin secretion in the rhesus monkey. *Recent Prog Horm Res* **30,** 1–46 (1974).

53. King JC, Arimura A, Williams T. Localization of luteinizing hormone-releasing hormone in rat hypothalamus using radioimmunoassay. *J Anat* **120,** 275–284 (1975).

54. Wheaton J, Krulich L, McCann S. Localization of luteinizing hormone releasing hormone in the preoptic area and hypothalamus of the rat using radioimmunoassay. *Endocrinology* **97,** 30–38 (1975).

55. Palkovits M, Arimura A, Brownstein M, et al. Luteinizing hormone-releasing hormone (LHRH) content of the hypothalamic nuclei in rat. *Endocrinology* **95,** 554–558 (1974).

56. Kizer J, Palkovits M, Brownstein M. Releasing factors in the circumventricular organs of the rat brain. *Endocrinology* **98,** 311–317 (1976).

57. Besser GM, Mortimer CH. Hypothalamic regulatory hormones: A review. *J Clin Pathol* **27,** 173–184 (1974).

58. King J, Tobet S, Snavel F, Arimura A. LHRH immunopositive cells and their projections to the median eminence and organum vasculosum of the lamina terminalis. *J Comp Neurol* **209,** 287–300 (1982).

59. Witkin J, Paden CM, Silverman A. The luteinizing hormone releasing hormone (LHRH) systems in the rat brain. *Neuroendocrinology* **35,** 429–441 (1982).

60. Krey LC, Silverman A. Luteinizing hormone-releasing hormone. In *Brain Peptides,* D Krieger, MJ Brownstein, JB Martin, Eds., J Wiley and Sons, New York, NY, 1983, pp 687–709.

61. King JC, Elkind KE, Gerall AA, Millar RP. Investigation of the LHRH system in the normal and neonatally steroid treated male and female rat. In *Brain Endocrine Interaction* **3:** *Neural Hormones and Reproduction,* D Scott, K Knigge, Eds., Karger, Basel, 1978, pp 97–107.

62. Millar RP, Aehnelt C, Rossier G. Higher molecular weight species of luteinizing hormone releasing hormone: Possible precursors of the hormone. *Biochem Biophys Res Commun* **74,** 720–731 (1977).

63. Krieger D. Brain peptides: What, where and why? *Science* **222,** 975–985 (1983).

64. Jonas HA, Burger HG, Cumming IA, et al. Radioimmunoassay for luteinizing hormone-releasing hormone (LHRH): Its application to the measurement of LHRH in ovine and human plasma. *Endocrinology* **96,** 384–393 (1975).

65. Jeffcoate SL, Fraser HM, Holland DT, Gunn A. Radioimmunoassay of luteinizing hormone-releasing hormone (LHRH) in serum from man, sheep and rat. *Acta Endocrinol (Copenhagen)* **75,** 525–635 (1974).

66. Nett TM, Akbar AM, Niswender GD, et al. A radioimmunoassay

for gonadotropin releasing hormone (GnRH) in serum. *J Clin Endocrinol Metab* **36**, 880–885 (1973).

67. Kawamura Y, Miyake A, Aoni T, Kurachi K. Plasma luteinizing hormone-releasing hormone levels in normal women and patients with amenorrhea. *Fertil Steril* **34**, 444–447 (1980).

68. Elkind-Hirsch K, Ravnikar V, Schiff I, et al. Determinations of endogenous immunoreactive luteinizing hormone-releasing hormone in human plasma. *J Clin Endocrinol Metab* **54**, 602–607 (1982).

69. Dierschke DJ, Bhattacharya A, Atkinson L, Knobil E. Circhoral oscillations of plasma LH levels in the ovariectomized rhesus monkey. *Endocrinology* **87**, 850–853 (1970).

70. Yen SSC, Tsai C, Naftolin F, et al. Pulsatile patterns of gonadotropin release in subjects with and without ovarian function. *J Clin Endocrinol Metab* **34**, 671–675 (1972).

71. Gay VL, Sheth NA. Evidence for a periodic release of LH in castrated male and female rats. *Endocrinology* **90**, 158–162 (1972).

72. Butler WR, Malven PV, Willett LB, Bolt DJ. Patterns of pituitary release and cranial output of LH and prolactin in ovariectomized ewes. *Endocrinology* **91**, 793–801 (1972).

73. Carmel PW, Araki S, Ferin M. Pituitary stalk portal blood collection in rhesus monkeys: Evidence of pulsatile release of gonadotropin-releasing hormone (GnRH). *Endocrinology* **99**, 243–248 (1976).

74. Knobil E. The neuroendocrine control of the menstrual cycle. *Recent Prog Horm Res* **36**, 53–88 (1980).

75. Pohl CR, Knobil E. The role of the central nervous system in the control of ovarian function in higher primates. *Annu Rev Physiol* **44**, 583–593 (1982).

76. Belchetz PE, Plant TM, Nakai Y, et al. Hypophysial responses to continuous and intermittent delivery of hypothalamic gonadotropin-releasing hormone. *Science* **202**, 631–633 (1978).

77. Comite F, Cutler GB Jr, Rivier J, et al. Short-term treatment of idiopathic precocious puberty with a long acting analogue of luteinizing hormone-releasing hormone: A preliminary report. *N Engl J Med* **305**, 1546–1550 (1981).

78. Wildt L, Hausler A, Marshall G, et al. Frequency and amplitude of gonadotropin releasing hormone stimulation and gonadotropin secretion in the rhesus monkey. *Endocrinology* **109**, 376–385 (1981).

79. Knobil E, Plant TM, Wildt L, et al. Control of the rhesus monkey menstrual cycle: Permissive role of hypothalamic gonadotropin-releasing hormone. *Science* **207**, 1371–1373 (1980).

80. Wildt L, Marshall G, Knobil E. Experimental induction of puberty in the infantile rhesus monkey. *Science* **207**, 1373–1375 (1980).

81. Marshall JC, Harsoulis P, Anderson DC, et al. Isolated pituitary

gonadotropin deficiency: Gonadotropin secretion after synthetic luteinizing hormone and follicle stimulating hormone releasing hormone. *Br Med J* **iv**, 643–645 (1972).

82. Mortimer C, Besser GM, McNeilly AS, et al. The LH and FSH releasing hormone test in patients with hypothalamic–pituitary–gonadal dysfunction. *Br Med J* **iv**, 73–77 (1973).

83. Taymor ML. The use of luteinizing hormone releasing hormone in gynecology. *Obstet Gynecol Annu* **7**, 285 (1978).

84. Wentz AC. Clinical applications of luteinizing hormone-releasing hormone. *Fertil Steril* **28**, 901–912 (1977).

85. Kastin AJ, Schally AV, Gual C, et al. Stimulation of LH release in men and women by LH-releasing hormone purified from porcine hypothalami. *J Clin Endocrinol Metab* **29**, 1046–1050 (1969).

86. Kastin AJ, Schally AV, Gual C, et al. Administration of LH-releasing hormone to selected subjects. *Am J Obstet Gynecol* **108**, 177–182 (1970).

87. Kastin AJ, Zarate A, Midgley AR Jr, et al. Ovulation confirmed by pregnancy after infusion of porcine LHRH. *J Clin Endocrinol Metab* **33**, 980–982 (1971).

88. Ferin M, Bogumil J, Drewes J, et al. Pituitary and ovarian hormonal response to 48 h gonadotropin releasing hormone (GnRH) infusions in female rhesus monkeys. *Acta Endocrinol (Copenhagen)* **89**, 48–58 (1978).

89. Keller DJ. Induction of ovulation by synthetic luteinizing hormone releasing factor in infertile women. *Lancet* **ii**, 570–571 (1972).

90. Zarate A, Canales ES, Soria J, et al. Further observations on the therapy of anovulatory infertility with synthetic luteinizing hormone-releasing hormone. *Fertil Steril* **25**, 3–10 (1974).

91. Leyendecker G, Wildt L, Hansmann M. Pregnancies following chronic intermittent (pulsatile) administration of Gn-RH by means of a portable pump (Zyklomat)—a new approach to the treatment of infertility in hypothalamus and amenorrhea. *J Clin Endocrinol Metab* **51**, 1214–1216 (1980).

92. Crowley WF, McArthur JW. Stimulation of the normal menstrual cycle in Kallmann's syndrome by pulsatile administration of luteinizing hormone-releasing hormone (LHRH). *J Clin Endocrinol Metab* **51**, 173–175 (1980).

93. Ory S. Clinical uses of luteinizing hormone-releasing hormone. *Fertil Steril* **39**, 577–591 (1983).

94. Valk TW, Corley KP, Kelch RP, Marshall JC. Hypogonadotropic hypogonadism: Hormonal response to low dose pulsatile administration of gonadotropin-releasing hormone. *J Clin Endocrinol Metab* **51**, 730–738 (1980).

95. Hoffman A, Crowley WF. Induction of puberty in men by long-

term pulsatile administration of low dose gonadotropin releasing hormone. *N Engl J Med* **307**, 1237–1241 (1982).

96. Speroff L, Glass RH, Kase NG. Regulation of the menstrual cycle. In *Clinical Gynecologic Endocrinology and Infertility,* Williams and Wilkins Co., Baltimore, MD, 1983, pp 75–100.

Habitual Abortion

Robert J. Carpenter, Jr.

Spontaneous Abortion

The most common cause of pregnancy loss after the clinical vertification of pregnancy is spontaneous abortion during the first 14 weeks of gestation. This process, which occurs in 15 to 18% of pregnancies, is first marked by the onset of bleeding, often unaccompanied by cramping. Thirty percent of all pregnancies will experience bleeding during the first trimester; however, only 50% will proceed to spontaneous loss. Losses occur most frequently during the first seven days after the onset of bleeding. If cramping occurs, the incidence of loss increases to 80%; if bleeding is heavy, 90% will miscarry.

Several groups have investigated these losses in an effort to determine the incidence of loss of normal vs abnormal conceptuses. They have confirmed that 50 to 60% of these pregnancies are chromosomally abnormal; a further 15% have nonchromosomally derived malformations (1, 2).

These abnormal karyotypes may be placed into one of four major categories: autosomal trisomy, polyploidy, monosomy X, and structural rearrangements. I shall briefly consider each of these major groups and the more common abnormalities.

Autosomal Trisomy

In 50% of all spontaneous abortions the fetuses have a full extra chromosome. Given an average of 2000 genes per chromosomes, these conceptuses have a tremendous excess of genetic material, the most common being in group D (no. 13–15), E (no. 16–18), and G (no. 21 and 22) chromosomes. Hassold et al. (3) in a study of 1000 consecutive losses found 20.6% to be trisomic, of which 60% belonged to either the D, E, or G group. If a fetus/embryo could be identified, 33% of these had abnormal karyo-

51

types; this proportion increased to 50% when only amnion, chorion, or villi were identified. The most common trisomy involved chromosome 16, which accounted for 25% of all trisomies and 11% of all chromosomal abnormalities. These data confirmed earlier work done on nonbanded karyotypes.

Polyploidy

The addition of one or more haploid sets of chromosomes, known as triploidy (69 chromosomes) or tetraploidy (92 chromosomes) make up 20% of abnormalities. Hassold et al. *(3)* identified 70 triploid and 33 tetraploid conceptions as 22.2% of all abnormals. Most polyploid pregnancies are lost in the first trimester; however, the pregnancies lost later often involve a combination of severe retardation of fetal growth, chorionic cysts or intraplacental hydatidiform changes, and pregnancy-induced hypertension (pre-eclampsia). Five of six patients with culture-proven triploidy have presented with this triad in our center.

Hassold et al. *(3)* also reported a 3:1 ratio of XXY to XXX sex chromosome constitution. Dispermy, fertilization of the ovum by two separate sperm, is the most common mechanism recognized for this *(4)*.

Monosomy X

The most frequently identified chromosome abnormality is XO (45, X), formerly known as Turner's syndrome. These fetuses are often grossly edematous, have cystic hygromas of the neck, and have associated cardiac defects *(5)*. This group makes up 24% of Hassold's abnormalities *(3)*. Despite the frequency of this karyotype at conception, the incidence of live births with this abnormality is 1 in 2500 to 3000. Therefore, at least 98% of these conceptions are lost, most during the first trimester.

Structural Rearrangements

In Hassold's series, 4.3% of abnormal fetuses had rearrangements of some type, supporting reports from other series *(6)* of a 5% incidence. This group includes some fetuses from parents who are carriers of a balanced translocation but who are phenotypically normal. Chromosomal studies of couples who have had habitual abortions indicate a 3.6 to 7.0% incidence of bal-

Table 1. **Incidence of Balanced Translocations in Habitual Abortion**

No. of spontaneous abortions per couple	Translocations No./total	%
2	4/48	8.4
3	1/37	2.7
4	2/20	10.0
5	1/17	5.9

anced translocations. Table 1 shows the range in frequency of balanced translocations, stratified for increasing number of spontaneous abortions, as described by Virginia Michels and her colleagues *(7)*.

Habitual Abortion

Habitual abortion, as classically defined, is used to designate a couple who have had three or more consecutive pregnancy losses. More recently, many physicians have redefined this to include any couple who have lost two or more pregnancies. Losses may occur during the first, second, or third trimester and as a rule must include spontaneous abortions or the delivery of a stillborn infant with or without malformations. Because of this change in definition, more women are being evaluated earlier in their reproductive life in an effort to identify correctable causes of recurrent pregnancy loss. Under the revised definition, the frequency of couples with habitual abortion is 0.5% (1/200).

Causes of habitual abortion (Table 2) may be relatively common or distinctly unusual. Because of their increased probability for

Table 2. **Etiology of Habitual Abortion**

Chromosomal	20–25%
Uterine	12–15%
Endocrine	20–25%
Medical	1%
Infection	4%
Immunologic	1%
Unknown	40%

subsequent loss, knowledge of the various causes of this problem should be known to all providers of women's health care *(8–10)*.

Chromosomal Abnormalities

Chromosomal abnormalities make up the largest recognizable group in habitual abortion. As discussed in the preceding section, at least half of the losses are chromosomally abnormal. During the evaluation of such couples, variable frequencies of individuals with balanced translocations are detected. These individuals may have offspring who are normal, who carry the balanced chromosomal complement, or who were aborted spontaneously or born with malformations.

Given a pregnancy loss associated with a balanced rearrangement, the probability of a subsequent normal outcome varies widely, depending upon the specific chromosomal rearrangement *(10, 11)*. An example would be the translocation of chromosome 21 to either chromosome 14 or its homolog 21. Given a Robertsonian 14/21 translocation, the theoretical frequency of abnormalities is 33%, because no infant with monosomy 21 would survive. The observed occurrence of an abnormality is 2 to 3% if the father is the carrier, and 10% if the mother is. If there is a 21/21 translocation, e.g., 45,XY,t (21q21q), however, no normal offspring can be anticipated: all viable offspring would have 46 chromosomes but three 21's, 46,XX,t (21q21q) *(11)*.

If all abortions occur in the first or early second trimester, the couple often ask, "What is our chance of having another loss?" Many studies *(3, 7, 12, 13)* have demonstrated a 25% risk of recurrence in any subsequent pregnancy. Hassold et al. *(3)* found these figures also to be applicable to prior pregnancies in those couples who had normal and abnormal karyotypes for their presenting abortions. Furthermore, Hassold has shown in a separate study *(14)* that if the chromosomal complement of the first pregnancy loss was normal, then 80% of subsequent losses would be normal. However, if an abnormal karyotype was identified, 70% of the subsequent abortions also would have an abnormal complement.

Uterine Factors

Uterine causes associated with habitual abortion can be divided into three separate groups: Müllerian fusion abnormalities, incompetent cervix, and acquired abnormalities such as leiomyomata. Approximately 3.5% of all women have some fusion abnormality, but only a small percentage of these have repetitive losses. Numerous studies *(15, 16)* report a high incidence of pregnancy wastage associated with the septate uterus and, in more recent literature, with the T-shaped uterus caused by in utero exposure to diethylstilbestrol (DES) *(17, 18)*.

Müllerian abnormalities. Recently, Buttram and Gibbons *(16)* proposed a classification of Müllerian abnormalities to standardize reporting so data from different researchers could be compared. The six classes are as follows: agenesis/hypoplasia, unicornuate, didelphys, bicornuate, septate, and DES-induced. In their group of 144 patients, 58 had 104 pregnancies. Only 24 children, a 23% fetal salvage rate, were living. Women with a septate uterus (group V) had a total of 17 survivors in 78 pregnancies (21%).

Kaufman et al. *(17)* reported 616 pregnancies in 327 women exposed to DES. Their data were divided into two groups: an experimental group of women who had DES exposure documented from review of medical records, and a group of patients who either were walk-ins, referred, or otherwise admitted to the DES study. The incidence of uterine malformations in the first group was 41.6%, 61.5% in the second group. Filling defects of the uterus were seen in 34.8% and 52.1% of the respective groups. Although these data are complex, one consistent feature was some form of unfavorable pregnancy outcome in women who had an abnormal uterus. If only pregnancies in the unbiased records-review group are considered, the difference in rate of unfavorable outcome between women with and without a normal cavity is significant (Table 3). Overall, 42% of this group with abnormal uterine cavities experience pregnancy wastage, compared with 22% of women with a normal cavity.

As a subset of this group, women who had McDonald cerclages placed for "incompetent cervix" did not do any better than the untreated group. Currently, routine cerclage placement cannot be recommended for DES-exposed women, including those with an abnormal cavity.

Leiomyomata. Leiomyomata (fibroids), benign growths of uterine smooth muscle that vary dramatically in size, are more frequent in women over age 30 and in black women. These tumors grow in three distinct locations. The submucosal fibroid often

Table 3. Pregnancy Outcome Related to Changes in the Shape of the Uterine Cavity

		Outcome of pregnancies, % of total					
HSG findings	No. of pregnancies	Term	Pre-term	SAB	Ectopic	Still-born	All
DES-exposed women (n = 169)[a]							
Abnormal	138	58	17	15	8	1.4	42
Normal	217	78[b]	6[b]	14	4[b]	4	22[b]
All women studied (n = 327)							
Abnormal	281	49	22	17	9	2	50
Normal	335	68[b]	10[b]	18	3[b]	0.2[c]	32[b]

HSG = hysterosalpinography, SAB = spontaneous abortion.
[a] Exposure documented by review of medical records.
[b] Significantly ($p \leqslant 0.01$ or $^{c}p \leqslant 0.05$) different from women with abnormal HSG findings.

protrudes into the uterine cavity, where it may deform the cavity. If the conceptus is implanted in the endometrium overlying a leiomyoma, placental development may be decreased, depriving the fetus of required nutrients; occasionally the cavity may be so confining that there is no room for expansion of the amniotic sac and fetal growth.

The second type of myoma is intramural, enclosed within the myometrium. These may become very large and grow outward to become subserosal myomas, which produce an irregular surface contour to the uterus.

The third type, or subserosal form, is of two types: sessile and attached to the uterus by a large flat base, or pedunculated and attached to the uterus by a narrow stalk.

Incompetent cervix. Cervical incompetence presents with painless dilatation of the cervix, followed by spontaneous rupture of membranes and often rapid delivery of a premature infant. Patients frequently remember no uterine contractions and, unless carefully monitored with either manual or electronic techniques, may present no obvious contractions in the labor suite. The critical problem with the "incompetent cervix" is whether it actually exists in a particular patient. Unless contractions can be demonstrated by objective techniques, many of the patients are labeled incorrectly. Including in the incompetent cervix group a patient in labor will bias the success of the subsequent cerclage procedures.

The causes of incompetent cervix proposed by Palmer and Lacomme—traumatic, congenital, and functional etiologies—have withstood the test of time *(19)*. Tumultuous labor, followed by lacerations of the cervix, whether induced by the products of conception or by rigid instruments such as forceps that disrupt cervical fibrous tissue, impairs the ability of the cervix to withstand the normal intra-uterine pressure of progressing gestation.

Congenital abnormalities are exemplified by the hypoplastic cervix often found after DES exposure, or by a short cervix associated with other uterine malformations. Other types of congenital abnormalities as described by Roddick et al. *(20)* may occur, in which muscle tissue replaces fibrous tissue within the cervix. Early dilation of the distensible muscular cervix results in loss of the fetus.

As previously implied, functional changes result from the onset of unrecognized preterm labor and have significant implications for therapy. As Dr. Gant will discuss next, the etiology of labor, whether term or preterm, has yet to be fully elucidated. When better understood, preterm labor may be avoided or prevented, to improve pregnancy outcome.

Many attempts to diagnose the incompetent cervix by various techniques have been reported. Balloons, sound, and contrast injection (hysterography) *(21)* have been used to study the progressive dilatation of the internal os. However, these methods do not satisfactorily determine whether the defect is present. My own experience, as well as that of others, suggests that only repetitive examinations in a subsequent pregnancy can diagnose an incompetent cervix when the patient lacks a classical history.

There are several methods for treatment of "incompetent cervix." In 1950 Lash and Lash *(22)* reported excision of cervical tissue with approximation of the fresh edges as one technique to decrease the size of the defect. Shirodkar *(23)* described the first cerclage procedure in 1955; he placed a fascia lata strip submucosally around the cervix. This technique, which required cesarean delivery, was modified in 1957 by McDonald *(24)*, who utilized a large nonabsorbable suture that could be removed later in pregnancy and thus allow vaginal delivery. Later, Marshall and Evans *(25)* used 5-mm Dacron tape instead of thinner, round sutures.

Salvage rates after any of the cerclage procedures are 85–90%. However, as described by Marshall and Evans *(25)*, many patients included in these series probably did not have true cervical incompetence. They estimate that 45–50% of patients subjected to this surgery did not require the cerclage.

Because of the possibility that unrecognized preterm labor might result in a diagnosis of "incompetent cervix," Rivera-Alsina et al. *(26)* utilized beta-mimetic agents (terbutaline, ritodrine, and isoxsuprine) to inhibit uterine contractions. Their series, although small and biased by the inclusion of patients with pregnancy complications such as premature labor, bleeding, and ruptured membranes, suggests the need for a randomized controlled prospective trial of cerclage vs tocolysis. They found that the drug-treated patients had a better pregnancy outcome than did patients, both their own and referred patients, who had had cerclages. The cerclage patients had higher incidences of premature rupture of membranes, chorioamnionitis, and premature labor.

The universally good results, regardless of the type of cerclage procedure, may make their study difficult to duplicate because many patients are instructed after a loss to accept a cerclage in any and all subsequent pregnancies *(27–29)*. When a patient experiences a good outcome after cerclage, she often will not accept any other procedure.

Systemic Disease

Systemic medical disorders are relatively rare causes for habitual abortion. Destruction or involvement of major branches of the uterine arteries perfusing the intervillous space does not normally occur—even in severe hypertension, regardless of etiology, or in diabetes mellitus. However, systemic lupus erythematosus has been reported in association with repetitive first- and second-trimester losses. Abramowsky et al. *(30)* performed histologic and immunofluorescent studies on placentas from 10 patients with systemic lupus and one with discoid lupus. Five of the 11 placentas revealed necrotizing or inflammatory lesion of the decidua. Seven multiparas produced 23 pregnancies with nine spontaneous abortions (39%) and five stillbirths (22%). Five patients, all multiparas with one or more losses, had decidual vessels that demonstrated necrosis and either mononuclear or polymorphonuclear inflammation. Of these five patients, two had large deposits of IgM and C3 complement within the vessels. Similar lesions have been seen in severe diabetes, eclampsia, and hypertension. Antinuclear antibody was eluted from several of the placentas; however, the authors suggested that these might have been contaminated with maternal serum. Other studies involving lupus patients show similar high loss rates.

Older publications frequently cite diabetes and thyroid disorders as two common causes of habitual abortion. Although some women with these disorders may repeatedly lose pregnancies, most observers do not believe that these are causally related (31). Normal laboratory results are usually found when these patients are screened. However, hypothyroid women are often infertile, and thyroid-hormone replacement therapy often results in pregnancy.

Immunologic Aspects of Pregnancy

The immunology of pregnancy is currently undergoing evaluation in many laboratories. Although this aspect is still poorly understood, some data suggest that some patients currently in the "unknown" or idiopathic group for recurrent abortion may have an immunologic etiology (32). The human fetus is known to develop blocking factors that apparently prevent rejection by the maternal immune system. These factors may block the production of a migration-inhibiting factor by maternal lymphocytes, which are stimulated by alloantigens from the father of the fetus. In some women with habitual abortion, this blocking factor of maternal origin is not present and the pregnancy is rejected. Rocklin et al. (33), in their description of this relationship, described one women with multiple losses who was deficient in this factor; however, in her fourth pregnancy, which resulted in a term live delivery, blocking antibody was present both during the third trimester and at retesting two months postpartum.

Beer et al. (34) studied two groups of women with habitual abortion. The control group consisted of women with a known etiology for their losses; the experimental group was women with no known etiology for their losses. Study of the major histocompatibility complex antigens (A, B, C, and D) showed that the couples in the experimental group shared a significant degree of HLA antigens. Testing the responsiveness of mixed lymphocyte culture to stimulation by mitomycin showed poor stimulation induction in six of 10 couples in the experimental group; however, good responses were induced in HLA-incompatible donors.

An additional example of immunologic association with abortion involves the PP blood group reported by Levine et al. in 1951 (35). Numerous individuals with pp-genotype who develop anti-PP antibodies have been reported to have a high frequency of abortion. One group of 11 pp-women had a 43% abortion rate; two sisters with the anti-PP antibody had nine missed abortions and only two live births (36). Other ABO groups are not usually associated with early pregnancy wastage; however, couples with Rh-system incompatibilities, especially when the women are anti-D producers, are known to be at risk for pregnancy loss and require special care including amniocentesis and bilirubin determination.

These data suggest that some couples do have impaired pregnancy outcome secondary to immunologic factors. Over the next several years, studies of immunologic involvement in the completion of term pregnancies will help us better understand the pathology involved in this area of pregnancy wastage.

Infection

Despite a large number of papers (37–40) on the influence of chronic infection, i.e., from Chlamydia or Mycoplasma, in habitual abortion, no prospective controlled double-blind study has been published supporting this concept. Acute infections with Listeria, group B streptococcus, *Escherichia coli,* and anaerobic agents causing chorioamnionitis are involved in many losses.

Evaluation of the Couple

The evaluation of a couple with habitual abortion involves the sequential assessment of the multiple factors that may be involved (41–43).

A detailed family history (pedigree) is reviewed to determine incidences of birth defects, transmittable genetic disease, and frequency of abortion. Both partners undergo chromosomal studies with banding techniques to determine whether translocation is involved (44).

A detailed history and physical examination are taken with special attention to the vagina, cervix, and uterus. A hysterosalpingogram may be used to evaluate the internal anatomy of the uterine cavity. Inspection of the cervix may reveal lacerations, ' which may suggest the presence of an incompetent cervix *(45)*.

If no other etiology is demonstrated, the couple may then be tested for medical problems. Appropriate laboratory tests may include a 3-h glucose tolerance test to screen for diabetes mellitus, and thyroid studies, such as assays for triiodothyronine, thyroxin, and triiodothyronine resin uptake, and (or) an assay for thyrotropin (thyroid-stimulating hormone, TSH). Occasionally, testing for systemic lupus erythematosus with an antinuclear antibody test and LE-prep may be performed. Most women with lupus will often have some positive history or physical finding, although some women with laboratory-diagnosed systemic lupus erythematosus present with habitual abortion as their first complaint.

Least likely to be used are histocompatibility testing for HLA and testing with mitogen-induced mixed lymphocyte cultures. Such tests are extremely expensive and indicated only if all other tests are nonproductive.

Cervical or seminal cultures for Mycoplasma, Chlamydia, toxoplasmosis, or Listeria are probably nonproductive, given the paucity of data concerning these infectious agents as causes of habitual abortion. In our unit, instead of doing expensive cultures for Mycoplasma and Chlamydia, we treat both partners with tetracycline 250 mg four times daily for 14 days.

Lastly, many patients with habitual abortion may be referred by endocrine-infertility specialists who have been successful in obtaining a pregnancy after a diagnosis of luteal-phase defect. The treatment of these women with 25-mg progesterone suppositories twice daily is reasonable through the tenth gestational week. Beyond that time, placental production of progesterone should be sufficient to maintain the pregnancy.

Although many patients will demonstrate a cause for habitual abortion, no etiology will be found for many patients. In these cases careful management is associated with a 75–80% subsequent good outcome *(46)*.

Psychosocial Management

All of the information presented so far touches on the purely medical, nonpersonal side of a problem that has dramatic overlying psychological and social interactions. After multiple losses, regardless of whether the couple has a living child in their home, feelings of self-failure or partner failure often cloud other areas of their daily interactions *(13, 47, 48)*. The desire to have a "scapegoat" for the losses or bad outcome is an expression of the attempt to fulfill the phases of a normal grief process. Often, after multiple losses, with or without a previous evaluation for etiologic factors, the couple is referred for genetic evaluation. Besides the medical evaluation and therapeutic options that are necessary to present, the major role of the counselor is to attempt to instill hope, to remove guilt, and to provide correct information about the potential for a good pregnancy outcome.

In many instances the original caregiver removed hope or gave information that had no basis in fact. Like cancer patients trying to believe that there will be a cure, the couple with chronic pregnancy wastage desire a good outcome but begin to sense that it will not occur. After a thorough evaluation, medical facts presented compassionately often will convey to these couples that hope is still present. With few exceptions, most habitual aborters will carry and deliver a living, normal child. Because of the often intense emotional components in this area of medicine, some couples may need professional psychiatric or psychological evaluation and care. Individuals proficient in the art as well as the science of medicine should be available to help the obstetrician-gynecologist or the medical geneticist with this.

With the infusion of hope and the possibility of a good outcome, therapy can be initiated without administering medications or performing diagnostic tests or "therapeutic" operations that may not be appropriate.

It is hoped that the art of medicine, which has been largely supplanted recently by the science of medicine, can take its rightful place as one of the dynamically interactive tools of the physician. When that occurs, the practice of medicine will have reached its zenith and become complete.

References

1. Boue J, Boue A, Lazar P. Retrospective and prospective epidemiological studies of 1500 karyotyped spontaneous human abortions. *Teratology* **12,** 11 (1975).
2. Glass RH, Golbus MS. Habitual abortion. *Fertil Steril* **29,** 257 (1978).

3. Hassold T, Chen N, Funkhouser J, et al. A cytogenetic study of 1000 spontaneous abortions. *Ann Hum Genet* **44**, 151 (1980).

4. Beatty RA. The origin of human triploidy: An integration of qualitative and quantitative evidence. *Ann Hum Genet* **41**, 299 (1978).

5. Bergsma D. *Birth Defects Compendium*, 2nd ed., The National Foundation–March of Dimes, Alan R. Liss, Inc., New York, NY, 1979.

6. Martin AO. Genetics of spontaneous abortion. In *Reproductive Endocrinology, Infertility, Genetics*, **5**, JJ Sciarra, Ed., Harper & Row, New York, NY, 1981, Chapter 91.

7. Michels VV, Medrano C, Venne VL, Riccardi V. Chromosome translocation in couples with multiple spontaneous abortions. *Am J Hum Genet* **34**, 507 (1982).

8. Funderburk SJ, Guthrie D, Meldrum D. Suboptimal pregnancy outcome among women with prior abortions and premature births. *Am J Obstet Gynecol* **126**, 55 (1976).

9. Bigelow B. Abortion. In *Pathology of the Female Genital Tract*, A Blaustein, Ed., Springer-Verlag, New York, NY, 1977, Chapter 32.

10. Boue JG, Boue A, Lazar P, Gueguen S. Outcome of pregnancies following a spontaneous abortion with chromosomal anomalies. *Am J Obstet Gynecol* **116**, 806 (1973).

11. Lubs HA, Ing PS. Human cytogenetic nomenclature. In *Principles and Practice of Medical Genetics*, **1**, AH Emery, L Rimoin, Eds., Churchill Livingston, New York, NY, 1983, Chapter 14, pp 162–169.

12. Warburton D, Fraser FC. Spontaneous abortion risks in man: Data from reproductive histories collected in a medical genetics unit. *Am J Hum Genet* **16**, 1 (1964).

13. Berezin N. *After a Loss in Pregnancy*, Simon and Schuster, New York, NY.

14. Hassold TJ. A cytogenetic study of repeated abortions. *Am J Hum Genet* **32**, 723 (1980).

15. Simpson JL, Golbus MS, Martin AO, Sarto GE. Spontaneous abortion and fetal wastage. In *Genetics in Obstetrics and Gynecology*, Grune & Stratton, New York, NY, 1982, Chapter 7.

16. Buttram VC, Gibbons WE: Müllerian anomalies: A proposed classification (an analysis of 144 cases). *Fertil Steril* **32**, 40 (1979).

17. Kaufman RH, Noller K, Adam E, et al. Upper genital tract abnormalities and pregnancy outcome in DES-exposed progeny. *Am J Obstet Gynecol* **148**, 973 (1984).

18. Richart RM. Uterine anomalies of DES progeny. *Contemp Obstet Gynecol* **16**, 143 (1980).

19. Rovinsky J. The incompetent cervix. In *Medical, Surgical, and Gynecologic Complications of Pregnancy*, 2nd ed., JJ Rovinsky, AF Guttmacher, Eds., Williams and Wilkins, Baltimore, MD.

20. Roddick JW Jr, Buckingham JC, Danforth DN. The muscular cervix, a cause of incompetency in pregnancy. *Obstet Gynecol* **17**, 562 (1961).
21. Greenhill JP, Friedman EA, Eds. Habitual abortion. In *Biological Principles and Modern Practice of Obstetrics,* W.B. Saunders Co., Philadelphia, PA, 1974, pp 372–379.
22. Lash AF, Lash SR. Habitual abortion: The incompetent internal os of the cervix. *Am J Obstet Gynecol* **59**, 68 (1950).
23. Shirodkar VN. A new method of operative treatment for habitual abortions in the second trimester of pregnancy. *Antiseptic* **52**, 299 (1955).
24. McDonald IA. Suture of the cervix for inevitable miscarriage. *J Obstet Gynecol Br Emp* **64**, 346 (1957).
25. Marshall BR, Evans TN. Cerclage for cervical incompetence. *Obstet Gynecol* **29**, 759 (1967).
26. Rivera-Alsina ME, Saldana LR, Arias JW. Nonsurgical treatment of cervical incompetence. *Tex Med* **79**, 40 (1983).
27. O'Brien DP, Murphy JF. Value of cervical cerclage in the treatment of cervical incompetence. *Ir J Med Sci* **147**, 197 (1978).
28. Harger JH. Comparisons of success and morbidity in cerclage procedures. *Obstet Gynecol* **56**, 543 (1980).
29. Schwartz RP, Chatwani A, Sullivan P. Cervical cerclage. A review of 74 cases. *J Reprod Med* **29**, 103 (1984).
30. Abramowsky CR, Vegas ME, Swinehart G, Gyves MT. Decidual vasculopathy of the placenta in lupus erythematosus. *N Engl J Med* **303**, 668 (1980).
31. Dickey RP. Evaluation and management of threatened and habitual first-trimester abortion. *Adv Clin Obstet Gynecol* **2**, 7–33 (1984).
32. Smith RT. The immunobiology of abortion. *N Engl J Med* **295**, 1249 (1976).
33. Rocklin RE, Kitzmiller JL, Carpenter CB, et al. Absence of an immunologic blocking factor from the serum of women with chronic abortions. *N Engl J Med* **295**, 1209 (1976).
34. Beer AE, Quebbeman JF, Ayers JWT, Haines RF. Major histocompatibility complex antigens, maternal and paternal immune responses, and chronic habitual abortions in humans. *Am J Obstet Gynecol* **141**, 987 (1981).
35. Levine P, Bobbitt OB, Waller RK. Isoimmunication by a new blood factor in tumor cell. *Proc Soc Exp Biol Med* **77**, 403 (1951).
36. Dodson MG. Immunology of abortion and preeclampsia. *Compr Ther* **8**, 59 (1982).
37. Harrison HR, et al. Cervical *Chlamydia trachomatis* and mycoplasmal infections in pregnancy: Epidemiology and outcomes. *J Am Med Assoc* **250**, 1721 (1983).

38. Quinn PA, et al. Serologic evidence of *Ureaplasma urealyticum* infection in women with spontaneous pregnancy loss. *Am J Obstet Gynecol* **145,** 245 (1983).
39. Kundsin RB, Driscoll SG, Monson RR, et al. Association of urea-plasma urealyticum in the placenta with perinatal morbidity and mortality. *N Engl J Med* **310,** 941 (1984).
40. Gump DW, Gibson M, Ashikaga T. Lack of association between genital mycoplasmas and infertility. *N Engl J Med* **310,** 937 (1984).
41. Stenchever MA. Genetic clues to reproductive wastage. *Comtemp Obstet Gynecol* **17,** 37 (1981).
42. Stenchever MA. Habitual abortion. *Comtemp Obstet Gynecol* **21,** 162 (1983).
43. Stenchever MA. Managing habitual abortion. *Contemp Obstet Gynecol* **16,** 23 (1980).
44. McDonough PG, Tho PT. Etiology of recurrent abortion. *Op. cit.* (see ref. *6*), Chapter 92.
45. DeCherney AH, Polan ML. Helping habitual aborters. *Contemp Obstet Gynecol* **20,** 241 (1982).
46. Goldzieher JW, Benigno BB. The treatment of threatened and recurrent abortion: A critical review. *Am J Obstet Gynecol* **75,** 1202 (1958).
47. Bruhn DF, Bruhn P. Stillbirth. A humanistic response. *J Reprod Med* **29,** 107 (1984).
48. Borg S, Lasker J. *When Pregnancy Fails. Families Coping with Miscarriage, Stillbirth, and Infant Death,* Beacon Press, Boston, MA, 1981.

The Role of the Fetus in the Initiation of Parturition

Paul C. MacDonald, John Johnston, M. Linette Casey,
Murray D. Mitchell, Janice Okita, Takeshi Okazaki, Gian
Carlo DiRenzo, Norimasa Sagawa, Daniel Strickland, and
Norman F. Gant

It is now popular to accept the theory that the human fetus is involved in the initiation of parturition; however, this idea is not a new one. Speigelberg put forward this proposition in 1882 (cited by Thorburn in 1983) *(1)*. Indeed, the ovine fetus and the human fetus appear to participate in the onset of labor *(2)*, in that certain anomalies interfere with the timing of the onset of labor. For example, if in early pregnancy a ewe eats the foliage of the plant, *Veratrum californicum,* her fetus develops a characteristic cyclopean deformity associated with abnormal vascularization between the hypothalamus and the pituitary. The resulting fetal adrenal hypoplasia is accompanied by prolonged gestation, lasting far beyond term, and the sheep fetus ultimately dies in utero *(1)*.

Among nonhuman species, the biochemical events of parturition have been best described for sheep. Even though the exact sequence of events and the nature of the signal(s) that leads to the onset of parturition in ewes appear to differ from those in women, many of the fundamental biochemical events appear to be similar in most, if not all, species. In sheep, the signal for the initiation of parturition likely emanates from the fetus; in fact, the normal onset of labor requires a functional fetal hypothalamus, pituitary gland, and adrenal gland, as well as a functional placenta *(3, 4)*. The earliest biochemical marker of the onset of ovine parturition is a sharp increase in fetal production of adrenal cortisol. Fetal cortisol acts on the placenta in a manner that decreases progesterone formation and possibly also augments estrogen secretion. The increased estrogen production almost certainly results in an increased production of prostaglandins *(5)*.

Effect of Adrenal Status

The functional integrity of fetal brain, pituitary, and adrenal in the spontaneous onset of labor in the sheep is demonstrated by several observations: *(a)* hypophysectomy, transection of the pituitary stalk, or adrenalectomy in the fetal sheep prolongs pregnancy, and *(b)* infusion of corticotropin (ACTH) or a glucocorticosteroid into the sheep fetus causes premature parturition. Liggins et al. *(3)* reported that the rate of secretion of these hormones increases before the onset of parturition.

Flint proposed *(5)* that cortisol acts on the placenta to increase the activities of steroid 17α-hydroxylase (EC 1.14.99.9) and steroid 17,20-lyase. Increased activities of these enzymes increase the conversion of progesterone to 17α-hydroxyprogesterone and then to androstenedione, a C_{19}-steroid that can serve as substrate for estrogen biosynthesis in the placenta. Thus, the actions of cortisol in sheep placenta decrease progesterone secretion and produce a sharp increase in estrogen secretion.

In 1898, Rae *(6)* reported an association between anencephaly in the human fetus and prolonged gestation. Malpas *(7)*, in 1933, extended these observations and concluded that this association seemed to be the consequence of anomalous brain–pituitary–adrenal function. In humans, as in sheep, the fetal adrenal may serve an important role in the onset of labor. The adrenals of the anencephalic fetus at term may weigh only 5–10% of those of a normal fetus, largely because of failure of the fetal zone to develop.

There is another similarity between the biochemical events of parturition in humans and those in sheep. A human fetus with adrenal hypoplasia may also undergo prolonged gestation *(8)*. Humans, however, unlike sheep, exhibit no apparent increase in cortisol concentration in fetal blood before the onset of parturition and give no evidence of a decrease in the concentration of progesterone in the maternal plasma.

The initiation of labor in humans does not appear to result from an increased fetal production of cortisol. In fact, infusion of glucocorticosteroids or corticotropin into the human fetus or amnionic fluid does not produce premature labor as it does in sheep (9). Also, in instances in which augmented production of fetal cortisol is blocked, e.g., in various forms of congenital adrenal hyperplasia, labor begins on time. Thus in humans, fetal cortisol does not appear to be the trigger that initiates parturition. The common occurrence, however, of prolonged gestation in women pregnant with an anencephalic fetus or with a fetus with adrenal hypoplasia cannot be ignored. The role of the fetal adrenals in the normal onset of labor is probably via placental production of estrogen from fetal adrenal precursors, with the estrogen then leading to an increased capacity to produce prostaglandins, as presumably occurs in sheep.

Prostaglandins

The rate of formation and inactivation of prostaglandins, or related compounds, before parturition is not fully understood. Apparently, however, major endocrine changes, such as increased cortisol secretion by the adrenals of the lamb fetus, lead to decreased placental secretion of progesterone and increased production of estrogen and, in turn, an increase in the prostaglandin concentrations in intra-uterine tissues and in uterine venous blood. Of these hormones, estrogen appears to be most closely related to the increased synthesis and release of prostaglandins within the uterus. Within 24 h after estrogen (as stilbestrol, 20 mg in oil) is administered to the pregnant ewe, the concentration of prostaglandins in the uterine venous blood markedly increases (3). In women, treatment with estradiol-17β also appears to facilitate cervical softening and effacement and thereby enhances responsiveness to oxytocin (10).

Prostanoids serve a critical role during human pregnancy and in the final events that lead to the initiation of parturition. For example, prostaglandin E_2 (PGE_2) and prostaglandin $F_{2\alpha}$ ($PGF_{2\alpha}$) cause uterine concentrations at any stage of pregnancy and also cause cervical softening and effacement.[1] Inhibition of prostaglandin synthase (EC 1.14.99.1) activity in pregnant women prolongs gestation and lengthens the induction–abortion time interval in women who undergo therapeutic termination of pregnancy by intra-amniotic instillation of hypertonic saline. Inhibitors of pros-

---

[1]Abbreviations used: PGE_2, prostaglandin E_2; $PGF_{2\alpha}$, prostaglandin $F_{2\alpha}$; PGDH, 11-hydroxyprostaglandin dehydrogenase.

taglandin synthetase (specifically, inhibitors of arachidonic acid cyclooxygenase activity) also are effective in suppressing preterm labor. There are striking increases in concentrations of prostaglandins in amniotic fluid and in maternal plasma during labor (2).

Luukkainen and Csapo (11) reported that the intravenous infusion of a lipid emulsion into pregnant rabbits caused an increase in the responsiveness of the myometrium to oxytocin. The active component of these emulsions was shown to be phosphatidylcholine enriched with linoleic acid, the precursor of arachidonic acid (the obligate precursor of PGE_2 and $PGF_{2\alpha}$). Nathaniels et al. (12) found that the intra-aortic infusion of arachidonic acid into pregnant rabbits induced labor, and Hertelendy (13) found that the intra-uterine injection of arachidonic acid induced premature oviposition in quail. van Dorp et al. (14) and Bergstrom et al. (15) demonstrated that arachidonic acid is the obligate precursor for the biosynthesis of prostaglandins of the 2-series. Furthermore, Lands and Samuelsson (16) and Vonkeman and van Dorp (17) demonstrated that it is free arachidonic acid that is utilized for prostaglandin formation. Thus knowledge of the mechanism(s) that serve to regulate the rate of synthesis of prostaglandins and their precursors is critical for an understanding of the nature of the signal that initiates labor.

Amnion Communication

It is reasonable to assume that the mature fetus signals its mother by way of an "organ communication system" in a manner that will result ultimately in accelerated formation of prostaglandins. Recall, however, that human pregnancies involve several unique anatomical features. Specifically, the human fetus lives in an aqueous environment of amniotic fluid that is contained within the fetal membranes, i.e., the *avascular* amnion and the *avascular* chorion laeve.

Anatomically, the amnion is placed to receive the initial fetal signal and to transmit a response to such a signal. The amnion is bathed by the amniotic fluid on one side; on the other side it is contiguous with the fetal chorion laeve, which, in turn, is contiguous with the maternal decidua vera. Direct communication between the fetus and avascular amnion is established by way of the amnionic fluid, which is composed principally of fetal excretions or secretions from kidney (fetal urine), lung, and skin. Thus, the fetus is in communication with its mother by way of the large surface area of fetal membranes that are contiguous with the maternal decidua. Moreover, because PGE_2 and $PGF_{2\alpha}$ are potent vasoconstrictive agents and could cause abruption of the placenta, this arrangement favors prostaglandin formation at a site removed from the placental implantation site.

Rupture, stripping, and infection of the fetal membranes, as well as instillation into the amniotic fluid of hypertonic solutions of NaCl, glucose, or urea, are well known to result in premature onset of labor. We hypothesize, therefore, that fetal membranes might transmit or mediate signals from a mature fetus to the mother that labor should begin; moreover, the fetus–amniotic fluid–fetal membranes–decidua complex may constitute a metabolically active unit that can transmit and respond to signals that lead to the onset of labor in normal human pregnancy.

Prostaglandin biosynthesis in amnion, chorion laeve, and uterine decidua vera has been demonstrated by several techniques. The biosynthesis and metabolism of prostaglandins in these tissues, however, are unique. By far, the major prostaglandin produced in amnion is PGE_2. Moreover, the amnion tissue contains little or no 15-hydroxyprostaglandin dehydrogenase (PGDH; EC 1.1.1.141), the enzyme that catalyzes the first and rate-limiting step in prostaglandin inactivation. Thus, PGE_2 can be formed in amnion in large quantities, but is not metabolized further in that tissue. In chorion, PGE_2 also is the major prostaglandin produced, but this tissue contains PGDH activity. On the other hand, PGE_2 and $PFG_{2\alpha}$ are synthesized in large quantities in uterine decidua vera tissue, and PGDH activity is present in cytosolic fractions prepared from homogenates of this tissue. All of these findings are compatible with the theory that fetal membranes are the source of arachidonic acid and of the prostaglandin biosynthesis that occurs during labor (2, 18).

In support of the theory that fetal membranes play a crucial role in the generation of prostaglandins during the initiation of human parturition is the following evidence:

• The specific activity of prostaglandin synthetase in amnion is greater than that in chorion laeve, decidua vera, myometrium, or placenta.

• The glycerophospholipids of amnion and chorion laeve are enriched with arachidonic acid, the obligate precursor of prostaglandins of the 2-series, probably as the result of estrogen stimulation, which increases throughout gestation.

• The concentrations of free arachidonic acid, as well as those of PGE_2 and $PGF_{2\alpha}$, in amniotic fluid increase during labor and as labor progresses.

• During early labor, there is a specific decrease in the arachidonic acid content of diacyl phosphatidylethanolamine and phosphatidylinositol in the amnion and chorion laeve.

• Phospholipase A_2 (EC 3.1.1.4), which has substrate specificity for phosphatidylethanolamines with arachidonic acid in the sn-2 position, is present in fetal membranes.

• Phosphatidylinositol-specific phospholipase C (EC 3.1.4.3) activity is present in human amnion and chorion laeve.

• A diacylglycerol lipase in amnion and chorion laeve catalyzes the release of the fatty acid from the sn-1 position of diacylglycerols; this enzyme may be relatively specific for diacylglycerols with arachidonic acid in the sn-2 position.

• Further, monoacylglycerol lipase in amnion and chorion laeve catalyzes the release of the fatty acid in the sn-2 position of monoacylglycerols (there may be relative substrate specificity of this enzyme in fetal membranes for sn-2 arachidonoyl monoacylglycerols). Thus, in this coordinated manner, by three enzymic reactions, arachidonic acid is released from phosphatidylinositol in the fetal membranes.

• The specific activities of phospholipases A_2 and C in human amnion increase strikingly late in gestation.

• Diacylglycerols, the human products of the reaction catalyzed by phosphatidylinositol-specific phospholipase C, accumulate in amnion during early labor.

• The activity of NAD^+-dependent PGDH, the enzyme that catalyzes the first reaction in the inactivation of prostaglandins, is not detectable in human amnion tissue (2, 18, 20).

The mechanism of regulation of phospholipase A_2, phosphatidylinositol-specific phospholipase C, diacylglycerol lipase, and monoacyglycerol lipase activities in amnion and chorion has been studied in detail (20). In addition to the substrate specificity of phospholipase A_2 of amnion for phosphatidylethanolamine that contains arachidonic acid in the sn-2 position, the activity of the enzyme in vitro is highly dependent on the concentration of Ca^{2+}. The activity of phosphatidylinositol-specific phospholipase C also is Ca^{2+}-dependent, as is the activity of diacylglycerol lipase (20). In this latter sequence of reactions, arachidonic acid is released, ultimately, from sn-2 arachidonoylglycerol in a reaction catalyzed by monoacylglycerol lipase. On the other hand, the activity of diacylglycerol kinase, an enzyme in amnion, chorion, and decidua vera tissue that catalyzes the conversion of diacylglycerol to the glycerophospholipid precursor phosphatidic acid, is inhibited by Ca^{2+}. The action of diacylglycerol kinase inhibits the release of arachidonic acid from diacylglycerols by recycling the diacylglycerols back into phospholipids. Thus, Ca^{2+} may serve an important function in the regulation of arachidonic acid and therefore of prostaglandin production in amnion and possibly chorion laeve and decidua vera. We envision that an increase in the intracellular concentration of Ca^{2+} could increase the rate of release of arachidonic acid from phosphatidylethanolamine, by way of the reaction catalyzed by phospholipase A_2, as well as from phosphatidylinositol, in a series of reactions catalyzed by phosphatidylinositol-specific phospholipase C, diacylglycerol lipase, and monoacylglycerol lipase. In addition, an increase in the intracellular concentration of Ca^{2+} could inhibit the utilization of diacylglycerol for glycerophospholipid biosynthesis by inhibiting the activity of diacylglycerol kinase, thus favoring the release of arachidonic acid. Additional evidence supports a role for Ca^{2+} in the regulation of PGE_2 synthesis in amnion. In enzymically dispersed human amnion cells, the production of prostaglandin was decreased in the absence of calcium or in the presence of calcium channel blockers (22) but was increased in the presence of calcium or calcium ionophore (20).

Okita et al. (22), using amnion cells maintained in monolayer culture, reported that these cells retained their morphological and biochemical characteristics. Specifically, PGE_2, almost the only prostanoid produced by these cells, is not metabolized by them; phospholipase A_2, phosphatidylinositol-specific phospholipase C, diacylglycerol lipase, and monoacylglycerol lipase are present in these cells, and their activities are similar to those in amnion tissue.

With this evidence available, Casey et al. (23) measured the effect of human fetal urine on synthesis of PGE_2 by amnion cells in monolayer culture. Fetal urine stimulated PGE_2 production by amnion cells in a tissue-specific and concentration- and time-dependent manner. They also reported *(23)* that the substance that stimulates PGE_2-synthesis in fetal urine was either proteinaceous, or else closely associated with a protein, and heat-stable. They also obtained evidence that the substance was synthesized in fetal kidney, not simply excreted by it (Casey, personal communication). Fetal kidney and fetal urine, therefore, appear to be important components in the organ communication system that is operative in the initiation and maintenance of labor in women.

There is, however, no clear-cut increase in the amount of stimulation of PGE_2 synthesis in fetal urine or amniotic fluid as term is approached. Also, the substance that stimulates PGE_2 synthesis acts independently of the flux of extracellular Ca^{2+}; however, the activity of PGE_2-synthesis stimulatory substance is facilitated if the Ca^{2+} flux is effected by another agent, e.g., a calcium ionophore. Therefore, during most of pregnancy, the fetal-renal substance that stimulates PGE_2 synthesis may act on amnion to synthesize PGE_2 in a manner that is principally involved in solute and water transport from amniotic fluid and thus in maintaining the homeostasis of amniotic fluid volume. At term, however, the coordinated action of the stimulatory substance with a calcium ionophore-like agent of fetal origin might result in an increase in prostaglandin formation that is characteristic of labor.

Increased synthesis of PGE_2 in amnion is probably the key event in the onset of labor. We also can envision that the increase of prostaglandin synthesis in amnion occurs in response to a signal or signals that emanate from the fetus by way of fetal urine and thence amnionic fluid. This fetal signal may act in amnion to increase the rate of release of arachidonic acid from glycerophospholipids or to increase the activity of prostaglandin synthetase *(24)*. Thus the human fetus may, indeed, be in control of its own destiny with respect to the onset of labor.

These studies were supported in part by NIH grant 5–P50–HD11149.

References

1. Thorburn GD. Past and present concepts on the initiation of parturition. In *Initiation of Parturition: Prevention of Prematurity* (Fourth Ross

Conference on Obstetric Research), PC MacDonald, JC Porter, Eds., Ross Laboratories, Columbus, OH, 1983, pp 2–11.

2. Casey ML, Winkel CA, Porter JC, MacDonald PC. Endocrine regulation of parturition. *Clin Perinatol* **10,** 709–721 (1983).

3. Liggins GC, Fairclough RJ, Grieves SA, et al. The mechanism of initiation of parturition in the ewe. *Recent Prog Horm Res* **29,** 111–159 (1973).

4. Liggins GC. Fetal influences on myometrial contractility. *Clin Obstet Gynecol* 16, 148–165 (1973).

5. Flint APF. Regulation of placental enzymes. In ref. *1,* pp 27–34.

6. Rae C. Prolonged gestation, acrania, monstrosity and apparent placenta praevia in one obstetrical case. *J Am Med Assoc* 30, 1166–1169 (1898).

7. Malpas P. Postmaturity and malformation of the fetus. *J Obstet Gynaecol Br Emp* **40,** 1046–1053 (1933).

8. Anderson ABM, Turnbull AC. Comparative aspects of factors involved in the onset of labor in ovine and human pregnancy. In *Endocrine Factors in Labour,* A Klopper, J Gardner, Eds., Cambridge University Press, London, 1973, pp 141–162.

9. Katz Z, Lancet M, Levani E. The efficacy of intra-amniotic steroids for induction of labor. *Obstet Gynecol* **54,** 31–38 (1979).

10. Pinto RM, Leon C, Mazzocco N, Scasserra V. Action of estradiol-17β at term and at onset of labor. *Am J Obstet Gynecol* **98,** 540–544 (1967).

11. Luukkainen TU, Csapo AI. Induction of premature labor in the rabbit after pretreatment with phospholipids. *Fertil Steril* **14,** 65–72 (1963).

12. Nathaniels PW, Abel M, Smith GW. Hormonal factors in parturition in the rabbit. Foetal and neonatal physiology. *Proc Sir J Bancroft Centenary Symp,* Cambridge University Press, London, 1973, pp 594–602.

13. Hertelendy F. Prostaglandin-induced premature oviposition in the coturnix quail. *Prostaglandins* **2,** 269–279 (1972).

14. van Dorp DA, Beerthuis RK, Nguteren DH, Vonkeman H. The biosynthesis of prostaglandins. *Biochim Biophys Acta* **90,** 204–206 (1964).

15. Bergstrom S, Danielson H, Samuelsson B. The enzymatic formation of prostaglandin E_2 from arachidonic acid: Prostaglandins and related factors. *Biochim Biophys Acta* **90,** 207–210 (1964).

16. Lands WEM, Samuelsson B. Prospholipid precursors of prostaglandins. *Biochim Biophys Acta* **164,** 426–429 (1968).

17. Vonkeman H, van Dorp DA. The action of prostaglandin synthetase on 2-arachidonoyl-lecithin. *Biochim Biophys Acta* **164,** 430–434 (1968).

18. Casey ML, MacDonald PC. Initiation of labor in women. In *The Biochemistry and Physiology of the Uterus and Labor,* G Huszar, Ed., CRC Press, 1984, in press.

19. MacDonald PC, Porter JC, Schwarz BE, Johnston JM. Initiation of parturition in the human female. *Semin Perinatol* **2,** 273–286 (1978).
20. Bleasdale JE, Okazaki T, Sagawa N, et al. The mobilization of arachidonic acid for prostaglandin production during parturition. In ref. *1,* pp 129–137.
21. Olson DM, Opavsky MA, Challis JR. Prostaglandin synthesis by human amnion is dependent upon extracellular calcium. *Can J Physiol Pharmacol* **61,** 1089 (1983).
22. Okita JR, Sagawa N, Casey ML, Snyder JM. A comparison of amnion cells in monolayer culture and amnion tissue. *In Vitro* **19,** 117 (1983).
23. Casey ML, MacDonald PC, Mitchell MC. Stimulation of prostaglandin E₂ production in amnion cells in culture by a substance(s) in human fetal urine. *Biochem Biophys Res Commun* **114,** 1056 (1983).
24. Strickland DM, Saeed SA, Casey ML, Mitchell MD. Stimulation of prostaglandin biosynthesis by urine of the human fetus may serve as a trigger for parturition. *Science* **220,** 521 (1983).

Discussion—Session I

DR. GOLDZIEHER: Dr. Gant, in the past your department has done a lot of work with assays for fetal prolactin. Has fetal prolactin been put into your assay system and does it have any relationship with parturition?

DR. GANT: John Porter and Paul MacDonald have been curious about the possibility that prolactin might be a second trophic agent for the adrenals. Apparently you can pour prolactin into adrenal culture in great quantities but you can't drive the reaction any further. Maybe the role of prolactin here involves mediation of the availability of low-density lipoprotein cholesteryl esters as precursors for steroidogenesis. It's possible—and, in fact, Evan Simpson in Dallas is looking at this—that prolactin may in part be responsible for converting very-low-density lipoproteins into high-density lipoproteins, which bind with cholesterol and then enhance steroidogenesis in the adrenals. If prolactin has any role, I think it would be there, in an indirect role, such that the more dehydroisoandrosterone sulfate produced by the fetal adrenal, the greater the production of estrogen. The more estrogen produced, the more there is loaded on the fetal membranes. At one time, we thought the effect of prolactin was more central than that but it appears to be secondary.

Q: Dr. Ross, does the progesterone in the antral fluid have a local effect at the ovary and can it be increased by exogenous administration of progesterone?

DR. ROSS: To both questions, I don't know. I would be surprised if the range of quantities achievable in peripheral circulation come close to the concentrations that exist in antral fluid already, i.e., hundreds of micrograms. This is near the limit of solubility of progesterone except that proteins are there to bind it.

Q: Dr. Elkind-Hirsch, is LHRH spray available for clinical use, and, if so, what dosage is recommended, and when in the cycle should it be used?

DR. ELKIND-HIRSCH: It's available for use, but I have never used it because it is not applicable for ovulation induction. Dr. Goldzieher, do you know about its dosage and use?

DR. GOLDZIEHER: It requires an special government investigational number at the present and for that particular use you would have to obtain a special investigational permit, I believe.

Q: How useful is acetylcholinesterase as an enzyme marker in conjunction with alpha-fetoprotein (AFP) for neural tube defects?

DR. CARPENTER: Acetylcholinesterase is used now as the most specific marker for the presence of neural tube defects. In the presence of fetal abdominal wall defects, whether gastrochisis (a complete opening of the ventral wall) or omphalocele, which is usually covered by a thin layer of peritoneum, above-normal concentrations of AFP may be present in amniotic fluid or maternal serum. In a number of other conditions, such as Turner's syndrome (45, XO), the Finnish form of congenital nephrosis, AFP may likewise be increased. However, in the absence of acetylcholinesterase in amniotic fluid, one must explain the high AFP by something other than an open neural tube defect. Before the availability of testing for acetylcholinesterase, some fetuses were aborted for neural tube defects who, in fact, did not have them. With the use of high-resolution ultrasound equipment, the vast majority of neural tube defects will be detected, and in the absence of a neural tube defect, an intact spine will be seen. Therefore, with the combination of AFP, acetylcholinesterase, and high-resolution ultrasound examination, only rarely will an abnormal fetus be missed or a normal fetus be terminated. A second item of importance concerning monitoring of maternal serum AFP is the evidence that a high concentration of AFP in maternal serum, in the absence of a fetal neural tube defect, places that patient at a significantly increased risk for an adverse outcome of pregnancy. Approximately 20% of these patients will undergo preterm delivery and 20–25% will have associated severe intra-uterine fetal growth retardation. The finding of an increased concentration of AFP in maternal serum calls for a change in the quality and intensity of surveillance by the obstetrician. This single benefit may justify the application of screening maternal serum AFP in the United States. However, a maternal serum AFP screening program

77

must be set up only when strictly coordinated with an experienced prenatal diagnostician, a genetic counseling service, and laboratory quality control.

Q: What would be the best marker in maternal plasma for the onset of labor in the period of 72 to 48 h preceding labor?

DR. GANT: For humans I know of no accurate marker. In sheep, if you're interested in sheep, it's an increase in cortisol with a decrease in progesterone, as documented by Peter Nathaniels while he was still at Cambridge, and by Jeffery Dawes and Murray Mitchell at Oxford. But in humans there is no plasma marker. I wish there were—I would then know when to leave town instead of waiting around for a week-late delivery.

Q: DR. Ross, your data showing the relationships between estradiol and progesterone in the maturing follicle and the correlation with the size of the follicle were presumably true for normal women. Do these relationships hold in women stimulated with clomiphene or Pergonal? If not, are there any data on the relationships of hormone concentrations and follicle size in women so stimulated?

DR. Ross: In the first place, the relationships between hormonal concentrations in antral fluid and follicle size in induced cycles are variable, I believe, with respect to everything except progesterone. The progesterone concentrations do, in fact, probably match up. A very recent paper [November or December 1983, *Journal of Endocrinology,* from the Steptoe Edwards official group] shows that progesterone concentrations in antral fluid are in fact an adequate indicator of the fertilizability of the oocyte, irrespective of how that oocyte was obtained.

Second, the hormone concentrations and follicle size relationships in stimulated women are distinctively different from those in unstimulated women. Follicles from the ovaries of women in which Pergonal has been used to stimulate multiple ovulations tend to be smaller at the time of follicle maturity than their counterparts would be in a spontaneous or a Clomid-induced cycle.

Q: What kinds of women are candidates for the pulsatile LHRH administration and what kind of success has there been?

DR. ELKIND-HIRSCH: We have just set that up at Baylor. Basically, our patient population consists of Clomid-resistant patients, because the pulsatile pump is a somewhat more costly method of ovulation induction. We stipulate that the patient be resistant to Clomid after at least six months of therapy with Clomid (150–250 mg daily) and hCG, and that tubal factors have been ruled out. Also, the patient has to wear this pump—even sleep with it, which has its limitations; and the therapy requires more monitoring, with ultrasound and blood tests. Leyendecker [Nillius SJ, *IPPF Med Bull* **17,** 1983] in Europe has used the pump in about 108 treatment cases; the ovulation rate is about 100% and the pregnancy rate is better than 60%. So, it has been very effective.

Q: Dr. Carpenter, why are your figures for the incidence of Down's syndrome higher than ones I have heard before?

DR. CARPENTER: I'm not sure that they should be high. The birth incidence of Down's syndrome (trisomy 21), is approximately 25% lower (Hooker JG, et al., *Prenatal Diag* **5:** 29–33, 1984) than the rates I mentioned. Hooker, in 1979, published several studies indicating that approximately 25% of fetuses recognized by genetic amniocentesis as having Down's syndrome will die in utero before delivery. Because of that estimate of fetal loss, different figures are available for application in genetic counseling as to the probability of risks of Down's syndrome. The figure most often quoted is, in fact, the risk in live births. Technically, to be fair to the patient in counseling information, the risk for detection of an abnormal karotype at the time of genetic amniocentesis would be the proper figure quoted.

DR. ROSS: Dr. Gant, why does it take so much estrogen to act during pregnancy since even patients with adrenal hypoplasia have measurable estrogen?

DR. GANT: Of course they have measurable estrogen—but we're talking about almost an order of magnitude, a tremendous amount, of difference. In these conditions, there is estrogen, to be sure; but the amount is only a fraction of the amount of estrogen in pregnancy and is also almost constant throughout gestation, very, very low. We're talking about milligram concentrations of urinary estrogens during pregnancy—40 or 50 mg vs 5 mg a day in other conditions. These are tremendous amounts of estrogen. We've wondered for years how anyone could tolerate such an assault of hormone and what it was there for, other than the cardiovascular effects in the mother. We now think it's there to enrich the fetal membranes with glycerophospholipids containing arachidonic acid.

DR. GOLDZIEHER: Interestingly, estriol is limited to humans and gorillas and chimpanzees. Lower down the primate ladder this particular flood of estrogen does not occur. This raises an interesting question of species differences in the endocrinology of this stage of pregnancy.

II

PREGNANCY TESTING

Yff a woman be with childe, take hyr to drynke mede whan she shal wende to bedde. And yf she haue moche wo in her wombe, it is a signe that she is with childe.

If a woman is pregnant, get her to drink mead when she goes to bed. And if she has much discomfort in her belly, it is a sign that she is with child.

—ROWLAND, pp 120–121

Early and Routine Testing for Pregnancy

Laurence M. Demers and James I. Heald

"Pregnancy tests" conventionally measure human choriogonadotropin (hCG) in urine or serum. Ordinarily utilized clinically to confirm the presence of normal pregnancy, these tests become particularly important in assessing the probability of pregnancy in a woman about to undergo radiologic studies, receive drugs that are potentially teratogenic, be immunized, or undergo surgery. Pregnancy tests are also useful in the accurate assessment of early gestation in the hormonally treated infertile patient, in the evaluation of missed or threatened spontaneous abortion, in the diagnosis of ectopic pregnancy, and in the diagnosis and evaluation of trophoblastic disease or other germ-cell malignancies secreting hCG. Other kinds of "pregnancy tests" still being evaluated involve other pregnancy-associated plasma proteins produced by the placenta and secreted into the maternal circulation in detectable amounts. Determinations of human placental lactogen and estriol have been used as tests of placental function later in pregnancy, and as an index of fetal well-being when the measurement of hCG is not diagnostically useful.

Choriogonadotropin

hCG, synthesized by the syncytiotrophoblast cells of the placenta, consists of two dissimilar, noncovalently linked polypeptides designated as alpha- and beta-subunits. There are extensive homologies of amino-acid sequence between the alpha-subunit of hCG and those of the pituitary glycoprotein hormones follitropin (FSH), lutropin (LH), and thyrotropin (TSH). The beta-subunits of these hormones, however, differ in both amino-acid sequence and antigenicity and thus provide the characteristic biological effect of each individual hormone. Although the beta-subunits of hCG and LH also have significant amino-acid homology, a unique 30-amino-acid carboxyterminal sequence of hCG allows for the generation of specific antibodies directed at the hCG beta-subunit.

hCG is first detectable in the blood six to 10 days after ovulation at the time of implantation *(1, 2)*. The concentration of hCG in serum increases exponentially during the first 60 days of gestation *(3)*, doubling about every two days *(4)*. As Table 1 indicates, peak concentrations of hCG in serum (about 100 000 int. units/L) are reached six to 10 weeks after ovulation, thereafter declining

Table 1. **Range of Expected Concentrations of hCG in Pregnancy**

Time post-conception	hCG, int. units/L
1 week	5–50
2 weeks	40–200
3 weeks	100–500
4 weeks	700–2000
2–3 months	12 000–200 000
2nd trimester	24 000–55 000

to 10 to 15% of the peak value for the remainder of gestation *(2, 3, 5, 6)*. Braunstein et al. *(7)* found that four of seven women with multiple gestations had serum concentrations of hCG exceeding the 90% confidence limits of singleton pregnancies.

hCG functions to maintain the corpus luteum of pregnancy and, until the fetal pituitary secretes LH, stimulates the Leydig cells in male fetuses to secrete testosterone during the critical period of sex differentiation. In fact, in response to hCG, testosterone concentrations in the blood of the male fetus reach adult male values at about 16 weeks of gestation, then decrease to prepubertal values after 24 weeks of gestation *(8)*.

The Development of Pregnancy Tests

Bioassays. The first pregnancy tests developed were bioassays. Serum or urine containing hCG was injected into laboratory animals (mice, rats, rabbits, toads, frogs), which were then examined for the presence of corpora lutea; ovulation *(9)*; hemorrhagic follicles *(10)*; ovarian hyperemia *(10)*; sperm release *(11)*; changes in the weight of the ovaries, uterus, seminal vesicles, or prostate; or depletion of ovarian ascorbic acid. These bioassays were technically difficult, time consuming, expensive, and imprecise; had low analytic sensitivity; and produced a significant number of false positives. The bioassays generally detected pregnancy four to six weeks after ovulation (two to four weeks after the missed period), when the concentration of hCG is at least 2000 int. units/L (see Table 2).

Table 2. **Sensitivity of Tests for hCG**

Kind of test	Sensitivity, int. units/L
Bioassay	2000
Immunoassay	
LAI	1500–3500
HAI	250–2500
Radioreceptor assay	200
Radioimmunoassay	2–100
Enzyme immunoassay	2–100

Although not in general use today, bioassays *(12)* have been used with immunoassays to generate a ratio of bioassay (B) to immunoassay (I) activity. A low B/I ratio in the presence of malignant trophoblastic disease is reportedly associated with a poor prognosis for this disease.

Immunoassays. In the 1960s, the tools for antibody recognition became available and immunoassays for hCG were developed *(13)*. The direct agglutination assays, no longer widely available, involved the adsorption of antibodies to hCG onto tanned sheep erythrocytes or latex particles. In the presence of sufficient hCG in the urine specimen, the erythrocytes or latex particles responded by agglutination and macroflocculation. More sensitive latex-agglutination-inhibition (LAI) and hemagglutination-inhibition (HAI) procedures soon became available and formed the basis of the urine pregnancy test used widely for many years and still used in many laboratories to this day.[1]

---

[1] Abbreviations used (not already defined on p. xviii): LAI, latex-agglutination inhibition; HAI, hemagglutination inhibition; RIA, radioimmunoassay; ELISA, enzyme-linked immunosorbent assay; IRP, International Reference Preparation; SPI, Schwangerschaftsprotein I; PAPP-A, pregnancy-associated plasma protein-A.

The LAI pregnancy tests performed with urine specimens on slides are classically rapid (2 min). Latex particles carry covalently bonded hCG antigen and are incubated with antiserum to hCG and the urine specimen. If sufficient hCG is present in the urine, macroflocculation of the latex particles is inhibited. Analytic sensitivity for hCG ranges from 1500 to 3500 int. units/L, concentrations in circulation by three to four weeks after ovulation. More sensitive LAI tube tests (e.g., Sensitex; Hoffmann-La Roche Inc., Nutley, NJ) are capable of detecting as little as 250 int. units of hCG per liter (14, 15).

HAI methods usually involve test tubes and take 1 to 2 h. hCG-coated erythrocytes are mixed with antiserum to hCG and the urine sample. Sufficient hCG in the urine will neutralize the anti-hCG, preventing erythrocyte agglutination, and the erythrocytes settle into a ring pattern. Analytical sensitivity of HAI methods for hCG range from 250 to 2500 int. units/L, values usually reached two to three weeks after ovulation (16).

False-positive test results. A major drawback of urine pregnancy tests that has persisted from the days of bioassay testing is the incidence of false positives. False-positive results for pregnancy tests occur with both the LAI and HAI methods. Both of these methods, which generally do not involve specific antibodies, respond to the presence of pituitary LH in the urine, in addition to hCG. LH markedly increases in nonpregnant women at the time of ovulation (200–400 int. units/L) and during menopause (as much as 400–500 int. units/L). Urine from a patient experiencing an early menopause can easily generate a positive test result in the conventional LAI and HAI pregnancy tests.

Several drugs are also associated with false-positive results for pregnancy tests. The phenothiazines promethazine and carbamazepine (17) increase pituitary secretion of LH, thus increasing the urinary LH in these patients. Methadone and proteinuria (protein of 1000 mg/L) may also cause false-positive results. False-negative results with the agglutination-based immunoassays for hCG can occur when the urine is too dilute (24-h urine volumes in excess of 3 L), or when the urine sample is contaminated with semen (18, 19), which contains an agglutination factor. For these methods, specimens of first-morning urine provide the greatest sensitivity, having about the same concentration of hCG as serum does (16). Schroeder and Halter (20), however, recently observed an hCG fragment in urine that was reactive with the more specific radioimmunoassay (RIA) for beta-subunit hCG—contributing more than 70% of the hCG immunoreactivity of urine samples—but was not present in serum.

Radioreceptor assays. The sensitivity of tests for hCG began to increase in the 1970s, when Saxena and Landesman *(21)* introduced the concept of radioreceptor assays. This technology, though still limited by cross reactivity with LH, was heralded as an advance in sensitivity and specificity. Radioreceptor assays are based upon competition between serum hCG and radioactively labeled hCG for binding to specific receptor sites on cell membranes prepared from bovine corpora lutea. Cross reactivity of the receptors with LH, however, requires that the cutoff level for a positive result be set at 200 int. units/L, to minimize the interference by physiological concentrations of LH. With this technology, among the first tests for pregnancy that involved blood samples, one could now detect pregnancy as early as about two weeks after conception, or about the time of the first missed period.

Radioimmunoassays for the beta-subunit of hCG. Perhaps the single most important advance in pregnancy testing in the last decade occurred with the introduction of antibodies specific for the beta-subunit of hCG. These antibodies showed none of the interferences inherent with the alpha-subunit similarities of other pituitary glycoprotein hormones, except for LH, and had the specificity and sensitivity to detect pregnancy

Vaitukaitis et al. *(22)* first reported a highly sensitive (5 int. units/L) and specific double-antibody RIA for hCG in blood, in which antiserum specific for the beta-subunit of hCG was used. In this assay, serum hCG competes with radiolabeled hCG for binding to an antibody specific for the beta-subunit of hCG. Using an antibody directed against the unique carboxyterminal region of the beta-subunit avoids problems of cross reactivity with LH and the other glycoprotein hormones. Until recently, most commercial RIA reagents for beta-hCG testing involved a polyclonal antiserum raised in rabbits. However, with the introduction of hybridoma technology for the commercial production of antibodies, we now have available highly specific monoclonal antibodies for use with both beta-hCG RIA and nonisotopic immunoassays.

In the initial studies with the RIA for beta-hCG, radiolabeled beta-hCG exhibited nonparallelism of results in diluted serum samples from a small but significant number of patients having choriocarcinoma. This does not appear to occur with the intact (alpha plus beta) radiolabeled hCG, which uniformly exhibits parallelism; thus total hCG is commonly used as the tracer *(23)*. Various RIA kit reagents yield widely differing results for hCG concentrations, which may be partly explainable by differences in the purity of the hCG standards used in some kits and by differences in the specificity of the antisera for different hCG preparations.

In contrast to the original double-antibody RIA developed by Vaitukaitis et al. *(22)*, which required 36 h of analytical time, most RIA procedures today take less than 3 h, without loss of specificity or sensitivity, and their cross reactivity with LH is minimal, varying from 0 to 5.7%. LH cross reactivity with monoclonal antibodies to beta-hCG is reportedly less than 0.3%, which makes these recently available antibodies the most specific to date. One of the commercial suppliers of an immunoassay for beta-hCG uses two different monoclonal antibodies directed against two different antigenic sites on hCG. Both antibodies must bind to the hCG molecule for the assay to work, which further increases the specificity of the measurement.

Standardization of hCG Reference Material

One of the major questions frequently asked in the standardization of hCG testing is, which international reference preparation to use for the primary standard? The international unit of hCG was determined in 1964 as the biological activity contained in 1.279 μg of a 2nd International Standard of hCG (2nd IS), as defined by six bioassay techniques *(24)*. The 2nd IS hCG (IS no. 6116), recognized as the primary standard for hCG, was prepared from human urine obtained during the first three months of pregnancy. It is a heterogeneous preparation containing, on the basis of its biological potency, about 20% intact hCG, free hCG subunits, and other substances.

After the development of more-specific assays for the beta-subunit of hCG, the wHO Committee on Biological Standardization established in 1974 a new International Reference Preparation (IRP) of hCG for immunoassay and called it the 1st International Reference Preparation (IRP no. 75/537). This "1st IRP" is a "secondary standard" of highly purified hCG, containing insignificant amounts of the free subunits; it was prepared for conventional immunoassays, in which cross reactivity with the 2nd IS primary standard is significant. IRPs have also been prepared for purified alpha (75/569) and beta (75/551) subunits.

Although the 1st IRP was intended to replace the 2nd IS, most manufacturers continued to use calibrators standardized against the 2nd IS, contending that wholesale confusion would be generated by changes in "normal" hCG values and in the sensitivity threshold of the pregnancy test kits then available *(25)*. Although results by the bioassay and the radioreceptor assay were about the same for the 1st IRP (mean, 650 int. units per ampule), the immunoassays, because of differences in antibody specificity, gave markedly heterogeneous results *(26)*. Stuart and Lazarus *(27)* used an RIA specific for the beta-subunit of hCG to show that 24 int. units of the 2nd IS equaled 1 int. unit (1 μg) of the 1st IRP beta-subunit of hCG. In a recent report *(28)* on a preparation of highly specific monoclonal antibodies, in which the calibrators were standardized against the 1st IRP, the quantitative results for hCG beta-subunit were about double the values reported for a conventional RIA standardized against the 2nd IS.

Thus an element of confusion still exists among manufacturers as to the best reference preparation for immunoassay quantification. Results of methods with monoclonal antibodies will probably support use of the 1st IRP as the new primary standard in the near future.

Although the use of RIA for measuring the beta-subunit of hCG in serum has dramatically lowered the incidence of false-positive results in the face of a markedly enhanced sensitivity, a few investigators have reported false-positive RIA results that could not be attributed to heterophilic antibodies or to low concentrations of protein in the serum.

Newer Nonisotopic Immunoassays for hCG

Recently, nonisotopic enzyme immunoassays *(32, 33)* and fluoroimmunoassays *(34, 35)* for the beta-subunit of hCG have been developed. These appear to provide a decided advantage over RIA and yet retain the specificity and sensitivity so attractive in RIA.

The prolonged shelf-life of nonisotopic reagents, their easy adaptibility to automation, and the rapidity of assay performance, in addition to the increasing concerns about disposal of low-radioactive waste, have propelled the nonisotopic immunoassay into today's modern clinical laboratory. Two-site "sandwich" enzyme-linked immunosorbent assays (ELISA) are available, in which antibody to the beta-subunit of hCG immobilized on polystyrene beads, and a conjugate of horseradish peroxidase with antibody to the alpha-subunit of hCG, form a link around the serum hCG. A colorimetric signal is generated as the bead containing the anti-hCG–anti-peroxidase "sandwich" comes in contact with the substrate o-phenylenediamine in the presence of hydrogen peroxide. An ELISA method for urine samples, also involving monoclonal antibodies, has been developed by at least two different commercial manufacturers.

In nonisotopic immunoassays that do not involve monoclonal antibodies, the cross reactivity with LH appears to be greater (4–8%) than in RIA, even when both assays use the same antibodies (32).

A recently described fluoroimmunoassay for hCG with monoclonal antibodies (35) was very rapid (20 min) and highly sensitive (2 int. units/L). At a cutoff level of 25 int. units/L for positive pregnancy, the sensitivity of the fluoroimmunoassay was 92%, its specificity 73%, and its predictive value 84% for the diagnosis of ectopic pregnancy in a population of 130 women with lower abdominal pain or uterine bleeding.

Clinical Utility of hCG as a Pregnancy Test

The clinical utility of measuring hCG in blood has been markedly enhanced by the improvements in methodology since the days of bioassays. Used solely as a pregnancy test when the sensitivity of the assay precluded its use for other clinical diagnoses, the measurement of hCG (especially its beta-subunit) is now widely applied—not only to confirm pregnancy but also to diagnose and manage a large number of pregnancy-related clinical disorders. Examples of these uses are as follows: to confirm the presence of early pregnancy 24–48 h post-implantation, to diagnose ectopic pregnancy, to predict spontaneous abortion in asymptomatic patients, to estimate gestational age, to determine induction of ovulation in infertile patients, to evaluate tubal surgery patients, and to monitor patients who have had recurrent miscarriages.

Because pregnancy can be specifically detected within a few hours of implantation, obstetricians are using the serum assay in early pregnancy to predict spontaneous abortion. About 70% of women who spontaneously abort have abnormally low concentrations of hCG in their serum 14 or more days after ovulation. Masson et al. (6) using an RIA for this purpose, determined nonviability with a diagnostic sensitivity of 84%, a specificity of 91%, and a predictive value of 93% in 54 women admitted with first-trimester vaginal bleeding, who were suspected of having had a spontaneous abortion.

Corson et al. (4), using the urine test for the beta-subunit of hCG, correctly predicted spontaneous abortion in symptomatic women 63% of the time as compared with 78% with the RIA for the beta-subunit of hCG in serum. If daily sequential sampling is used, decreases in serum concentrations of beta-subunit hCG enhance the predictive value of this test in those patients whose pregnancy has failed. Use of exogenous hCG in infertile patients who subsequently undergo spontaneous abortion does not pose a problem with testing done six or seven days later (16, 36).

Ectopic pregnancies are another clinical condition for which a sensitive and specific test for beta-subunit of hCG markedly improves the clinician's ability to diagnose and treat. Ectopic pregnancies frequently (75–86%) have lower serum concentrations of hCG than do intra-uterine pregnancies after a comparable gestation period (36–40). Whereas LAI or HAI tests for hCG in urine are negative in about half of the surgically proven ectopic pregnancies (7, 36), 99–100% of these cases show detectable concentrations of hCG in serum by RIA or radioreceptor assay (7, 29, 41). Because accurate timing of pregnancy (dating from either the last menstrual period or the date of ovulation) is frequently not available, Kadar et al. (42) have proposed using the percentage increase in hCG over 48 h to detect ectopic pregnancy; they save the first sample and run it with the second sample in the same assay, to minimize interassay variation. If the increase exceeds 66%, the specificity of the test for ectopic pregnancy is 86% and the diagnostic sensitivity is 83%. The population that would benefit most from sequential testing are the clinically stable patients without hemoperitoneum on culdocentesis, whose serum hCG is less than 6000 int. units/L and for whom ultrasound findings are not diagnostic. Determinations of the beta-subunit of hCG have been recently used to assess the adequacy of conservative surgery for ectopic gestations (43).

Determinations of both hCG and human placental lactogen have been used to estimate the gestational age of the fetus between the 10th and 20th week of gestation (44), according to the formula: gestational age in days $= 97.3 + 24.8$ ln[placental lactogen] $- 14.5$ ln[hCG]. When applied at the above-mentioned time in gestation, this formula has an error of about ± 2.5 weeks, based on the result for a single blood sample. Determination of hCG alone is limited to the first eight to 10 weeks of gestation; after that, its concentrations begin to decrease (3). Westergaard et al. (44) used concentrations of hCG alone to estimate the gestational age and found an error (2 SD) of 16.8 days. Lagrew et al. (3) reported that the mean difference in estimated dates of confinement as predicted by the date of the last menstrual period and by changes in hCG concentrations was 3.1(SD 2.3) days.

Finally, Whittaker et al. (45) recently reported that measurement of placental lactogen alone may be useful for estimating gestational age up to 14 weeks of gestation.

Other Pregnancy Tests

The gynecologic endocrinologist uses the hCG test slightly differently than the obstetrician does, focussing more on gynecological problems that cause infertility and habitual abortion. The beta-subunit of hCG is measured to establish early pregnancy within hours of implantation in essentially four types of patients: those undergoing ovulation induction with agents such as Pergonal (follitropin and lutropin) and Clomid (clomiphene); those who have had tubal surgery who develop tubal anastamosis, 10% of whom have ectopic pregnancies; patients with prior failed pregnancies who have recurrent miscarriages; and infertile patients with luteal-phase defects who are being treated with progesterone suppositories. In all of these patients, it is important to confirm pregnancy as quickly as possible so that the patient can be treated accordingly. Once the gynecologic endocrinologist has established a positive pregnancy, the patient usually will be turned over to a high-risk obstetrician for the remainder of the pregnancy.

The need for a specific and sensitive test for hCG is also useful in a few circumstances to rule out pregnancy, especially when the patient may be undergoing a procedure or placed on medication that may be potentially harmful to the fetus.

Although hCG and human placental lactogen are the most well-known analytes in pregnancy tests, other proteins associated with pregnancy have been proposed as potentially useful for this: the Schwangerschaftsprotein I (SPI), pregnancy-specific β_1-glycoprotein (PAPP-C), and the pregnancy-associated plasma protein-A (PAPP-A). An RIA has been developed for SPI (6), the mean concentration of which increases from 4 to 12 ng/L between seven and 14 weeks' gestation (counted from the last menstrual period). In evaluating the likelihood of spontaneous abortion, by using as a cutoff value − 2 SD, measurement of this protein is 97% predictive of nonviability in these patients. The mean plasma concentrations of PAPP-A, a glycoprotein produced by the placenta and decidua, increase from 0.2 to 6.0 ng/L between seven and 14 weeks from the last menstrual period. Again at the − 2 SD cutoff, this test correctly predicted nonviability 84% of the time. Patients with an ectopic pregnancy have slightly lower concentrations of PAPP-A.

The use of these placental-specific proteins in pregnancy testing has been limited essentially to clinical research. The assays for these measurements are not readily available and, given the improved sensitivity and specificity of tests involving the beta-subunit of hCG, do not appear ready to displace the use of the latter in establishing the presence of pregnancy.

Both infertility specialists and high-risk obstetricians use a wide variety of other tests before and during pregnancy to focus primarily on the well-being of the fetus itself. Estradiol and progesterone are more useful in evaluating the infertile patient, particularly in monitoring the success of medications for inducing ovulation and in establishing whether a functional corpus luteum is present. Estriol and human placental lactogen are used by the obstetrician as an index of fetal well-being in the third trimester of pregnancy.

Diagnostic Use of hCG Testing Other than for Pregnancy

Measurements of the beta-subunit of hCG has another important place in the obstetrician's armament of laboratory testing, aside from conventional early and routine pregnancy testing. hCG is persistantly increased in patients with various hCG-secreting tumors. Trophoblastic neoplasms (hydatidiform mole and chorionepithelioma) are associated with a significant output of hCG in the second trimester of pregnancy. The beta-subunit of hCG has been measured to diagnose and monitor these patients postoperatively. Similarly, oncologists have come to rely on the beta-hCG test as a tumor marker in males who develop testicular germ cell tumors such as a choriocarcinoma, teratoma, seminoma, and embryonal cell carcinoma—all of which may elaborate vast quantities of hCG.

References

1. Braunstein GD, Rasor J, Adler D, et al. Serum human chorionic gonadotropin levels throughout normal pregnancy. *Am J Obstet Gynecol* **126**, 678–681 (1976).
2. Lindstedt G, Lundberg PA, Janson PO, Thorburn J. Biochemical diagnosis of ectopic pregnancy. *Scand J Clin Lab Invest* **42**, 201–210 (1982).
3. Lagrew DC, Wilson EA, Jawad MJ. Determination of gestational age by serum concentrations of human chorionic gonadotropin. *Obstet Gynecol* **62**, 37–40 (1983).
4. Corson SL, Batzer FR, Schlaff S. A comparison of serial quantitative serum and urine tests in early pregnancy. *J Reprod Med* **26**, 611–614 (1981).
5. Smith DH, Sinosich MJ. Saunders DM. Pregnancy-specific β_1-glycoprotein and chorionic gonadotropin levels following conception. *J Reprod Med* **26**, 555–557 (1981).
6. Masson GM, Anthony F, Wilson MS, Lindsay K. Comparison of serum and urine HCG levels with SPI and PAPP-A levels in patients with first-trimester vaginal bleeding. *Obstet Gynecol* **61**, 223–226 (1983).
7. Braunstein GD, Karow WG, Gentry WE, et al. First trimester chorionic gonadotropin measurements as an aid in the diagnosis of early pregnancy disorders. *Am J Obstet Gynecol* **131**, 25–32 (1978).
8. Kaplan SL, Grumbach MM. Pituitary and placental gonadotropins and sex steroids in the human and sub-human primate fetus. *J Clin Endocrinol Metab* **7**, 487 (1978).

9. Friedman MH, Lapham ME. A simple, rapid procedure for the laboratory diagnosis of early pregnancies. *Am J Obstet Gynecol* **21**, 405–410 (1931).

10. Frank AT, Berman RL. Twenty-four hour pregnancy test. *Am J Obstet Gynecol* **42**, 492–496 (1941).

11. Wiltberger PB, Miller DF. The male frog, *Rana pipiens*, as a new test animal for early pregnancy. *Science* **107**, 198 (1948).

12. Delfs E. Quantitative chorionic gonadotrophin. Prognostic value in hydatidiform mole and chorionepithelioma. *Obstet Gynecol* **9**, 1–24 (1957).

13. Wide L, Gemzell CA. An immunological pregnancy test. *Acta Endocrinol (Copenhagen)* **35**, 261–267 (1960).

14. Corson SL, Batzer FR. Early urinary pregnancy testing correlation with serum beta-HCG radioimmunoassay. *J Reprod Med* **27**, 725–728 (1982).

15. Ryder KW, Munsick RA, Oei TO, et al. An evaluation of four serum tests for pregnancy. *Clin Chem* **29**, 561–563 (1983).

16. Wang CF, Gemzell C. Neocept. A simple, sensitive urine test of early pregnancy in women undergoing ovulation induction. *J Reprod Med* **27**, 193–195 (1982).

17. Lindout D, Meinardi H. False negative pregnancy test women taking carbamazepine. *Lancet* **ii**, 505 (1982).

18. Bastiaans L, Geelen L. False pregnancy tests caused by semen contamination. *Lancet* **i**, 356 (1983).

19. Kammeraat C, Van Elburg-Kuipers A, Langejan L. False pregnancy tests caused by semen contamination of urine. *Lancet* **ii**, 1162 (1982).

20. Schroeder HR, Halter CM. Specificity of human β-subunit choriogonadotropin assays for the hormone and for an immunoreactive fragment present in urine during normal pregnancy. *Clin Chem* **29**, 667–671 (1983).

21. Saxena BB, Landesman R. Diagnosis and management of pregnancy by the radioreceptor assay of human chorionic gonadotrophin. *Am J Obstet Gynecol* **131**, 97–107 (1978).

22. Vaitukaitis JL, Braunstein GD, Ross GT. A radioimmunoassay which specifically measures human chorionic gonadotropin in the presence of human luteinizing hormone. *Am J Obstet Gynecol* **113**, 751–758 (1972).

23. Tyrey L, Hammond CB. The HCG-beta-subunit radioimmunoassay: Potential error in HCG measurement related to choice of labeled antigen. *Am J Obstet Gynecol* **125**, 160–165 (1976).

24. Banghan DR, Grab B. The second International Standard for chorionic gonadotropin. *Bull WHO* **31**, 111–125 (1964).

25. Hager H, van Weemen BK. Standardization of human chorionic

gonadotropin, HCG subunits, and pregnancy tests. *Lancet* **i**, 629 (1982).

26. Banghan DR, Storring PL. Standardization of human chorionic gonadotropin, HCG subunits, and pregnancy tests. *Lancet* **i**, 390 (1982).
27. Stuart MC, Lazarus L. Standardization of human chorionic gonadotropin, HCG subunits, and pregnancy tests. *Lancet* **i**, 1123 (1982).
28. College of American Pathologists. *Ligands Assays,* Series 1, CAP, Skokie, IL, 1983.
29. Filstein ME, Cullinan JA, Strauss JF. Aberrant results of serum beta-human chorionic gonadotropin assays: An infrequent but vexing problem. *Fertil Steril* **39**, 714–416 (1983).
30. Vladutiu AV, Sulewski JM, Pudlak KA, Stull CG. Heterophilic antibodies interfering with radioimmunoassay. *J Am Med Assoc* **248**, 2489–2490 (1982).
31. Regester RF, Painter P. False-positive radioimmunoassay pregnancy test in nephrotic syndrome. *J Am Med Assoc* **26**, 1337–1338 (1981).
32. Wada HG, Danisch RJ, Baxter SR, et al. Enzyme immunoassay of the glycoprotein tropic hormones-choriogonadotropin, lutropin, thyrotropin with solid-phase monoclonal antibody for the beta-subunit and enzyme-coupled monoclonal antibody specific for the beta-subunit. *Clin Chem* **28**, 1863–1866 (1982).
33. Mehta HC, MacDonald DJ. A sensitive enzyme immunoassay specific for human chorionic gonadotropin. *Clin Chim Acta* **121**, 245–250 (1982).
34. Petterson K, Siitari H, Hemmila I, et al. Time-resolved fluoroimmunoassay of human choriogonadotropin. *Clin Chem* **29**, 60–64 (1983).
35. Stenman UH, et al. Ultra-rapid and highly sensitive time resolved fluoroimmunometric assay for chorionic gonadotropin. *Lancet* **ii**, 647–649 (1983).
36. Rasor JL, Braunstein GD. A rapid modification of the beta-HCG radioimmunoassay. Use as an aid in the diagnosis of ectopic pregnancy. *Obstet Gynecol* **50**, 553–558 (1977).
37. DeCherney AH, Minkin MJ, Spangler S. Contemporary management of ectopic pregnancy. *J Reprod Med* **26**, 519–523 (1981).
38. Bischot P, Reyes H, Herrman WC, Sizonenko PC. Circulating levels of pregnancy-associated plasma protein-A (PAPP-A) and human chorionic gonadotropin (HCG) in intrauterine and extrauterine pregnancies. *Br J Obstet Gynaecol* **90**, 323–325 (1983).
39. Braunstein GD, Asch RH. Predictive value analysis of measurements of human chorionic gonadotropin, pregnancy specific $beta_1$-glycoprotein, placental lactogen, and cystine aminopeptidase for the diagnosis of ectopic pregnancy. *Fertil Steril* **39**, 62–67 (1983).
40. Kosasa TS, Levesque LA, Goldstein DP. Early detection of implanta-

tion using a radioimmunoassay specific for human chorionic gonado-tropins. *J Clin Endocrinol* **36**, 622–626 (1973).

41. Bryson SCP. Beta-subunit of human chorionic gonadotropin, ultra-sound, and ectopic pregnancy: A prospective study. *Am J Obstet Gyne-col* **146**, 163–165 (1983).

42. Kadar N, Caldwell BV, Romero R. A method of screening for ectopic pregnancy and its indications. *Obstet Gynecol* **58**, 162–165 (1981).

43. Peeters LK, Lemons JA, Niswender GD, Battaglia FC. Serum levels of human placental lactogen and human chorionic gonadotropin in early pregnancy: A maturational index of the placenta. *Am J Obstet Gynecol* **126**, 707–711 (1976).

44. Westergaard JG, Teisner B, Grudzinskas JG, Chard T. Accurate mea-surement of early gestational age by measuring serum HCG and SPI. *Lancet* **ii**, 567–568 (1983).

45. Whittaker PG, Aspillaga MO, Lind T. Accurate assessment of early gestational age in normal and diabetic women by serum human placental lactogen concentration. *Lancet* **ii**, 304–305 (1983).

III

INDUCED (CONTRACEPTIVE) AND ENDOGENOUS INFERTILITY

Ad restringuendum coytum: R_x: olei 3 iiii. camphore 3 iii. pul-
uerizata camphora; & misceantur et unge renes & castitatem
seruabit. Item, si quis comedit florem salicis uel populi omnem
ardorem libidinis in eo refrigerabit bene hoc longo usu. Item
veruena portata uel portata non sinit uirgam erigi donec depona-
tur & si sub seruicali posueris non potest erigi uirga uii diebus,
quod si probare uolueris da gallo mixtam cum furfure & super
gallinas non ascendet.

> *To restrain sexual intercourse.* Take 4 drachms of oil, 3 drachms
> of camphor, crushed camphor; let them be mixed and anoint
> the kidneys, and the preparation will preserve chastity. Again,
> if anyone eat the best part of the willow or poplar he will
> effectively cool all the lust in himself by continued usage. Again,
> vervain carried or drunk will not permit the penis to go stiff
> until it is laid aside, and vervain placed under the pillow makes
> an erection impossible for seven days, which prescription, if
> you wish to test, give to a cock mixed with bran, and the cock
> will not mount the hen.
>
> ROWLAND, pp 156–157

Yff so be a woman desire to conceyue of a man that she wold
conceyue of, it muste first be wyst yf she be able to haue her
desire, that is for to wyten yf ony defaute be of one of hem or
of bothe. Thus it may be wist: take twey litell pottes as hit

were mustard pottes & in yche of the pottes putte whete branne:
& put of the mannes uryne in that oon potte and of the
womannes uryne in that other potte & so late the pottes stonde
ix dayes or more. And yf cas be that the man be not
able, thou shalt fynde after tho ix daies wormes in the uryne
and foule stynkyng. And yf the defaute be in the woman, thou
shalt fynde the same proof. And yf wormes appere not in
neyther uryne, thorough medecynes they mow be amendid &
haue her desyre with the grace of God . . .

If a woman desires to conceive, it must first be ascertained
whether she is able to have her wish, to know if there is any
fault in either one of them or both. It may be ascertained thus:
Take 2 little pots like mustard pots, and in each of the pots
put wheat bran; and put the man's urine in one pot and the
woman's in the other pot, and so let the pots stand nine or
more days. And if the fault is in the man, after those nine
days you will find worms in the urine and a terrible smell.
And if the fault is in the woman, you will find the same proof.
And if worms appear in neither pot of urine, the condition of
the man and the woman can be remedied, and they may have
their wish with the grace of God through medicines. . .

—ROWLAND, pp 168–169

Some Aspects of Contraception by Oral Steroids and the Potential for Contraception by Immunological Approaches

Joseph W. Goldzieher and Melvin G. Dodson

Oral Steroid Contraceptives

The utilization of synthetic ethynyl estrogens in oral contraceptive (OC)[1] steroid formulations was a fortunate accident *(1)*. In the early 1950s the 19-norprogestins available for clinical use were contaminated with small amounts (about 10 mg/g) of mestranol; in fact, most of the early animal and clinical studies had been carried out with such material. Later, when use of chemically pure norethynodrel or norethindrone did not maintain adequate menstrual-cycle control, mestranol in amounts up to 150 μg per tablet was added back into the formulations. Only much later were ethynyl estrogens recognized as more potent inhibitors of pituitary gonadotropins than any other estrogens; and even later, the pituitary-inhibiting actions of 19-norsteroid and ethynyl estrogen were found to be synergistic, so that the total amount of steroid needed for consistent inhibition of ovulation could be greatly reduced.

Little attention was given to the metabolism, clinical pharmacology, and pharmacokinetics of the estrogen because mestranol differed only trivially from ethynyl estradiol, which had been used therapeutically for many years; thus there was no apparent reason to scrutinize it intensely, aside from the intrinsic interest in a compound being used for years by millions of women. However, its pharmacokinetics became increasingly important as consider-

---

[1] Abbreviations used (not already defined on p. xviii): OC, oral contraceptive; PASA, *p*-aminosulfonic acid; TT, tetanus toxoid; LDH, lactate dehydrogenase.

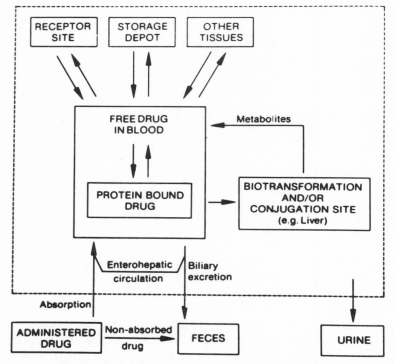

Pharmacokinetics: factors which regulate body levels and time-course of pharmacological effects of drugs.

Fig. 1. Pharmacokinetics of a drug with enterohepatic circulation

ations of safety led to the determination of the minimum clinically effective dose.

The intermediate metabolism of mestranol and ethynyl estradiol (2), particularly the formation of catechol estrogens from these and other estrogens, and the possible relation of these compounds to mutagenesis is an entirely separate topic, which has been reviewed elsewhere (3).

Claims of cardiovascular hazards (4) associated with the estrogenic (and later, with the progestational) component of the OCs produced great pressure to lower the drug dosage to a minimum. A knowledge of the pharmacokinetics of these compounds thus became essential to an understanding of which factors influence bioavailability and efficacy. In Figure 1, note particularly the phe-

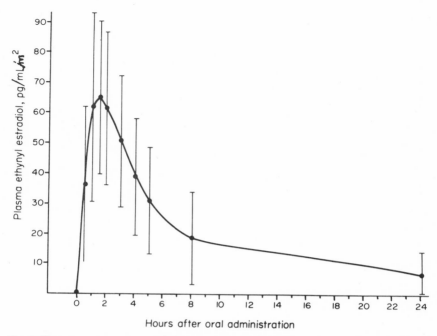

Fig. 2. Plasma concentration of unconjugated ethynyl estradiol after oral administration of 50 μg of the hormone

Note the great variability, shown by the large 95% confidence limits (*bars*)

nomena of biotransformation and enterohepatic circulation of these hormones.

Mestranol is biologically inactive until the 3-methyl group is removed and the compound is transformed into ethynyl estradiol. The efficiency of this demethylation reaction varies from individual to individual and, more importantly, from species to species. Thus, studies in rodents, some of which demethylate very poorly, are apt to give low estimates of potency for mestranol that are not reflected in studies with humans. This has been a source of some confusion.

When ethynyl estradiol is given orally, its concentrations in plasma are as shown in Figure 2. In spite of meticulous attention to the experimental conditions, there is a very wide variability in its concentration in plasma, as is typical for a drug with substantial enterohepatic circulation (the so-called "first-pass" effect). The decrease in bioavailability related to the first-pass effect is clearer in Figure 3; the ordinate is logarithmic, so that the differ-

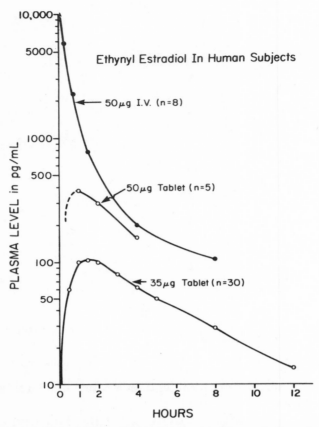

Fig. 3. Comparison of plasma concentrations of ethynyl
estradiol after oral vs intravenous administration

ence in the areas under the curves is even larger than it first
appears.

Most orally administered ethynyl estradiol is absorbed in the
stomach. When the estrogen is in a weakly alcoholic solution,
its absorption produces a rapid increase in its concentrations in
blood to relatively high values; this, in turn, is responsible for
some of the side effects of the drug, such as nausea, a central
effect. For various reasons, we attempted to formulate a slow-
release OC pill and found that in addition to the first-pass effect,
estrogen that reaches the intestine is very rapidly sulfated, thereby
further decreasing its bioavailability. Between hepatic extraction

and duodenal sulfation, it was impossible to prepare a formulation that gave satisfactory concentrations in blood at an acceptably low dosage.

When much individual variation is seen, the experimental protocol is always suspect. Variables thought to be unimportant—such as duration of fasting, volume of fluid ingested, etc.—have to be evaluated as sources of the problem. Replicate oral studies with a group of 10 women clearly showed that the K_m values obtained on both occasions were very similar: 0.119 ± 0.039 and 0.123 ± 0.049 (not significantly different by Student's paired t-test). The coefficient of variation *within* subjects was a satisfactory 13%, but variation *between* subjects (CV = 37%) accounted for the differences—i.e., the differences are real. This was our first quantitative insight into this problem. A subsequent study performed with single-tablet doses under exacting conditions in a group of volunteers shows this feature in greater detail (Figure 4). There is extraordinary variability in the peak height, time to peak height, and differences in plasma concentrations 10 h after drug intake. These differences may be genetically conditioned, as has previously been seen in other studies of antipyrine and coumarin in identical and fraternal twins, the latter group showing much greater variability in drug half-lives than the former group.

In studies in several developing countries—Singapore, Thailand, Nigeria, Sri Lanka—and in the U.S., we were able to investigate this problem in depth *(5, 6)*. There were marked differences in the proportions of conjugates (glucuronides and sulfates), and in the plasma concentrations of estradiol and of various oxidative metabolites of ethynyl estradiol and mestranol. The peak plasma concentrations of free estrogen and the half-life of the elimination phase differed markedly between countries (Figure 5), even when we corrected for body weight differences by expressing the plasma concentrations after adjustment for body weight.

Such observations are not confined to ethynyl estrogens. Some years later, studies of two socioeconomic groups in India also showed substantial differences in the plasma kinetics of norethindrone, the other constituent of a widely used OC. In both cases the data for first-cycle users and for long-term users were similar.

These differences obviously represent differences in hepatic and renal conjugation and in hepatic oxidative metabolism, not just

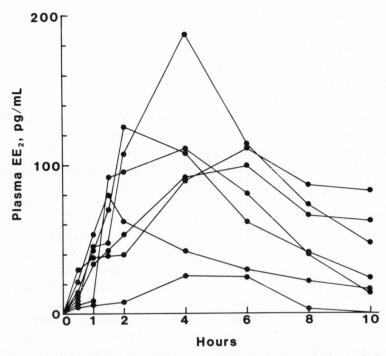

Fig. 4. Individual curves for plasma concentrations of ethynyl estradiol in a carefully monitored trial, with control of previous food and liquid ingestion

Note variability in peak height, time to peak, and area under the curve

a difference in digestive-tract bacteria, or some other relatively trivial matter. The implications are considerable: because different geographic groups metabolize these drugs differently, one may anticipate geographic differences in bioavailability, potency, and adverse reactions. This fully justifies the need for multinational comparative studies, which have been an important part of the agenda of the Human Reproduction Unit of the World Health Organization.

It is clear, therefore, that variation between human beings is much greater than within inbred strains of laboratory animals. Projections from animals to humans must take this into account, as must the determination of a therapeutically effective dose. If an OC is to provide at least 98% protection from conception, most users will of necessity be overdosed to ensure the necessary margin of safety. Not only variations between groups of individu-

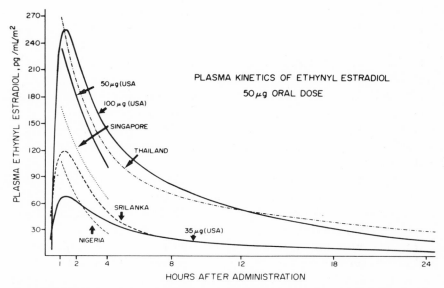

Fig. 5. Plasma concentrations of ethynyl estradiol after a single dose, in previously untreated women, in various countries

Values are adjusted for differences in body weight

als, but also variations within an individual must be considered to account for occasional circumstances such as diarrhea or the concomitant use of antibiotics or enzyme-competitive drugs that may alter bioavailability.

Immunocontraception

An "ideal" contraceptive would be one that, among other properties, confined its activity exclusively to a critical point in the process of conception. However, even mechanical contraceptives such as condoms and diaphragms have extra-contraceptional activities, e.g., significant effects on sexually transmitted disease. The unexpected effects of steroidal contraceptives include the reported reduction in the incidence of rheumatoid arthritis in OC users. In any event, one of the overriding considerations in the acceptability of a contraceptive modality is its freedom from unwanted or hazardous side effects. The more ubiquitous the sites of action of a chemical substance, the more likely it is to run afoul of problems.

The attempt to use prostaglandins for contraception is an excellent example. It could have been (and was) predicted that this modality would be too trouble-ridden for general contraceptive use. Nevertheless, one U.S. agency invested several million dollars in unproductive research on contraception with prostaglandins.

The effects of steroidal sex hormones on nontarget tissues, e.g., the cardiovascular system and the coagulation mechanism, are too well known to require description. Concern about these hazards (whether justified or not) has discouraged millions of potential users of this modality.

Many antispermatogenic compounds have proved to be hepatotoxic or cytotoxic in doses adequate to produce aspermia. Even vasectomy was thought, at one time, to have deleterious effects on the concentrations of plasma lipids.

The lesson to be learned from these experiences is that a potential contraceptive agent should have as restricted and specific a locus of action as possible. This constraint is indeed a strict one: one would think that an antigonadotropic substance, e.g., long-acting gonadoliberin (gonadotropin-releasing hormone, GnRH), would meet these specifications; however, it suppresses steroidogenesis (and therefore libido) as well as spermatogenesis—clearly an unacceptable "side effect." Again, this was entirely predictable, but money and effort are still being expended in some quarters in the hope that the research investment in developing GnRH analogs can be recouped by the development of a usable contraceptive. In our view, this effort, like the effort with prostaglandins, is headed for failure.

These experiences underscore the potential advantages of using a mechanism as highly specific as an immunological one. Indeed, this situation has not gone unnoticed, although professional immunologists as a group have shown little interest. However, the antigenic determinant—i.e., that portion of the antigen that participates in the antigen–antibody reaction—is only large enough to bind about four to five amino acid residues. Because there are a finite number of these amino acid residues and therefore a finite number of combinations of them, it is not surprising that cross reactivity can occur, and indeed this phenomenon is well known to clinical chemists and others experienced in radioimmunoassay. Considering that about 25% of all proteins have allotypic variants in different individuals, the potential for problems from cross reactivity should not be underestimated.

Let us first consider the methods, advantages, and limitations of immunization as applied to fertility control, and then discuss the status of specific research efforts.

Immunization Concepts

The immunization process, which may be either active or passive, may be directed toward self antigens, "foreign antigens," or pregnancy-related antigens. Examples of self antigens would be the zona pellucida antigens of the ovum in the female or sperm antigens in the male. Examples of foreign antigens would include sperm in the female. Pregnancy-related antigens have some of the characteristics of foreign antigens, in that paternal antigens may be expressed, but they are generally well tolerated by the host and therefore behave like self antigens. Such antigens would include choriogonadotropin and placental antigens. All of these agents have been considered in fertility control, yet each involves a unique set of problems. Self antigens have an important disadvantage—they are "tolerated"—and it is often difficult to evoke an immune response to them. This limitation is often bypassed by chemically modifying the antigen. Such modified antigens are then recognized as "foreign" and evoke an immune response; however, the immune response is directed toward the modified antigen, so that the response against the target self antigen is in reality a form of cross reactivity. Although the immune response to the modified antigen may be strong, the response to the target antigen is often much more limited. Adjuvants are often used to enhance the immune response. Foreign antigens, like sperm in the female, are immunogenic. But sperm present a different problem—the repeated exposure to a massive amount of antigen in a very short time. Immune responses, even secondary responses, often require days to produce enough antibody to neutralize the offending antigen. Sperm have been noted in the fallopian tube as quickly as 5 min after intercourse; therefore, antisperm antibody would have to be "in place" to be effective—there would not be enough time to generate a secondary immune response. Even if a suitable sperm antigen is found, the problem of completely and consistently neutralizing 50 to 100 million sperm in just a few minutes is asking a lot of the immune system—perhaps too much.

Pregnancy-related antigens present many of the problems of self antigens. Choriogonadotropin is very similar to lutropin (luteinizing hormone, LH) and is not immunogenic per se.

Passive immunization involves the passive transfer of immunogically active components, usually antibodies (no antigen). One advantage of passive immunization is that it does not require or depend upon individual immune responses.

In 1975 Kohler and Milstein introduced the technique of cell fusion (hybridoma production), by which almost limitless quantities of highly specific antibodies can be produced. However, even hybridoma antibodies may have some limitations. There are a considerable number of immunoglobulin allotypes in the human population, for example, Kappa Gn (gamma) allotypes in the heavy chain of IgG and Inv allotypes in the κ light chains. Although such allotypic variants have not been a major problem in passive immunization with anti-$Rh_0(D)$, it is less clear how important (i.e., immunogenic) they would be in long-term repeated exposures after multiple injections over a period of years.

Passive immunization generates a transient immune response. The short half-life of immunoglobulin (about 23 days for IgG) is also an inevitable constraint to the application of this technology.

Although hybridomas provide a method for generating cheap, abundant, and highly specific antibodies and have certainly increased the prospect of a passive immunotherapy strategy for fertility control, a considerable number of problems still exist, including the finding of a suitable antigen, the short half-life of immunoglobulin, and the presence of antibody allotypes that might also provoke an immune response to the passively transferred antibodies.

Active immunization involves inoculation or exposure to an antigen or immunogen that provokes an immune response: the production of antibodies and the development of cells specifically sensitized to the immunogen. Active immunization has the advantage that it is a "continuing" immune reaction with a secondary response on re-exposure to antigen. This can also be a considerable disadvantage, if an individual develops an autoimmune disease secondary to a cross-reactive antigen. Active immunization with self antigens is difficult because of the body's tolerance to them. Because active immunization requires participation of each individual's immune system, variations in immune responsiveness can present problems when large populations are involved.

Another important aspect of active immunization is that once stimulated, an active response is difficult to control and may be irreversible. Thus, active immunization may be limited to sterilization rather than contraception.

Use of Choriogonadotropin as an Antigen

Because human choriogonadotropin (hCG) is manufactured by the blastocyst very early in gestation and plays an essential role in early gestation, it has become a focal point for efforts an immunologic contraception.

The structure of hCG has been well defined, consisting of an alpha and a beta chain. Because the alpha chain is almost identical in structure to the alpha chain of LH, follitropin (follicle-stimulating hormone, FSH), and thyrotropin (TSH, thyroid-stimulating hormone), problems of cross reactivity make the alpha chain a poor candidate as a target for immunization. Although there are some similarities in the structure of the beta chain of hCG with that of FSH and TSH, the greatest homology is with human LH (hLH). hCG and hLH share 94 of the first 110 amino acid residues (85% homology), but hCG is larger (145 vs 115 amino acids) and has a unique sequence of 35 amino acids on its carboxyterminus. This situation presents both an immunologic dilemma and an opportunity. The dilemma is the problem of cross reaction between β-hCG and β-hLH (on the order of 10%), and the fear that immunization with β-hCG would result in immune reaction against hLH and the anterior pituitary, with induction of anovulation and menstrual changes. The opportunity is the potential of developing a "fertility vaccine" contraceptive by using the unique C-terminus of β-hCG. As might be expected, hCG and its β-subunit are not immunogenic in humans, and the 35 amino-acid C-terminus of hCG is at best weakly immunogenic. Therefore, researchers have attempted to conjugate hCG or portions of it to immunogenic substances or to modify it chemically, e.g., by conjugating the whole hCG molecule or the β-chain to p-aminosulfonic acid (PASA) or by conjugating the β-chain to puri-

111

fied tetanus toxoid (β-hCG-TT), flagellin, or diphtheria toxoid. Conjugating the C-terminus or fragments of it to large immunogenic carriers is a particularly appealing strategy, and, in fact, antisera to the C-terminus have not shown cross reactivity with hLH or other pituitary hormones.

Although a choriogonadotropin-like substance is present in rats, mice, hamsters, and hares, it is not clear whether this plays the same essential physiological role in supporting pregnancy in these animals as in humans. Although the animals will respond immunologically when injected with hCG, their antisera have a low cross reactivity with the animals' endogenous choriogonadotropins. Consequently, studies in rodents and rabbits of the efficiency and safety of immunization with this hormone are difficult to interpret in terms of a comparable human situation, and must be viewed with some skepticism. Although true, it is almost irrelevant that fertility has been somewhat inhibited without toxicity in these species. This is not a criticism of early studies, it being quite natural, considering cost, convenience, etc., to begin such studies with rodents, which in many experimental systems have substituted admirably for humans. This subject has been discussed in detail quite nicely by Jones (7) and Stevens (8).

Even subhuman primates present problems in practical discussions of the feasibility, effectiveness, and safety of immunofertility regulation with choriogonadotropin. For example, baboons immunized with the β-chain of hCG produce antisera that react with hCG and also baboon CG, but to a much lesser degree with baboon CG than with hCG. Such antisera also cross react with hLH, but not with baboon LH. The differences between such experimental models and the human situation should not be underestimated. β-hCG is not immunogenic per se in the human, and the baboon immune response means that it is "seeing" something foreign and different in the molecule than what the human immune system will "see" and respond to. Antifertility effects in such animal systems are therefore based on cross reactivity to antigenic determinants of baboon CG that may not even exist in the human; moreover, the lack of reactivity to baboon LH limits interpretations of toxicity and of the effect on ovulation and menses, which are of considerable importance.

The critical nature of the immunizing antigen can be appreciated by the fact that the antisera to the C-terminus 37-amino-acid residue of β-hCG react with hCG in vitro and neutralize its physiologic activity in vivo, whereas antisera to less than the terminal 35-amino-acid residues react with hCG but do not block its biological function.

Despite their limitations, subhuman primates remain the best model system available for experimentation, provided we appreciate their limitations. Consider the following experiments with these animals.

Stevens [8] actively immunized eight baboons with β-hCG and eight with PASA-β-hCG. As might be expected, there was considerable cross reactivity with hLH but minimal reactivity with baboon LH, and the animals menstruated normally. None of 10 animals (mated a total of 30 times) conceived. Pregnant marmosets immunized by Hearn [9] before the eighth day of pregnancy aborted or absorbed their fetuses and remained infertile for up to 16 months; late immunization did not affect the outcome of the pregnancy. Interestingly, after an abortion, the menstrual cycles were normal until antibody titers began to decline, at which time cycles became progressively longer; repeated abortion occurred for several years. Humans immunized with β-hCG-TT had markedly varied antibody responses, with only 25% of women developing adequate antibody response; as a consequence, 10 pregnancies were reported in eight immunized women [10].

Two mechanisms have been suggested to explain the antifertility effect of immunization with hCG: a neutralization of the luteotropic effect of the hormone, and a direct cytotoxic effect. Experimental evidence regarding the mechanism is conflicting. The zona pellucida of blastocysts washed from the marmoset uterus was intact, with no evidence of a direct cytotoxic reaction, thus suggesting a luteotropic rather than a direct cytotoxic effect; however, four out of five marmosets given progesterone implants, which would presumably compensate for any loss of luteotropic effect, aborted. The other animal delivered a normal offspring. Hysterectomies in marmosets done before they aborted also showed no placental pathology, and their concentrations of estradiol-17β and progesterone were normal. It is therefore not clear whether a luteotropic, cytotoxic, or other as yet unidentified mechanism(s) is involved.

The potential for toxicity from immunization is of obvious interest, especially considering the relatively good safety record of other contraceptive methods.

Eight rhesus monkeys immunized with β-hCG-TT and repeatedly challenged with hCG and hLH showed no gross or microscopic anomalies and no evidence of immune complex disease *(10)*. No toxicity has been reported in immunized baboons or chimpanzees. Women immunized with β-hCG-PASA *(11)* showed cross-reactive antibodies to hLH, and eight of 10 postmenopausal women showed a decrease of hLH; premenopausal women had a decrease in mid-cycle hLH. Despite the lack of a pre-ovulatory peak of hLH, two of four women had ovulatory patterns of serum progesterone. There were no changes in the menstrual cycle in premenopausal women. More than 60 women immunized with β-hCG-TT showed no clinical or laboratory evidence of toxicity or autoimmune diseases, and menstruation remained normal.

The experience to date suggests that hCG or some fragment involving the C-terminus might provide a safe and effective means of immunological fertility control, but considerably more work is needed to define the suitable antigen.

One extraordinary outcome of research on the immunological properties of hCG and similar molecules has been the discovery of the ubiquity of these materials. For example, some strains of bacteria make substances immunologically indistinguishable from hCG, and several human tumors and perhaps even normal human tissues make materials that apparently differ from hCG only in the degree of sialylation. The possible consequences of these exciting observations are just beginning to be explored.

Sperm Antigens

Immunological infertility resulting from antibodies to sperm has been suggested for some time. The potential for an immunologically mediated infertility is enhanced by the realization that IgA and IgG antibodies are present in the cervical mucus, as well as in the endometrial cavity and fallopian tubes. However, the picture is clouded by considerable controversy regarding the significance of antisperm antibodies in cervical mucus—fostered by the poor correlation between the presence of such antibodies (as demonstrated by indirect immunofluorescence) and fertility. The correlation between fertility and the presence of antisperm antibodies appears to be better when assayed with a sperm immobilization test. Reportedly, 5 to 10% of women with unexplained infertility have antisperm antibodies (12), whereas such antibodies are uncommon in fertile controls. The existence of a "naturally occurring" infertility raises the prospect for immunological fertility control based on immunization with sperm.

Interestingly, in 1932, Baskin (13) immunized 20 women with three intramuscular injections of 5 to 20 mL of whole semen. No complications from the injection were noted and cytotoxic antibodies persisted for as long as 12 months. None of the women became pregnant while antibody titers persisted. Although effective, whole semen is a "dirty" immunogen, and researchers have attempted to define in some way the antigen(s) that can be effectively used for immunological fertility control.

More than 20 enzymes in mammalian sperm might serve as a potential immunizing antigen. Acrosin (EC 3.4.21.10) and acrosomal hyaluronidase have been tested, and have no antifertility effect. The lactate dehydrogenase (EC 1.1.1.27) isoenzyme LDH-C4 has been the most effective antigen tested so far. This sperm-specific but not species-specific isoenzyme is located in the midpiece of mature sperm, and accounts for 95% of the LDH activity of sperm. Although primarily cytoplasmic, it is also present in the sperm membrane. Interestingly, although the primary mechanism of fertility inhibition occurs before fertilization—possibly mediated by sperm agglutination, cytotoxicity, sperm immobilization, or enhanced phagocytosis, or by blocking fertilization—there is also an increase in embryo loss in immunized animals after fertilization. Although immunization with LDH-C4 decreases fertility in rabbits and baboons, the pregnancy rates have been too high to consider the experiments anything but preliminary. Again, additional work is needed to develop LDH-C4 as a potential antifertility antigen.

Zona Pellucida Antigens

The zona pellucida plays an essential role in sperm recognition and in the attachment of sperm to the ovum. The zona is also involved in osmotic regulation and the mechanical protection of the egg. Interestingly, antigens isolated from the zona of several species are surprisingly similar.

115

The potential usefulness of the zona as a target antigen in immunological fertility regulation was suggested by clinical reports of infertility associated with the presence of anti-zona antibodies; unfortunately, the reliability of infertility secondary to anti-zona antibodies has been questioned because antibodies have also been found in fertile and postmenopausal women. Shivers and Dunbar (14), using porcine zona and immunofluorescent antibody techniques, first reported the presence of human anti-zona autoantibodies in infertile women, but Mori et al. (15) demonstrated cross reactivity of human serum heteroantibodies with porcine zona pellucida. The human serum anti-porcine zona activity could be removed by adsorption with porcine erythrocytes. Sacco and Moghissi (16) have noted no difference in the incidence of such antibodies in infertile or fertile women or in men. When positive human sera (reactive with porcine zona) were tested against human ova, they were only weakly reactive or negative (16). It would therefore appear that the antibodies initially described in human serum that react to porcine zona occur "naturally" and are a cross-reactive or heterophile antibody and do not correlate with infertility.

Experimental animal systems involving zona pellucida as an immunogen for fertility regulation have given much more encouraging results. It has been possible to raise by active immunization some highly specific antibodies to heterologous zona antigens that have blocked fertility in several species of rodents. Attempts at active immunization by homologous immunization (with zona pellucida from the same species) have had only limited success in the mouse, hamster, and rat. Passive immunization of mice with anti-zona antibodies via a single intraperitoneal injection has been contraceptive for as long as 30 days; interestingly, the effect was reversible. A return to normal fertility was also reported after successful contraception by active immunization with heterologous zona antigens.

Pig zona antigens cross react with antibodies from monkeys, baboons, chimpanzees, and humans, and immunization with crude pig zona pellucida preparations has prevented pregnancies in marmosets and baboons.

The mechanism of fertility inhibition is not clear. Perhaps the antibodies inhibit zona shedding or sperm binding and penetration (17). The short duration of effect may reflect the fact that antibodies react only with secondary oocytes having a zona pellucida, and not with immature non-zona-coated oocytes.

Although no single zona antigen has been fully identified and characterized, Bleil and Wasserman *(18)* have characterized three major glycoproteins (ZP_1, ZP_2, and ZP_3) from the mouse zona. ZP_3, a sperm receptor, is the object of some current efforts to develop a vaccine. This approach, which involves using a more purified antigen rather than whole zona, offers the potential for antigen modifications to increase the immune effect and to decrease potential cross reactivity with non-zona antigens. Clearly, research involving the use of zona antigens as a potential antifertility vaccine is not nearly as advanced as research with hCG, but it does offer some very interesting possibilities. Because the zona antigens are present in only very limited quantity, there might be an antifertility effect even with quite low antibody titers. The fact that zona antigens appear only in developed oocytes gives the potential for a more reversible "active" immunization. Additional research will be required.

References

1. Goldzieher JW. Hormonal contraception—whence, how, and whither? In *Clinical Use of Sex Steroids,* JR Givens, Ed., Year Book Medical Publishers, Chicago, IL, 1980, pp 31–43.
2. Helton ED, Goldzieher JW. Pharmacokinetics of ethynyl estrogens. A review. *Contraception* **15,** 255–284 (1977).
3. Purdy RH, Goldzieher JW, LeQuesne PW, et al. Active intermediates and carcinogenesis. In *Catechol Estrogens,* GR Merriam, MB Lipsett, Eds., Raven Press, New York, NY, 1983, pp 123–140.
4. Goldzieher JW. Oral contraceptive hazards—1981. *Tex Med* **77,** 61–64 (1981).
5. Williams MD, Goldzieher JW. Chromatographic patterns of urinary ethynyl estrogen metabolites in various populations. *Steroids* **36,** 255–282 (1980).
6. Goldzieher JW, Dozier TS, de la Pena A. Plasma levels and pharmacokinetics of ethynyl estrogens in various populations. II. Mestranol. *Contraception* **21,** 17–27 (1980).
7. Jones WR. *Immunological Fertility Regulation,* Blackwell Scientific, Boston, MA, 1982, pp 35–70.
8. Stevens VC. Perspectives of development of a fertility control vaccine from hormonal antigens of the trophoblast. In *Development of*

Vaccine for Fertility Regulation (WHO Symposium), Scriptor Publ., Copenhagen, 1976, p 93 ff.

9. Hearn TP. The immunobiology of chorionic gonadotropin. In *Immunological Aspects of Reproduction and Fertility Control*, TP Hearn, Ed., MTP Press, Lancaster, 1980, pp 229–244.

10. Stevens VC. Potential methods for immunological fertility control in the female. In *Comprehensive Endocrinology. Endocrine Mechanisms in Fertility Regulation*, G Benagiano, E Diczfalusy, Eds., Raven Press, New York, NY, 1983, pp 141–162.

11. Gupta PD, Natu I, Talwar GP. Immunofluorescence and electron microscopic studies on kidney, choroid plexus and pituitary in rhesus monkeys immunized with the anti-hCG vaccine PR-β-hCG-TT. *Contraception* **18**, 91–104 (1978).

12. Speroff L, Glass RH, Kane GN. *Clinical Gynecologic Endocrinology and Infertility*, 3rd ed., Williams and Wilkins, Baltimore, MD, 1983, 482 pp.

13. Baskin MJ. Temporary sterilization by the injection of human spermatozoa—a preliminary report. *Am J Obstet Gynecol* **24**, 892–897 (1932).

14. Shivers CA, Dunbar BS. Autoantibodies to zona pellucida: A possible cause for infertility in women. *Science* **197**, 1082–1084 (1977).

15. Mori T, Nishimoto T, Kohda H, et al. A method for specific detection of autoantibodies to the zona pellucida in infertile women. *Fertil Steril* **32**, 67–72 (1979).

16. Sacco AG, Moghissi KS. Anti-zona pellucida activity in human sera. *Fertil Steril* **31**, 503–506 (1979).

17. Jones WR. *Op. cit.* (ref. 7), pp 160–161.

18. Bleil TD, Wasserman PM. Structure and function of the zona pellucida: Identification and characterization of the proteins of the mouse oocyte's zona pellucida. *Dev Biol* **76**, 185-202 (1980).

Androgen Excess and the Infertile Female

Rogerio A. Lobo

In recent years there has been increased interest as well as a better understanding of the role of androgens in reproductive medicine, primarily because of improvements in our ability to accurately measure low concentrations of circulating steroids. With this technological advance we have been able to assess the glandular and extraglandular sources of androgen production. In addition, subtle defects in steroidogenesis that result in androgen excess are now being diagnosed more frequently. Identification of specific markers of androgen production has also led to more rational and effective methods for treating and monitoring patients with androgen excess. In this chapter I will stress the clinical use of biochemical markers and will discuss how these measurements aid in diagnosis and treatment of the various syndromes of androgen excess. Although many patients with androgen excess will present with infertility, this discussion is not limited to patients with infertility.

The Clinical Presentation of Androgen Excess

Patients with hyperandrogenism usually present with hirsutism and (or) virilism (1, 3), but other patients without hirsutism may also have increased concentrations of androgens, e.g., patients with acne (4, 5), anovulation (6, 7), luteal dysfunction (8), or amenorrhea (9). In addition, androgens may have an important role in the development of resistance to insulin (10–12), as well as resistance to the induction of ovulation (9, 13, 14).

Although androgen excess is clinically evident in patients with virilism and hirsutism, it is not always so clear that some of the other conditions may be associated with hyperandrogenism. Patients with acne, for example, particularly those who do not re-

119

spond well to conventional dermatologic measures, are well documented to have above-normal concentrations of androgens (4, 5); their conditions usually improve once these concentrations have been adjusted to more normal values (4).

Anovulation is found frequently in patients who have androgen excess, whether or not hirsutism is present (6, 7). Whether this is the result of follicular atresia (15) or the sequela of alterations in gonadotropin feedback mechanisms is not completely clear. Some have suggested that there is disparity between the effect of androgens at peripheral target tissue sites, e.g., the skin, and their effect on the hypothalamic–pituitary axis. Thus patients without hirsutism who have high concentrations of androgens may present with amenorrhea (9).

Although not as well documented, androgen excess may lead to luteal dysfunction as well (8). Because the latter is a syndrome of defective folliculogenesis (16) and because anovulation is so prevalent with androgen excess, this association is not unexpected. Evidence for such an association has been demonstrated in primates (17).

Although obesity and acanthosis nigricans are associated with insulin resistance, patients with polycystic ovary syndrome (PCO) who are not obese and lack acanthosis nigricans may also exhibit insulin resistance.[1] This resistance, although relatively mild, is reflected in the concentrations of insulin in fasting patients, and is clearly related to the concentrations of androgens (11, 12) (Figure 1).

Patients with anovulation who are treated with clomiphene usually respond well, despite increased concentrations of androgens (18). However, in a subgroup of patients who fail to ovulate and who are therefore resistant to the use of clomiphene, decreasing the androgen with dexamethasone (13) has resulted in presumptive ovulation (Figure 2). Similarly, in patients with PCO who do not respond well to human menopausal gonadotropins, the adjunctive use of dexamethasone to lower above-normal concentrations of androgens has improved the patients' responses and increased the pregnancy rate (14).

---

[1] Abbreviations used: PCO, polycystic ovary syndrome; DHEA-S, dehydroepiandrosterone sulfate; 3α-diol G, 3α-androstanediol glucuronide; SHGB, sex-hormone-binding globulin.

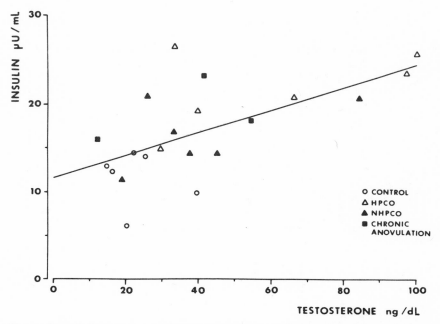

Fig. 1. Correlation between serum testosterone and concentrations of insulin (micro-int. units/mL) in serum from fasting control subjects, hirsute (HPCO) and non-hirsute (NHPCO) patients with polycystic ovary syndrome, and women with chronic anovulation

Androgen Production and Androgen Markers

The sources of glandular production of androgen have been somewhat controversial. Stimulation and catheterization studies intended to settle this issue have been fraught with problems in interpretation. Of potential merit in evaluation of the androgen source is the use of a GnRH agonist *(19)*, which will inhibit ovarian but not adrenal androgen production (Figure 3). In this way production of steroids by these two glands may be differentiated. In clinical practice, however, there is general agreement that serum testosterone best reflects ovarian production of androgen, with as much as two-thirds of circulating testosterone thought to originate in the ovaries. Most investigators also agree that the best marker of adrenal production of androgen is serum dehydroepiandrosterone sulfate (DHEA-S). DHEA-S circulates in large quantities (micrograms per milliliter), has a slow metabolic clearance rate (≤20 L/day), and in women is virtually exclusively a product of the zona reticularis of the adrenals *(20)*. The correlation of

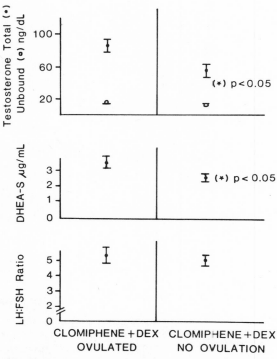

Fig. 2. Mean ± SE for serum total and unbound testosterone, DHEA-S, and the LH:FSH ratio of women sampled before treatment with clomiphene and dexamethasone (DEX)

Four women ovulated *(left panel)* and four did not *(right panel)*

serum DHEA-S with urinary excretion of 17-ketosteroids, corrected for creatinine, is excellent (Figure 4), but DHEA-S is a more sensitive marker for adrenal androgen than are urinary 17-ketosteroids. DHEA-S is only weakly androgenic itself, and may be most correctly considered a pre-hormone.

A long neglected source of androgen production is the extraglandular or peripheral compartment. As is well documented, peripheral tissues are capable of producing androgens and modulating androgen action. The mechanism for this most relevant to this review is via the action of 5α-reductase, which amplifies the effect of androgen. Until recently, there has been no marker for the peripheral compartment. However, some of our recent

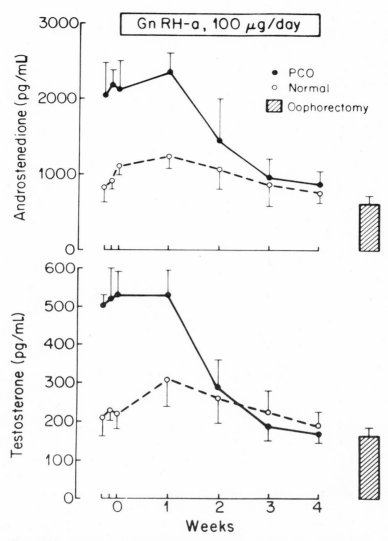

Fig. 3. Mean serum concentrations of androstenedione and testosterone in women with PCO and in normal ovulatory subjects before and after treatment with a GnRH agonist (GnRH-a) and in oophorectomized women

work indicates that an androgen metabolite in blood, 3α-androstanediol glucuronide (3α-diol G), is very reflective of activity within the peripheral compartment (21). Serum 3α-diol G, which is of extrasplanchnic origin, most probably is a product of 5α-

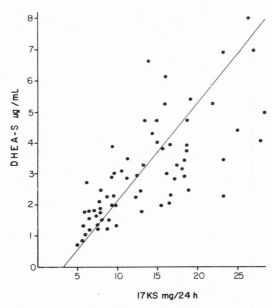

Fig. 4. Correlation between serum DHEA-S and total 17-ketosteroids (17-KS) in 71 women: $r = 0.7$; $p < 0.0005$

Total 17-ketosteroids corrected for creatinine excretion (assumed to be 20 mg of creatinine per kilogram of body weight)

and 3α-keto reduction of androgen in tissues. Although it is produced primarily as an androgen disposal mechanism, it is closely reflective of the clinical state (22, 23). Recent work by our group has confirmed the in vitro production of 3α-diol G by genital skin. In addition, there is a close correlation between 5α-reductase activity of skin in vitro and the measurement of 3α-diol G in serum. Serum concentrations of 3α-diol G correlate extremely well with the presence of hirsutism in women and, as Figure 5 shows, differentiate hirsute from nonhirsute patients with PCO who have similarly increased concentrations of glandularly produced androgens (testosterone and DHEA-S) (22). In summary, therefore, we have three markers of androgen production: testosterone primarly reflects ovarian production of androgen, DHEA-S represents adrenal production, and 3α-diol G reflects androgen production in the peripheral compartment.

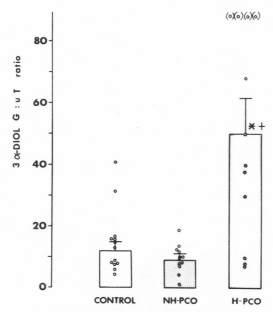

Fig. 5. Ratios of serum 3α-diol G:testosterone (uT) in controls, NH-PCO and H-PCO patients

Bars indicate mean ± SEM; the *asterisk* indicates higher ratios compared with controls ($p < 0.05$); and the *cross* indicates higher ratios compared with NH-PCO patients ($p < 0.05$). H-PCO, NH-CPO, see Fig. 1

Modulators of Androgen Action

A major modulator of androgen action is sex-hormone-binding globulin (SHBG). When androgen excess results in a decrease in SHBG (Figure 6), the concentration of non-SHBG-bound testosterone is usually increased. Increasing the concentration of androgens in serum decreases the ability of SHBG to keep androgens bound, and more of the androgen, such as testosterone, is free *(24)*. Non-SHBG-bound testosterone is the moiety of testosterone associated with albumin; nonetheless, it should be physiologically important and available to the androgen receptor *(25)*. Moreover, this has to differentiated from testosterone that is dialyzably "free." Salivary testosterone, a natural dialysate, is a third "analyte" used to increase the accuracy of testosterone measurements *(26)*. Despite some debate as to which of these three moieties

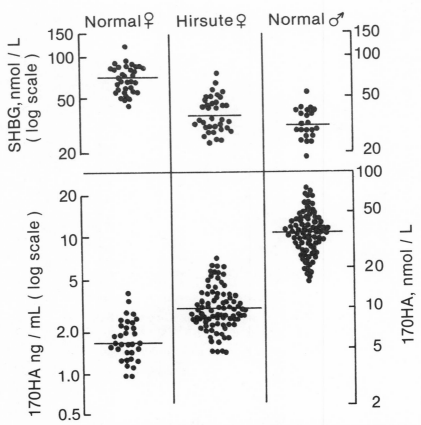

Fig. 6. Plasma concentrations of sex-hormone-binding globulin (SHBG) in individuals with relatively low, modest, and high concentrations of circulating, biologically potent androgens (17β-hydroxyandrogen, 17OHA) as found in normal women, hirsute women, and normal men

Note that SHBG concentrations in adult women are more than twice those in adult men. Adapted from Anderson (37)

of testosterone serves best to reflect hyperandrogenism, there is little difference in how measurements of these analyte fractions help clinically. Indeed, although all of these measurements increase the precision of diagnosing ovarian hyperandrogenism, they do not help greatly in the treatment of patients. Subtle increases in non-SHBG-bound testosterone, as might occur when serum concentrations of testosterone remain normal in certain patients, would be treated in much the same way, depending on the abnormalities in the other two compartments (see below). Alternatively, high concentrations of testosterone, which result in high concentrations of non-SHBG-bound testosterone, would also be treated in a fashion that is not dependent on knowing the magnitude of the increase in non-SHBG-bound testosterone. This viewpoint has been supported by recent data *(27)*.

Another major modulator of androgen action is 5α-reductase activity. Our present concept as to how androgen excess is manifest in peripheral tissues (hirsutism and virilism) is that the activity of 5α-reductase has a key role in tissue. Therefore, we have attempted to find a way to quantify this enzymic process. At present there is evidence that serum 3α-diol G reflects this activity, at least in part; however, in vitro incubations of skin tissue from patients offer the opportunity to study directly the way in which androgens are interconverted within individual patients. With such an approach we have developed a model system for diagnosing and treating hyperandrogenism in individual women who have increased activity of 5α-reductase in the peripheral compartment *(28)*.

Enzymic Defects in Hyperandrogenism

Although congenital adrenal hyperplasia may be diagnosed in a woman in her reproductive years who presents with androgen excess *(29)*, in such patients the concentrations of androgen are not discriminatory. However, the concentration of 17-hydroxyprogesterone in serum is increased both basally and, more especially, in response to corticotropin (Figure 7). We use a cutoff value for 17-hydroxyprogesterone of >3 ng/mL to screen for this disorder. Although a few patients may have exaggerated responses to stimulation with corticotropin, but basal 17-hydroxyprogesterone concentrations <3 ng, this is extremely uncommon; these patients, who have an extremely mild defect, are treated effectively according to the scheme described later. On the other hand, many patients whose concentrations of 17-hydroxyprogesterone exceed 3 ng/mL will have normal responses to corticotropin stimulation; in these patients, the source of increased 17-hydroxyprogesterone is the ovary. The decision to measure baseline values of this hormone to screen for this disorder has been somewhat arbitrary up to now. We stress, however, that a patient should be screened if she is shorter than other family members, has a

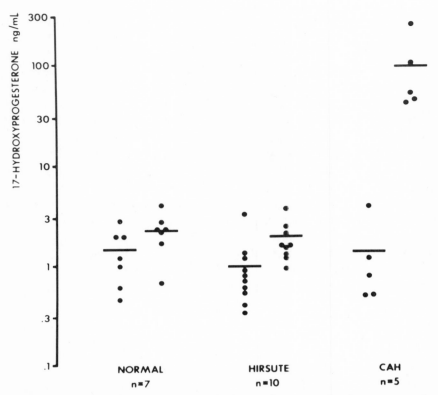

Fig. 7. Serum 17-hydroxyprogesterone before and 60 min after intravenous administration of a single bolus of 0.25 mg of corticotropin (ACTH) in seven normal female controls, 10 hirsute oligomenorrheic women, and five women with congenital adrenal hyperplasia (CAH)

strong family history for androgen excess, displays a significant degree of hirsutism and (or) virilization at a young age, or has higher than expected concentrations of testosterone and DHEA-S. Other patients with excess adrenal androgen, particularly some of those considered to have PCO, will have mild defects in 3β-ol dehydrogenase isomerase *(30)*. These patients have high concentrations of baseline serum DHEA-S and normal or low concentrations of testosterone, and may be diagnosed by finding exaggerated $\Delta^5:\Delta^4$ steroid ratios in response to stimulation with corticotropin (Figure 8). Serum DHEA-S and Δ^5-androstenediol are the most useful markers for this disorder. Adrenal production

128

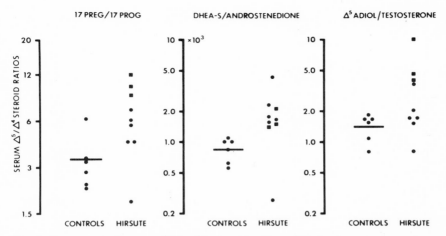

Fig. 8. Responses of serum Δ⁵ to Δ⁴ steroid ratios of 17-hydroxypregnenolone to 17-hydroxyprogesterone after 1 h, and of DHEA-S to androstenedione, and of Δ⁵-androstenediol (Δ⁵adiol) to testosterone after 3 h, in six control women and nine hirsute women after stimulation with corticotropin

Three hirsute women (■) have abnormal ratios for all of these Δ⁵ to Δ⁴ steroid pairs

of androgen is easily suppressed by administration of glucocorticoids.

Syndromes Resulting in Hirsutism

Although I will not discuss the clinical evaluation of patients with hirsutism, the candidates for differential diagnosis are listed in Table 1, the diagnosis of each being based on the clinical evaluation as well as the results of specific diagnostic tests. The most common causes of hirsutism are "idiopathic" hirsutism and PCO. Idiopathic hirsutism is somewhat of a misnomer; it has been reserved for those patients with normal menses who present with hirsutism and have relatively normal concentrations of serum androgens. However, the rate of androgen production and the proportion of free androgens may be abnormal in these patients. In addition, androgen production by the ovaries or the adrenals may not suffice to explain the abnormality, given that peripheral production (the third compartment) of androgen is heightened in virtually all of these patients (21).

PCO is not an ovarian abnormality; frequently, the adrenal is

Table 1. **Differential Diagnosis of Hirsute Women**

Iatrogenic
"Idiopathic": a misnomer
Polycystic ovary syndrome
Stromal hyperthecosis
Ovarian tumors
Adrenal tumors
Cushing's syndrome
Congenital adrenal hyperplasia
Abnormal sexual development

also involved. In addition, ovarian size per se is not a criterion for the diagnosis. Rather the characteristic marker for this disorder is biochemical. Inappropriate gonadotropin secretion is the cardinal feature of PCO *(31)* and is exemplified by an increased concentrations of lutropin (LH) in serum, a normal or low concentration of follitropin (FSH), an LH:FSH ratio > 3, and an exaggerated LH response to gonadoliberin (GnRH) stimulation (Figure 9). Whereas the serum concentrations of LH and the LH:FSH ratio may be increased in only 70% of patients, a relatively new marker, bioactive LH, is increased in virtually all patients (Figure 10). Serum bioactive LH, as measured by assay of mouse interstitial cells, appears to be an extremely useful marker for PCO, and in addition is highly correlated with glandular production of androgen in PCO *(32)*. However, hirsutism in PCO may not be related primarily to glandular production of androgen: in those 30% of patients with PCO who are not hirsute, despite increased concentrations of testosterone and DHEA-S, the peripheral production of androgen reflected by serum 3α-diol G is normal *(22)*.

Clinical Assessment of Androgen Excess

Regardless of the specific diagnosis, the clinical approach should to directed to determining the source(s) of androgen excess, so that specific therapy may be instituted. Therefore, after a careful history and physical examination, we stress the measurement of testosterone, DHEA-S, and 3α-diol G, in serum, to investigate the three compartments of androgen production. In addition, 17-hydroxyprogesterone may be measured, as indicated. Once conditions such as tumor, congenital adrenal hyperplasia, Cushing's

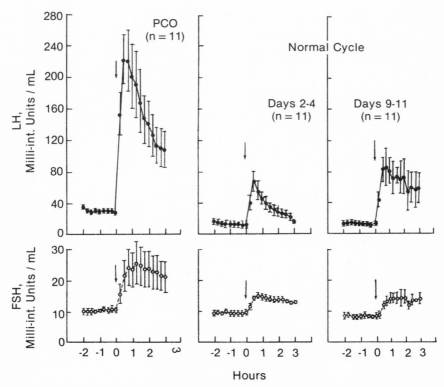

Fig. 9. Comparison of quantitative LH and FSH release in response to a single bolus of 150 μg of luliberin (injection indicated by *arrow*) in PCO patients and in normal women during low-estrogen (early follicular) and high-estrogen (late follicular) phases of their cycle

Adapted from Rebar et al. *(31)*

syndrome, etc. have been ruled out by careful history, physical examination, and adjunctive tests, if necessary, treatment may be instituted. Regardless of the presenting complaint of androgen excess (hirsutism, acne, anovulation), treatment should be dictated by the source of the androgen excess.

Concentrations of testosterone in excess of 1.5 ng/mL are suggestive of ovarian neoplasm and warrant further investigation. Similarly, serum concentrations of DHEA-S greater than 8 μg/ mL signify significant adrenal production of androgens and warrant investigating the possibility of an adrenal neoplasm. High concentrations of 3α-diol G suggest increased peripheral production of androgens. If testosterone and DHEA-S are also increased,

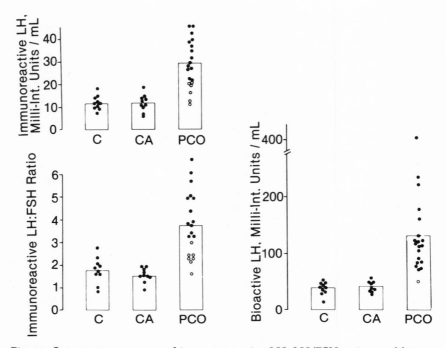

Fig. 10. Serum measurement of immunoreactive LH, LH/FSH ratios, and bioactive LH in control subjects (C), in women with cancer (CA), and in women with PCO

Closed circles for women with PCO indicate values exceeding 3 SD of mean control values

there are several therapeutic options: androgen production by the ovary or the adrenal may be hindered, androgen receptors may be blocked, or various combinations of the above may be tried. However, if concentrations of serum 3α-diol G are increased but those of testosterone and DHEA-S are normal (often called "idiopathic" hirsutism), specific receptor-blocking drugs should be used.

Treatment of Androgen Excess

Increased concentrations of testosterone suggest excess ovarian production of androgens; treatment with oral contraceptives may therefore be most effective (33). A specific benefit of such therapy is an increase in SHBG binding, which decreases the non-SHBG-bound or free moiety of testosterone. Estrogen at 35 μg is effective in this regard, so that "low-dose" oral contraceptives may be used. Spironolactone, which is used as an androgen-receptor blocking drug (see below), also lowers testosterone concentrations *(34, 35)*.

Corticosteroids are indicated only if excess androgen has an adrenal source, as documented by increases in DHEA-S. Concentrations as great as 4 μg/mL may be effectively treated with oral contraceptives containing norethindrone. If corticoids are used, give 0.5 mg or less of dexamethasone or 5–7.5 mg of prednisone each night.

If both testosterone and DHEA-S are significantly increased, a combination of corticosteroids and oral contraceptives may be effective *(36)*.

Increases in 3α-diol G suggest increased peripheral production of androgen; androgen-receptor-blocking drugs should be considered. Although cyproterone acetate has received much attention in Europe, it is not available in the United States. Of various receptor-blocking drugs tried in the United States, including cyproheptadine, cimetidine, and spironolactone, the last is the most effective. Treatment with it increases the metabolic clearance rate of testosterone and decreases the production rate (possibly through a reduction in cytochrome P450). However, serum concentrations of DHEA-S are not lowered, and we have not used spironolactone to treat those patients who have evidence only of adrenal-source androgen excess. In work in progress we have found that spironolactone blocks androgen receptors in addition to the above mechanisms and also reduces the activity of 5α-reductase in tissue (P Serafini and RA Lobo, unpublished). We have tried daily doses of 50 to 200 mg of spironolactone, of which 200 mg daily appears to be the most effective.

References

1. Mauvais J, Kuttenn F, Mowszowicz L. *Hirsutism,* Springer-Verlag, New York, NY, 1981, p 1.
2. Bardin CW, Lipsett M. Testosterone and androstenedione blood production rates in normal women and women with idiopathic hirsutism and polycystic ovaries. *J Clin Invest* **46**, 891 (1976).
3. Kirschner MA, Zucker IR, Jespersen D. Idiopathic hirsutism—an ovarian abnormality. *N Engl J Med* **294**, 637 (1976).

4. Marynick SP, Chakmakjian ZH, McCaffree DL, Herndon JH Jr. Androgen excess in cystic acne. *N Engl J Med* **308**, 981–986 (1983).

5. Darley CR, Kirby JD, Besser GM, et al. Circulating testosterone, sex hormone bindng globulin and prolactin in women with late onset or persistent acne vulgaris. *Br J Dermatol* **106**, 517 (1982).

6. Lobo RA, Goebelsmann U, Mishell DR Jr. Serum levels of DHEAS in gynecologic and endocrinopathy and infertility. *Obstet Gynecol* **57**, 607–612 (1981).

7. DeVane GW, Czekala MN, Judd JL, et al. Circulating gonadotropins, estrogens and androgens in polycystic ovarian disease. *Am J Obstet Gynecol* **121**, 496 (1975).

8. Sherman DM, Korenman SG. Measurement of serum LH, FSH, estradiol and progesterone in disorders of the human menstrual cycle: The inadequate luteal phase. *J Clin Endocrinol Metab* **39**, 145 (1974).

9. McKenna TF, Moore A, Magee F, Cunningham S. Amenorrhea with cryptic hyperandrogenemia. *J Clin Endocrinol Metab* **56**, 893 (1983).

10. Chang RJ, Nakamura RM, Judd HL, Kaplan SA. Insulin resistance in non-obese patients with polycystic ovarian disease. *J Clin Endocrinol Metab* **57**, 356 (1983).

11. Shoupe D, Lobo RA. Insulin resistance in polycystic ovary syndrome. *Am J Obstet Gynecol* **147**, 588–592 (1983).

12. Shoupe D, Lobo RA. Influence of androgens on insulin resistance. *Fertil Steril* (in press).

13. Lobo RA, Paul W, March CM, et al. Clomiphene and dexamethasone in women unresponsive to clomiphene alone. *Obstet Gynecol* **60**, 497–501 (1982).

14. Evron S, Navot D, Lanfer N, Diamant YA. Induction of ovulation with combined human gonadotropins and dexamethasone in women with polycystic ovarian disease. *Fertil Steril* **40**, 183 (1983).

15. Louvet JP, Harman SM, Schreiber JR, Ross GT. Evidence for a role of androgens in follicular maturation. *Endocrinology* **97**, 366 (1975).

16. DiZerega GS, Hodgen GD. Folliculogenesis in the primate ovarian cycle. *Endocr Rev* **2**, 27 (1981).

17. Castracane VD, Wright E, Czar PL. The effect of testosterone on human chorionic gonadotropin stimulated ovarian steroidogenesis in vivo in the baboon *(Papio cynocephalus)*. *Fertil Steril* **40**, 683 (1983).

18. Lobo RA, Gysler M, March CM, et al. Clinical and laboratory predictors of clomiphene response. *Fertil Steril* **37**, 168–174 (1982).

19. Chang RJ, Laufer RL, Meldrum RD, et al. Steroid secretion in polycytic ovarian disease after ovarian suppression by a long-acting gonadotropin releasing hormone agonist. *J Clin Endocrinol Metab* **56**, 897–903 (1983).

20. Lobo RA, Paul WL, Goebelsmann U. Dehydroepiandrosterone sulfate as an indicator of adrenal androgen function. *Obstet Gynecol* **57**, 69–73 (1981).
21. Morimoto I, Edmiston A, Hawks D, Horton R. Studies on the origin of androstanediol and androstanediol glucuronide in young and elderly men. *J Clin Endocrinol Metab* **52**, 772 (1981).
22. Horton R, Hawks D, Lobo R. 3α,17β-Androstanediol glucuronide in plasma: A marker of androgen action in idiopathic hirsutism. *J Clin Invest* **69**, 1203–1206 (1982).
23. Lobo RA, Goebelsmann U, Horton R. Evidence for the importance of peripheral tissue events in the development of hirsutism in polycystic ovary syndrome. *J Clin Endocrinol Metab* **57**, 393–397 (1983).
24. Lobo RA, Goebelsmann U. Effect of androgen excess on inappropriate gonadotropin secretion as found in the polycystic ovary syndrome. *Am J Obstet Gynecol* **142**, 394–401 (1982).
25. Pardridge WM. Transport of protein-bound hormones into tissues in vivo. *Endocr Rev* **2**, 103 (1981).
26. Smith RG, Besch PK, Bill B, Buttram V. Saliva as matrix for measuring free androgens: Comparison with serum androgens in polycystic ovarian disease. *Fertil Steril* **31**, 513 (1979).
27. Schwartz U, Moltz L, Brotherton J, Hammerstein J. The diagnostic value of plasma free testosterone in non-tumorous and tumorous hyperandrogenism. *Fertil Steril* **40**, 66 (1983).
28. Serafini P, Goebelsmann UT, Lobo RA. Increased 5α-reductase activity in hirsutism. *Fertil Steril* **41**, 3S–4S (1984).
29. Lobo RA, Goebelsmann U. Adult manifestation of congenital adrenal hyperplasia due to incomplete 21-hydroxylase deficiency mimicking polycystic ovarian disease. *Am J Obstet Gynecol* **138**, 720–726 (1980).
30. Lobo RA, Goebelsmann U. Evidence for reduced 3β-ol-hydroxysteroid dehydrogenase activity in some hirsute women thought to have polycystic ovary syndrome. *J Clin Endocrinol Metab* **53**, 394–400 (1981).
31. Rebar R, Judd HL, Yen SSC, et al. Characterization of the inappropriate gonadotropin secretion in polycystic ovary syndrome. *J Clin Invest* **57**, 1320 (1976).
32. Lobo RA, Kletzky OA, Campeau JD, DiZerega GS. Elevated bioactive luteinizing hormone in women with the polycystic ovary syndrome (PCO). *Fertil Steril* **39**, 674–678 (1983).
33. Givens JR. The effectiveness of two oral contraceptives in suppressing plasma androstenedione, testosterone, LH and FSH and in stimulating plasma testosterone-binding capacity in hirsute women. *Am J Obstet Gynecol* **124**, 333 (1976).
34. Boiselle A, Trenblay RR. New therapeutic approach to the hirsute patient. *Fertil Steril* **32**, 276 (1979).

35. Cumming DC, Yang JC, Rebar RW, Yen SSC. Treatment of hirsutism with spironolactone. *J Am Med Assoc* **247,** 1295 (1982).
36. Casey JH. Chronic treatment regimens for hirsutism in women: Effect on blood production rates of testosterone and on hair growth. *Clin Endocrinol* **4,** 313 (1975).
37. Anderson DC. Sex hormone binding globulin. *Clin Endocrinol* **3,** 69 (1974).

Male Infertility

William D. Odell

Introduction

Anatomic, biochemical, physiological, pharmacological, and psychological abnormalities all affect the fertility of men. Lecturers or writers discussing these abnormalities usually take one of two seemingly different viewpoints as a framework for discussion. The urologist frequently initiates evaluation of his patients with a sperm analysis, whereas the reproductive endocrinologist often begins by measuring serum testosterone, lutropin (luteinizing hormone, LH), and follitropin (follicle-stimulating hormone, FSH). Often, the selection or referral of a patient as well as which approach is chosen is related to the complaint the patient brings to the physician—e.g., infertility, decreased or absent libido, small testes, failure to undergo puberty, gynecomastia, and various other problems. Either of these entry points of analysis, if carried out with an understanding of endocrine physiology, can lead to a "best possible" (based on current knowledge) diagnosis and treatment. In this discussion, I shall present and briefly analyze both of these viewpoints. Because their proper use depends on an understanding of male reproductive physiology, I shall review that first.

Review of Male Reproductive Physiology

The male reproductive endocrine system may be schematically pictured as a "closed-loop" feedback control system (Figure 1), in which each component is connected to other components by means of neuronal or hormonal signals (1). Analysis of such a system can begin at any level; I will begin here with the testes.

The testes are composed of two anatomical compartments: the interstitial cells of Leydig, which secrete testosterone, and the

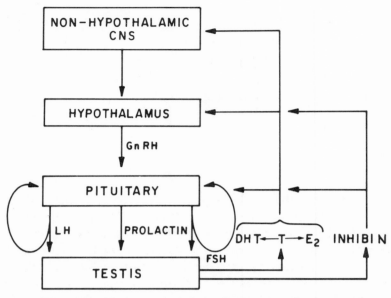

Fig. 1. Schematic presentation of the endocrine reproductive system in men

GnRH, gonadotropin releasing hormone; FSH, follicle-stimulating hormone; LH, luteinizing hormone; DHT, dihydrotestosterone; T, testosterone; E_2, estradiol; CNS, central nervous system. From Odell and Larsen *(1)*

testicular tubules. The tubules make up more than 90% of the volume or bulk of the testes. Hence, a man with small testes (<4 cm maximum length or <16 cm³ volume) has a loss of tubular volume and probably of function. Two cell types line the periphery of tubules: the Sertoli cell and the spermatogonia. The functions of the Sertoli cell, a particularly active cell, have recently been clarified by several studies of Sertoli cell cultures in vitro *(2–6)*, as follows:

Functions of the Sertoli cell

1. Steroidogenesis
2. Synthesis and secretion of androgen-binding protein
3. Synthesis and secretion of inhibin
4. Maintenance of the blood–testes barrier
5. Maintenance of potassium- and bicarbonate-rich tubular fluid
6. Nourishment of developing germ cells

The final controlling determinant of spermatogenesis is probably the steroid hormone, testosterone. Testosterone is generally believed to be secreted by the Leydig cells, transported across the tubular wall, bound by androgen-binding protein (ABP)[1] secreted by the Sertoli cell, and delivered in high concentrations to the spermatogonia. However, it is important to note that the Sertoli cell can also synthesize steroids: several investigators have shown that these cells can synthesize several steroids, including testosterone, from acetate (2, 3). However, Sertoli cells lack the enzyme 5-ane-3β-hydroxysteroid dehydrogenase, and hence cannot convert pregnenolone to progesterone. Synthesis of androgens must proceed via hydroxylation of 17-hydroxypregnenolone and dehydroepiandrosterone. Sertoli cells may thus contribute significantly to the concentrations of androgen in tubular fluid and at the spermatogonia.

FSH is the pituitary hormone that stimulates and controls secretion of ABP. However, testosterone from any source also stimulates ABP secretion, probably by mechanisms largely independent of regulation by FSH. Inhibin, a protein hormone secreted by Sertoli cells, acts in partial feedback control of FSH secretion. Despite extensive work (7–9), inhibin remains somewhat poorly characterized, and assay systems capable of quantifying it in blood have not been described. Its role in the reproductive physiology of both males and females remains to be clarified.

LH is the major regulator of testosterone synthesis and secretion by Leydig cells. During Leydig cell development, however, FSH is required to stimulate development of LH receptors. Studies from our laboratory (10) have shown that in the absence of FSH, the immature testes of rats are incapable of responding to LH, even when very large doses are used; pretreatment with FSH restores responsiveness to LH. During sexual maturation, the response to LH correlates with the number of LH receptors (10).

All of these observations on the effects of FSH can explain the sometimes confusing observations of *maintenance* of spermatogenesis in hypophysectomized adult rats with testosterone alone (11), and the requirement for FSH and LH to *initiate* spermatogen-

---

[1] Abbreviations used (not already defined on p. xviii): ABP, androgen-binding protein; DHT, dihydrotestosterone; MIF, Müllerian inhibiting factor; POEMS, acronym for polyneuropathy, organomegaly, endocrinopathy, M protein, skin abnormality.

esis in sexually immature animals or in hypophysectomized animals in which spermatogenesis was permitted to regress *(12)*. Let me suggest the following hypothesis: In the animal with established spermatogenesis, with Sertoli cells developed and secreting ABP, presumably large doses of testosterone can maintain production of ABP and deliver adequate testosterone to the spermatogonia. In the immature animal with the blood–testes barrier intact and little or no ABP available, FSH is required to stimulate Leydig cell responsiveness to LH, Sertoli cell development, and ABP synthesis. In support of this construction, Von Berswordt-Wallrabe and Mehring *(13)* have shown that even in animals with full regression of spermatogenesis after hypophysectomy, large doses of testosterone (25–50 mg/day per rat) can *initiate* and maintain spermatogenesis and fertility.

The major secretion of the testes is testosterone. In the sexually mature male, well over 90% of blood testosterone is derived from testicular (Leydig cell) secretion. The testes also secrete small amounts of estradiol and dihydrotestosterone (DHT), but most of the blood concentrations of these two steroids is derived from *peripheral* tissues (mainly muscle, adipose tissue, and liver), which produce them from testosterone *(14, 15)*. Figure 2 shows the relative sources of blood testosterone, estradiol, and DHT in normal men. Each of these sources contributes to the effects of each steroid on body tissues and on feedback control of LH and FSH secretion. Tissues derived embryonically from the genital tubercle require the action of DHT for their development, whereas tissues derived from the Wolffian duct respond to testosterone per se.

The DHT that regulates development of the genital tubercle is made predominantly in the genital tubercle cell itself by the enzyme 5α-reductase present in these cells. Thus, patients with congenital absence of 5α-reductase develop a peculiar form of localized tissue hypogonadism. Because testosterone synthesis and secretion are normal (as is testicular morphology), all body tissues responding to testosterone develop normally; in contrast, those tissues requiring DHT fail to develop. At birth, such males have abnormalities limited to the external genitalia. The phallus is small and clitoral-like, with no urethral orifice, and usually a urogenital sinus opens onto the perineum. Within the sinus are two orifices: an anterior one leading to the urethra, and a posterior one that

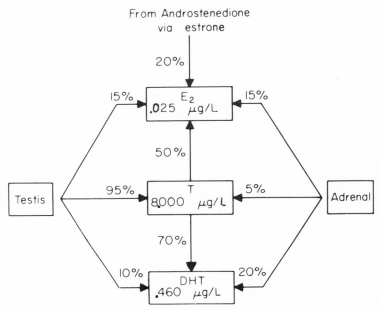

Fig. 2. Schematic representation of the sources of blood testosterone (T), dihydrotestosterone (DHT), and estradiol (E₂) in normal men

Adapted from Odell and Swerdloff *(34)*

ends in a blind vaginal pouch *(14)*. In addition to lacking the enzyme in tissues derived from the genital tubercle, such individuals also lack 5α-reductase in other tissues, so that blood concentrations of DHT are very low although testosterone concentrations and all body effects of testosterone per se are normal. This rare form of male infertility (male hypogonadism) has helped clarify the role of DHT during the development of the male phenotype *(16)*.

As mentioned above, estradiol is also predominantly formed in peripheral tissues in males *(15)*. Although only low concentrations of it circulate, these are likely of major importance in feedback regulation of LH and FSH secretion, estradiol being 50- to 100-fold more potent than testosterone in suppressing LH and FSH when administered to castrated male rats *(17)*. Indeed, the testosterone given in such studies may be acting predominantly as estradiol: the hypothalamus actively aromatizes testosterone to estradiol. Further evidence that estradiol may be the most important regulator of secretion of LH and FSH is the observation that normal men respond to the anti-estrogen drug, clomiphene, with increases of LH and FSH concentrations in their blood. My colleagues and I found that treatment of normal men with clomiphene for seven days produced an increase in blood LH and FSH similar to that seen seven days after castration (17, 18).

As indicated in Figure 1 and reviewed here, feedback regulation of FSH secretion is largely mediated by estradiol formed from testosterone locally within the hypothalamus, as well as in peripheral tissues such as liver, muscle, and fat. The feedback is an integrated effect of testosterone, estradiol, and DHT, but the major steroid acting in this feedback is probably estradiol. All three steroids act both at the pituitary and, as shall be discussed later, at the hypothalamus. In the male, these actions are predominantly negative (inhibitory) feedback control.

In addition to this steroid regulation of LH and FSH secretion, studies from our laboratory (19–21) have shown the existence of a sensitive and specific autoregulatory secretion for LH and FSH (also shown in Figure 1). LH acts directly on the pituitary to inhibit its own secretion. LH does not affect FSH secretion, and FSH does not affect LH secretion. In contrast to this specific system, the control mechanisms of testosterone and estradiol affect both LH and FSH. This autoregulatory system is adequately sensitive to control secretion at the concentrations of LH and FSH found in eugonadal men. Its role in pathophysiology remains to be defined.

Abundant data in many species, including humans, attest to the fact that the central nervous system is capable of modulating reproductive processes. In male reproduction, perhaps the most striking and, to the learner, often most confusing observations relate to the phenomenon of "androgen sterilization." Pfeiffer in 1936 (22) first recorded that, in male rats castrated at birth and given an ovarian graft at adulthood, such grafts functioned cyclically in a fashion characteristic of the female. If adult males were castrated and received an ovarian graft, the graft did not function cyclically—follicles developed, but ovulation did not occur. Later, Barraclough and Gorski (23, 24) and several other investigators (25–27) further studied this phenomenon.

Their findings may be summarized as follows: a single dose of testosterone given to a newborn female rat results, after growth and sexual maturation, in an adult who fails to ovulate; she remains in constant estrus. However, estradiol administered to newborn female rats produces an identical phenomenon, and this hormone is much more potent than testosterone. DHT, an androgen that is not aromatized to estradiol, is ineffective in producing "androgen sterilization." An electrolytic lesion placed in the anterior pre-optic area of the hypothalamus produces a similar phenomenon, suggesting that this area is the anatomic location of this phenomenon. Gorski (28) reported that a morphological difference is visible in male and female rats in this area of the hypothalamus, the volume of the medial pre-optic area being eightfold larger in the male rat brain than in the female. Interestingly, estrogens are present in both sexes of rats in the perinatal period, largely derived from maternal pregnancy secretion. Administering an anti-estrogen (tamoxifen) to neonatal female rats also produces permanent sterility after sexual maturation.

In interpreting these data, Dohler and Gorski (27) postulate that the brains of both sexes are undifferentiated at birth. High concentrations of maternal estrogens "program" the female hypothalamus to develop into the normal pattern, permitting cyclic positive feedback of estrogens and progestogens and producing the ovulatory LH/FSH surge. These same maternal estrogens added to testicular secretions in the neonatal male rat functionally alter the "cyclic center" in the anterior supra-optic area that produces the male hypothalamus. Figure 3 illustrates their model.

The functional counterpart of these observations in other species is being actively studied. In sheep, this steroid imprinting occurs during the first trimester of pregnancy rather than at birth. In rhesus monkeys, such imprinting may not occur at all; males castrated as adults respond to estrogen in positive feedback, and typical LH ovulatory surges are observed. However, in men who are castrated as adults, administration of estrogen, or of estrogen and progestogen, either fails to produce positive feedback or at best produces much less of a response than in the postmenopausal or castrated female. Estrogen and progesterone administered to castrated or menopausal women produce a typical LH/FSH ovulatory-type surge (29). Some hypogonadal men who have not been

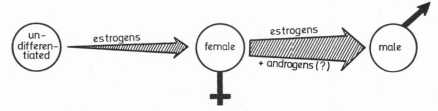

Fig. 3. Diagram summarizing the concept of progressive brain differentiation

The embryonic brain is undifferentiated. Female sexual differentiation is actively induced by moderate interaction with estrogens (of placental or maternal origin). Male sexual brain differentiation is induced by interaction of the embryonic brain with higher concentrations of estrogens which, in addition to those of maternal and placental origin, are derived from enzymic conversion of testicular androgens. Androgens per se may act synergistically with estrogens. From Dohler and Gorski *(27);* used with permission.

exposed neonatally to the effects of androgen can, as adults, respond to estrogen treatment with positive feedback.

The hypothalamic neurosecretory hormone that controls pituitary secretion of LH and FSH is a 10-amino-acid peptide, gonadotropin-releasing hormone (GnRH). (For an excellent review of this topic, see ref. *30.*) This hormone, synthesized by hypothalamic neurones, is secreted in a pulsatile fashion, which in turn produces pulsatile secretion by the pituitary of LH and FSH. Because of the difficulties in measuring GnRH in peripheral blood, most data consist of measurements of LH and FSH at 1- to 20-min intervals. The pulsations in LH are easily observed; pulsations in FSH often lie within the limits of assay variability, are smaller in amplitude, and frequently do not occur on a one-to-one basis with LH. The pituitary response to exogenous GnRH in normal men or women is a large secretion or release of LH and a small release of FSH, which may explain the difficulty in observing FSH pulsation. Figure 4 shows the pulsatile pattern in serum LH, FSH, and testosterone in two normal men. In hypogonadal men, however, the pulse amplitude and pulse frequency of LH and FSH are often abnormal; moreover, their response to single injections of GnRH is often different: the increase in serum FSH may exceed that of LH. Although it has usually been believed that each gonadotropin was synthesized and secreted by a specific cell type, this may not be true. Recent data *(26)* suggest that at least some gonadotrophs may secrete both LH and FSH.

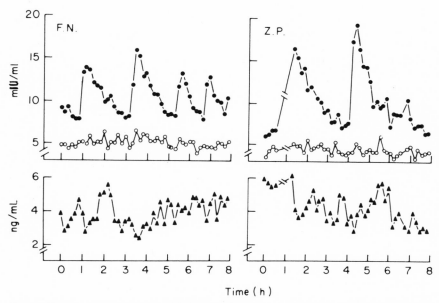

Fig. 4. Blood concentrations of LH (●), FSH (○), and testosterone (▲) measured at short intervals in two normal men

From Naftolin et al., *J Clin Endocrinol Metab* **36:** 285, 1973; used with permission

Genetic Control of Male Reproduction

For an excellent review of genetic control of male reproduction, see reference *16*.

Like the early hypothalamus, the early embryonic gonad is undifferentiated. Under the initial influence of the genetic mechanisms, the gonad differentiates into either an ovary or a testis. The development of the gonad and its secretory products then determines the phenotypic expression of sex. A 46XX complement of chromosomes is necessary for the development of a normal ovary with normal function at sexual maturity. However, the 46XX complement is not necessary to produce a *phenotypic* female. The Y chromosome, or at least a part of it, probably predominantly the short arm, is required for a *phenotypic* male and testicular development. The mechanisms by which the Y chromosome produces development of the testes is uncertain; presumably, it controls the synthesis and production of an organizing substance that stimulates development of the testes. The testes then secrete steroids and proteins to control sex accessory development (Figure 5). A

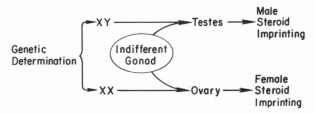

Fig. 5. Differentiation of the gonad: the embryonic gonad, which is neither male nor female, develops into a testis or an ovary under the genetic influence of the Y chromosome (XY karyotype) or the XX karyotype, respectively; the secretions of the testis or ovary then "program or imprint" the hypothalamus, resulting in the development of a male or a female hypothalamus

The secretions of the gonads also modulate sex accessory development. From Odell and Larsen *(1)*

protein hormone, Müllerian inhibiting factor (MIF), causes the Müllerian duct to regress. Congenital deficiency in this factor results in a phenotypically normal male who has normal testicular production of steroids and sperm, but who also has a uterus, usually in a hernial sack. Testicular secretion of testosterone stimulates differentiation of the Wolffian ducts, and formation of DHT from testosterone in the genital tubercle produces the normal male phenotype. If there is any defect in androgen action, the Wolffian ducts fail to develop and a subject with female phenotype is produced or, if the decrease in androgen action is partial, the individual will have ambiguous genitalia (Figure 6). Such a defect in androgen action may result from a biochemical resistance to androgen action in the presence of normal testicular secretion (androgen resistance syndromes), from an enzyme deficiency that prevents the biosynthesis of androgen, or from Leydig cell agenesis. Congenital absence of the testes, occurring early in embryogenesis, also produces a female phenotype.

Thus, decreased or absent androgen effects early in embryogenesis can produce an individual who appears to be a normal phenotypic female, but is in fact a 46XY genetic male. Depending on the severity of the androgen deficiency, the phenotypic alterations range from a normal female through all forms of ambiguous genitalia to a normal male with altered spermatogenesis (Figure 6).

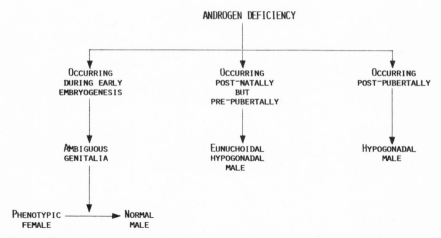

Fig. 6. Clinical presentation of androgen deficiencies that occur at different periods of life

Resistance to androgen action or 5α-reductase deficiency can also produce ambiguous genitalia. From Odell and Swerdloff *(34)*

Diagnosis of Male Hypogonadism or Infertility

History and Physical Examination

The complaints of the "infertile" man are not always those of infertility. Often, the complaint is one of impotence, gynecomastia, or failure to complete sexual maturation—or there may be no complaint at all. Occasionally, a pending divorce or a childless marriage without a specific complaint is the clue. Slag et al. *(31)* screened 1180 men presenting to an outpatient clinic for general medical problems. Of these, 401 men were impotent, of whom only 47% chose to be examined or evaluated for this problem. Breakdown of the causes of their impotence is of interest: medications, 25%; psychogenic, 14%; neurological, 7%; urologic, 6%; primary hypogonadism, 10%; secondary hypogonadism, 9%; diabetes mellitus, 9%; hypothyroidism, 5%; hyperthyroidism, 1%; hyperprolactinemia, 4%; miscellaneous, 4%; and unknown, 7%. As I will discuss later, these authors also found that measurements of serum LH, FSH, testosterone, and prolactin, as well as studies of thyroid function, were required to diagnose the etiology. The investigators did not evaluate the response to treatment in these patients, e.g., discontinuation of the implicated medication or treatment of the systemic illness such as hypo- or hyperthyroidism. Nevertheless, this diagnostic survey is an important reference study.

Swerdloff and Boyers (32) considered a different aspect of the problem, focusing on couples who complained of infertility per se. They developed a study algorithm for evaluation of the male, based on the initial examination of semen analysis. The men evaluated by Slag et al. (31) did not complain of infertility and obviously presented a different group problem than the men considered by Swerdloff and Boyers. Nevertheless, both groups are largely "infertile" and fall into the broad category under review. Collins et al. (33) analyzed a two- to seven-year follow-up of 1145 infertile couples. Pregnancy occurred in 246 of 597 treated couples (41%) and in 191 of 548 untreated couples (35%). Even in the treated couples, 31% of the pregnancies occurred more than three months after the last medical treatment, or more than 12 months after surgery, which suggests that the treatment had little to do with the pregnancy. These authors concluded that the potential for spontaneous cure of infertility is high, and treatment modalities should therefore be evaluated in randomized clinical trials.

Given that the complaints of males with infertility are varied and frequently are not even stated by the patient, how can physical examination assist? Swerdloff and I (34) have previously described the often subtle physical findings in men with infertility, which include:

• hypogonadal facies—fine, linear, radiating creases extending outward around the mouth and eyes—combined with alterations in beard distribution and density (as compared with the "norm" for the man's family and race or "strain")
• alterations in body hair distribution and density, again as related to race–strain norms
• arm-span/height and lower segment/upper segment ratios different from 1 (these are altered if hypogonadism was present during sexual maturation)
• hyposmia or anosmia (often present in congenital hypothalamic disorders)
• small testicular size (normal = >4 cm in length or >16 cm^3)
• abnormalities of the genitalia (e.g., hypospadias)

Diagnoses Based on Measurements of Hormones

Table 1 shows the extensive differential diagnosis of male hypogonadism. In evaluating any patient it is important to determine a complete history and physical examination, particularly as regards possible systemic illnesses and all medications used. In the absence of suspicious findings in these areas, one should measure LH, FSH, and testosterone in serum. Obtaining three independent blood samples 15 to 20 min apart avoids problems in diagnosis caused by the pulsatile nature of LH/FSH secretion (see above); these are pooled and sent as one serum specimen to a reliable laboratory for determination.

Table 1. **Differential Diagnosis of Male Hypogonadism**

I. *Hypothalamic abnormalities*

   A. LH-FSH deficiency (Kallmann's syndrome)
   B. Prader–Willi syndrome
   C. Vasquez–Hurst–Sotos syndrome
   D. Laurence–Moon–Biedl syndrome
   E. Cerebellar ataxia
   F. Hypothalamic mass lesions (e.g., craniopharyngioma)
   G. Many systemic illnesses
   H. Psychiatric disorders
   I. Obesity

II. *Pituitary abnormalities*

   A. Panhypopituitarism
   B. Isolated FSH deficiency
   C. Isolated LH deficiency
   D. Hyperprolactinemia syndromes
   E. Production of biologically inactive LH or FSH

III. *Primary gonadal abnormalities*

   A. Involving androgen production
      1. Klinefelter's syndrome
      2. XX males (sex reversal syndrome)
      3. True hermaphroditism
      4. Streak gonads–XY karyotype
      5. Testicular agenesis (vanishing testes syndrome)
      6. Noonan's syndrome
      7. Acquired testicular disorders: orchitis, surgical castration, etc.
      8. Chemotherapy
      9. Leydig cell agenesis
     10. Myotonia dystrophica

(continued on next page)

Table 1 *(continued)*.

    B. Involving sperm production or function only
       1. Adult seminiferous tubule failure (idiopathic oligospermia or azoospermia)
       2. Sertoli cell only syndrome
       3. Testicular mosaicism and infertility
       4. Kartagener's syndrome
       5. Partial androgen resistance

IV. *Enzymic defects in androgen synthesis*
    A. 20α-Hydroxylase deficiency (lipoid adrenal hypoplasia)
    B. 17,20-Desmolase deficiency
    C. 3β-Hydroxysteroid dehydrogenase deficiency
    D. 17-Hydroxylase deficiency
    E. 17-Ketosteroid reductase deficiency
    F. 5α-Reductase deficiency

V. *Defects in androgen action*
    A. Complete androgen insensitivity (testicular feminization)
    B. Incomplete androgen sensitivity

VI. *Miscellaneous causes*
    A. Persistent Müllerian duct syndrome
    B. Cystic fibrosis
    C. POEMS syndrome
    D. Drugs and medications
    E. Neurological abnormalities
    F. Renal failure

Assay artifact is an increasingly important problem in endocrine diagnosis. Occasionally, patients have antibodies to the hormone in question or to rabbit immunoglobulins; these directly interfere with the assay by binding the label, or interfere with the separation step in an immunoassay. The source of such antibodies is often obscure, but most likely is related to the patient's past exposure to injected protein hormones (e.g., bovine thyrotropin, pituitary extracts, choriogonadotropin), or contamination or cross reaction to immunization with gamma-globulin preparations (see refs. *35* and *36*). With the values for LH/FSH and testosterone in hand, no systemic illness present, and no medication being taken, the investigator can use the scheme in Figure 6. Many of the syndromes in Table 1 are rare, and I will not deal with each one in detail. For additional references, consult my previous reviews, in which I have emphasized descriptions of each disease *(1, 34)*.

1. *Hypothalamic abnormalities* (low testosterone, low or inappropriately "normal" LH/FSH, and positive response to GnRH if repetitively administered): This category can be differentiated from pituitary causes by the response to repetitive GnRH administration *(37)*. The prototype in this category is Kallmann's syndrome and the median cleft face syndrome. Kallmann's is a relatively common cause of hypogonadism consisting of hypothalamic hypogonadism, anosmia or hyposmia, and, as originally described, syndactyly, short fourth metacarpals, color blindness, nerve deafness, and mental retardation *(38, 39)*. Since the original description, most of these patients have been found to suffer less severe defects of hypothalamic hypogonadism and hyposmia. The median cleft face syndrome is often mistakenly called Kallmann's syndrome, but in fact is a congenital abnormality resulting from malfusion of the two embryonic halves of the brain. This results in a wide spectrum of deformities, ranging from grotesque, Cyclops-like individuals who may not survive, to nearly normal individuals who have a cleft chin ("dimple") and hypogonadism. In addition to the defect in LH/FSH secretion, hypothalamic abnormalities affecting secretion of other pituitary hormones may also occur *(40, 41)*.

The Prader–Willi syndrome consists of massive hypothalamic obesity, mental retardation, hypothalamic hypogonadism, and neonatal muscle hypotonia. These patients invariably die as young adults from complications of obesity *(42)*. The Vasquez–Hurst–Sotos syndrome is endocrinologically similar to the Prader–Willi syndrome; to date, only five patients have been described *(43)*, characterized by hypogonadism, gynecomastia, obesity, short stature, mental retardation, and X-linked inheritance. The Laurence–Moon–Biedl syndrome is characterized by retinitis pigmentosa, syndactyly or polydactyly, mental retardation, and hypothalamic hypogonadism *(44)*. Familial cerebellar ataxia is a syndrome characterized by nerve deafness, short fourth metacarpals, and hypothalamic hypogonadism. Hypothalamic mass lesions interfere with GnRH synthesis and (or) secretion. Neurological lesions that interfere with pulsatile GnRH secretion, but not with its synthesis, as well as amino acid substitutions of GnRH that alter bioactivity, will probably be described in the future. Many systemic illnesses (starvation, renal disease, psychiatric disorders, and extensive inflammatory bowel disease) associated with abnormalities of reproduction presumably produce abnormalities in the hypothalamic secretion of GnRH (45). Although 5 to 10% of hospitalized patients older than 50 years are hypothyroid, they often produce no overt symptoms that the physician relates to the thyroid. As reported by Slag et al. (31), some of these patients are also impotent. I consider it worthwhile to evaluate patients for hypothyroidism, although no prospective study of the effects of treatment for it on impotence has yet been performed.

2. *Disorders of the pituitary* (low or inappropriately "normal" LH/ FSH, low testosterone, no response to GnRH): Disorders of the pituitary gland itself may interfere with the endocrine processes of reproduction. At times, these may be selective (e.g., isolated LH or FSH deficiency) or nonselective (e.g., panhypopituitarism). Presumably, the rare disorders of isolated LH or FSH deficiencies are caused by processes affecting the gonadotroph cells. Recently, an interesting man with an immunologically active but biologically inactive LH has been described (46). His LH was slightly above normal by immunoassay, but below normal by bioassay; he responded to exogenous choriogonadotropin. Prolactin-secreting adenomas or hyperprolactinemia from other causes produces hypogonadism because of the effects of prolactin on several portions of the reproductive system. Studies from our laboratory and review of the available literature (47, 48) suggest the following effects of prolactin: (a) inhibition of gonadotropin action on the testes, thus producing low testosterone concentrations in serum; (b) prevention of the expected increase in LH/FSH in response to the low testosterone; and (c) decreasing of the frequency of the pulsatile secretion of LH.

3. *Disorders of the gonads* [increased FSH and (or) LH with low testosterone]: This category is a large one, comprising both congenital and acquired disorders. The most frequently occurring disorder is Klinefelter's syndrome, classically associated with profound hypogonadism, very small testes, and XXY karyotype. However, in our experience, the hypogonadism is often subtle and the testes are larger than expected; the subject may even be fertile (although this wanes later in life); and a mosaic karyotype XXY/XY with a wide percentage of mosaicism may be found. The XX males resemble Klinefelter's patients clinically, yet have an XX karyotype; when carefully studied with modern techniques, these individuals invariably have a portion of the Y chromosome

present, usually the short arm (see also ref. *34*). In true hermaphroditism, both ovarian and testicular tissues are present in the same individual. The karyotype of such individuals is varied. Benirschke et al. *(49)* analyzed 119 reported cases and found the following distribution: 51% XX, 19% XY, and 30% chimeras and mosaics. However, as was true for the so-called XX males, most studies show that these XX hermaphrodites have the H-Y antigen present. Clinically, these patients have a wide range of ambiguous genitalia.

Patients with the streak gonads-XY karyotype are eunuchoid phenotypic females with amenorrhea. None have abnormalities suggesting Turner's syndrome; indeed, many patients are tall. This appears to be an inherited disorder with X-linkage; the phenotypic appearance suggests that the testes disappear early in embryogenesis. Compare this clinical picture with the vanishing testes syndrome (testicular "agenesis"), in which a eunuchoidal individual, karyotype XY, has no testes, either inguinally or within the abdomen; these are phenotypic males, which indicates that the testes disappeared after embryogenesis was largely complete.

Noonan's syndrome is associated with hypogonadism in some affected subjects, both male and female; many subjects, however, have normal fertility. The original nine children studied suffered from pulmonary valve stenosis, short stature, hypertelorism, mild mental retardation, ptosis, various skeletal malformations, and undescended testes in boys *(50)*. In contrast to Klinefelter's subjects, the karyotype is 46XY. Char et al. *(51)* described 45 patients with this syndrome. The physical findings are variable, but facial characteristics are similar in many unrelated patients and short stature is common.

Acquired testicular disorders are usually evident by history or physical examination. Patients with Leydig cell agenesis, a rare syndrome first described by Berthezene et al. *(52)*, are phenotypic females who present with primary amenorrhea and lack of breast development, as would be expected if the Leydig cell maldevelopment occurred early in embryogenesis. The karyotype is 46XY, and appropriate evaluation demonstrated that an enzyme deficiency was not responsible for the findings. Myotonia dystrophica is a hereditary disorder, usually showing symptoms in the third or fourth decade and progressing slowly until death. The major finding is myotonia, a tonic spasm of muscles, followed by atro-

153

phy; other findings include cataracts, frontal balding, mental impairment, and gonadal atrophy. Sagel et al. *(53)* studied eight men with this syndrome and found concentrations of FSH in serum to be moderately increased, but LH was normal and testosterone low; response to GnRH was supranormal.

Several defects result in only abnormal sperm production or abnormal sperm function (Table 1). Adult seminiferous tubule failure and idiopathic oligospermia or azoospermia are, for the most part, disorders of unknown cause. These disorders, which are probably many disorders of various causes, are common and all result in oligoazoospermia. Younger men with these disorders present with a complaint of infertility; however, many older men do not complain of infertility and yet develop such a disorder. In severely oligospermic men, FSH concentrations may be moderately increased or at times normal; LH concentrations are normal. Lipshultz et al. *(54)* reported that men who had previously had an orchiopexy for unilaterally undescended testes are likely to have oligospermia as adults. Because the cryptorchidism was unilateral, the findings suggest a primary dysgenesis of the testes.

Some additional disorders involving gonadal abnormalities are as follows. The Sertoli-cell-only syndrome is characterized by azoospermia, normal Leydig cell function, modestly decreased testes size, and (on biopsy) spermatic tubules lined only with Sertoli cells (no spermatogonia). The karyotype is normal 46XY, although rarely 46XYY has been present. Serum concentrations of FSH are moderately increased and LH concentrations are normal.

A relatively common cause of male infertility is testicular mosaicism and infertility. About 5% of young infertile men have a chromosomal error detectable in peripheral blood; nearly half of these errors involve sex chromosomes *(55),* the remainder have translocations. This estimate may be low, in that current genetic techniques have not been used in such a survey. The genetic defect may reside in the testes alone. Jones et al. *(56)* described a man with normal serum concentrations of LH, FSH, and testosterone, with no chromosomal abnormalities in peripheral blood cells, but with azoospermia. Testicular biopsy showed that three clones of cells were present in the primary and secondary spermatocytes, but no discernible abnormalities were seen in spermatogonia.

Kartagener's syndrome, when fully expressed, consists of situs inversus, chronic sinusitis, bronchiectasis, and infertility; cilia of the respiratory tract and the sperm are immotile. Morphologically, the tails of the sperm lack the dynein arm, a structure found in normally contractile sperm tails *(57)*. Partial deficiency of androgen action may also result in a phenotypically normal male with only oligospermia. This category is discussed under androgen resistance syndromes.

4. Enzymic defects in androgen biosynthesis. As shown in Table 1, six enzymic abnormalities lead to a decrease in androgen synthesis and produce hypogonadism in men. As would be predicted from the above sections on physiology and genetics, these defects, if they are severe and occur early in embryogenesis, produce a phenotypic female with 46XY male karyotype. Partial defects are not commonly described but may occur unrecognized. Laboratory findings include a low serum concentration of testosterone, increased concentrations of LH and FSH and, depending on which enzyme is involved, above-normal concentrations of steroid precursors or products. Figure 7 illustrates which steroids must be measured. Each of these defects is autosomal recessive and affects genitalia to various degrees, depending on the severity of the enzyme block. Some of these defects also result in low cortisol production (deficiencies of 20α-hydroxylase, 17,20-desmolase, 3β-hydroxysteroid, and 17-hydroxylase), but two do not (deficiencies of 17-ketoreductase and 5α-reductase deficiency). Patients with low testosterone and high LH and FSH concentrations, and who do not fall into a clear syndrome of differential diagnosis (e.g., Klinefelter's), should probably have cortisol measured in the same specimens that were used for determining LH/FSH. If the concentration of cortisol is low or low normal, the possibility of an enzyme deficiency should be considered. If the cortisol concentration is normal, but no clear diagnosis is apparent in a man who has low testosterone and above-normal LH/FSH, deficiencies of 17-ketoreductase or 5α-reductase should be considered. The known cases of these enzyme deficiencies will not be reviewed here; many of the published cases have been presented in a previous review *(34)*.

5. Defects in androgen action. As would be predicted from the review of physiology and genetics, complete insensitivity to androgens results in genetic XY males who are phenotypic females.

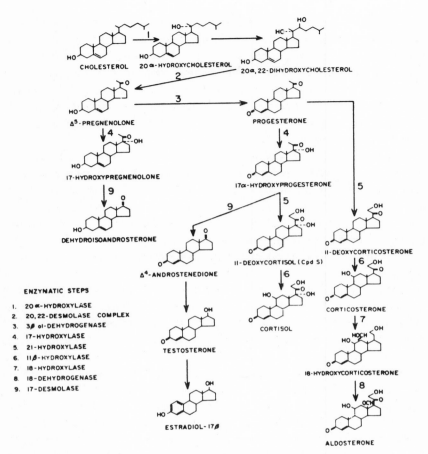

Fig. 7. Major biosynthetic pathways for steroid hormones

From Temple TE, Liddle GW. Inhibitors of adrenal steroid biosynthesis. *Annu Rev Pharmacol* **10:** 199, 1970; used with permission

Less severe defects result in lesser degrees of abnormal genitalia; minor degrees of androgen insensitivity result only in oligospermia *(58)* (see Figure 6). The syndrome of complete insensitivity to androgens appears as an X-linked recessive or male-limited dominant disorder, and it results from a complete defect in action of both testosterone and DHT. Subjects are phenotypically female with little or no body hair (but normal head hair), who undergo feminization at puberty with excellent estrogen effects on skin, body fat distribution, breast tissue, and voice. They are heterosexual and consider themselves to be normal females. Physical examination reveals a blind vaginal pouch with no cervix or uterus; testes are often palpable in the inguinal areas. Testosterone concentrations in blood are high normal or above normal, and serum LH is modestly increased; FSH concentrations are normal *(34)*.

The incomplete forms of insensitivity to androgen produce a wide range of ambiguous genitalia, ranging from phenotypic male to phenotypic female. In published literature, these patients are described under a large number of eponyms (e.g., Lubs, Gilbert–Dreyfus, Reifenstein, and Rosewater syndromes). However, Wilson et al. *(59)* described a large family with incomplete androgen resistance in which the affected members showed a broad spectrum of ambiguous genitalia encompassing many of the previous eponyms. These workers suggested that the various disorders all relate to various degrees of androgen resistance, a postulate now well accepted. Thus, the multiple eponyms are seldom used anymore.

6. *Miscellaneous disorders:*

a. Persistent Müllerian duct syndrome. This syndrome is caused by a defect in Müllerian duct regression in XY males *(60, 61)*. Patients usually present as phenotypic males with inguinal hernias, cryptorchidism, and otherwise normal external genitalia. During the hernia repair, the uterus and fallopian tubes are found in the inguinal canal. Wolffian duct derivatives are normal male in type, although in some the vas deferens courses through the uterus. Several families have been reported in which several males are affected, which suggests that this may be an autosomal recessive trait. The cause appears to be a deficiency in the elaboration of Müllerian duct regression factor.

b. Cystic fibrosis. Males with cystic fibrosis are infertile because of failure to develop the vas deferens *(62)*. In some patients, the seminal vesicles are absent and the epididymis is immature. Because the prostate and external genitalia develop normally, these would appear to be defects in differentiation of Wolffian duct derivatives, and it is uncertain whether this is an associated primary defect caused directly by the cystic fibrosis gene or an embryonic effect related secondarily to the prime gene action.

c. POEMS syndrome (Polyneuropathy, Organomegaly, Endocrinopathy, M protein, Skin abnormality). This interesting syndrome, described in several patients *(63–65)*, is associated with severe progressive polyneuropathy, organomegaly (usually hepatomegaly), and various endocrine abnormalities. In men, impotence and hypogonadism are commonly present. Other features of the syndrome usually include production of M protein, lymphadenopathy, and hyperpigmentation and thickening of the skin. The endocrine findings in men with hypogonadism include low serum concentrations of testosterone, and either inappropriately low (normal) or modestly increased concentrations of LH and FSH. For example, Bardwick et al. *(63)* described a 52-year-old man whose serum testosterone was 4054 ng/L (normal 5734 ± 1489 mean ± SD), serum LH 25 int. units/L, and serum FSH 22 int. units/L. Imawari et al. *(65)* described a 42-year-old man whose serum testosterone was 1850 ng/L (normal 400 to 1200), LH 3.4 int. units/L, and FSH 2.1 int. units/L. In these patients, who often present with impotence and gynecomastia, the prime disease of concern is usually the multiple myeloma and disabling peripheral neuropathy.

d. Drugs and medications. A wide variety of medications or drugs affect reproduction. A patient who complains of decreased libido, loss of potency, or infertility, who is also taking any type of medication, should have that medication considered as the cause of his complaints. For example, thiazides, which are commonly used for treating hypertension, caused impotence in 19.58 per 1000 subjects in a single-blind study of mild hypertension treatment *(66)*. In the same study, propranolol caused impotence in significantly greater numbers than the placebo. Sulfasalazine, used to treat ulcerative colitis, also has been reported to cause reversible infertility *(67)*.

It is beyond the scope of this chapter to review all of the medications that produce such symptoms in men; usually, the mechanisms involved are poorly understood. Some medications act on the hypothalamus to induce hyperprolactinemia and subsequent hypogonadism. Others may act directly on the gonads. The patients with sulfasalazine infertility had oligospermia with normal serum concentrations of LH, FSH, and testosterone; presumably, this is a direct gonadal interference with spermatogenesis. Some medications affect neurological control of penile erection or affect penile blood flow, thus preventing erection or ejaculation.

In summary, the mode of action of drugs affecting reproduction is varied; actions occur at all levels of the reproductive system shown in Figure 1. Therefore, all medications should be considered as potential anti-fertility substances.

e. Neurological abnormalities. Alterations in neuronal control of the hypothalamic modulation of GnRH secretion interfere with reproduction, as discussed in the section on the hypothalamus. In addition, alterations in neuronal control of blood flow to the genitalia and of the mechanisms causing erection and ejaculation cause impotence or infertility. Leriche syndrome, caused by terminal aortic occlusion, consists of hip, thigh, and buttock claudication and impotence. After some procedures such as complete prostatectomy, rectosigmoid surgery, and distal aortic bypass surgery, there is interference with the parasympathetic system and impotence may result. Spinal cord injuries frequently cause impotence. Diabetes mellitus is often associated with multiple neurological defects and commonly with impotence. Again, it is beyond the scope of this chapter to thoroughly review the neurological bases for impotence. Suffice it to say that all men with impotence and infertility deserve a thorough neurological evaluation.

f. Renal failure. Renal failure is commonly associated with decreased libido, potency, and testicular size (for an excellent review, see ref. *45*). Most patients with end-stage renal failure have azoospermia or severe oligospermia. Concentrations of testosterone and dihydrotestosterone in plasma are low, while LH is increased and FSH is increased or normal. Testicular production of testosterone in response to choriogonadotropin is commonly subnormal; the LH response to GnRH is accentuated, but the FSH response is indistinguishable from normal. Prolactin is also increased in many patients with renal failure, but its role in this pathophysiology is uncertain. Lim and Fang *(68)* reported that estrogen concentrations were increased in renal failure; after treatment with the anti-estrogen clomiphene citrate, LH and FSH concentrations rose further and testosterone returned to normal. The defect thus involves both the testes and the hypothalamus. Low concentrations of zinc have been reported in the plasma from some impotent patients on dialysis *(69);* treatment with zinc may reverse impotency in these subjects.

g. Obesity. Obesity is a common finding, and many obese men suffer from mild hypogonadotropic hypogonadism. In a careful study of the endocrine defect in obese men *(70),* the obese men

159

as a group had significantly lower concentrations in plasma of total testosterone, free testosterone, and FSH than did slender, age-matched controls. LH concentrations were inappropriately "normal," and libido and spermatogenesis were within the "normal range." The abnormalities are explained by the increased conversion of testosterone to estradiol in adipose tissue, with partial suppression of the hypothalamic–pituitary system, predominantly at the pituitary. Because the same increase in estradiol raises the serum concentration of sex-hormone-binding globulin, the finding of decreased testosterone has even greater significance (one would expect an increase in testosterone in the presence of increased sex-hormone-binding globulin).

Summary/Conclusion

As has been discussed, the most difficult step in diagnosis is often the initial suspicion of hypogonadism on physical examination. The diagnosis may be suspected before puberty by extragonadal manifestations such as anosmia, hypotonia, and family history. By using the classification scheme in Table 1, in conjunction with the simple biochemical investigations of blood LH, FSH, and testosterone determinations, one can correctly form the diagnosis or at least narrow it to two or three possibilities. In addition, karyotype determination is often indicated, particularly in patients with increased serum concentrations of gonadotropins; buccal smears are not recommended for screening, owing to their high false-negative rate. Defects in enzyme biosynthesis of testosterone may be difficult to distinguish from absent or streak gonads, although the presence of palpable gonads would exclude the latter cause. Measurements of selected steroids can assist in evaluation of the enzymic defects.

Using the differential diagnosis listed in Table 1, one can make a systematic approach to diagnosis. The flow chart in Figure 8 is entered by measuring serum LH, FSH, and testosterone. On the basis of the information obtained, the major diagnostic categories (I to VI) can be selected and further considered. In patients with low testosterone and LH/FSH, or low testosterone and "normal" LH/FSH, neoplasms of the central nervous system (e.g., craniopharyngioma) and pituitary tumors must be considered. Thus, all men in diagnostic categories I and II require a computerized

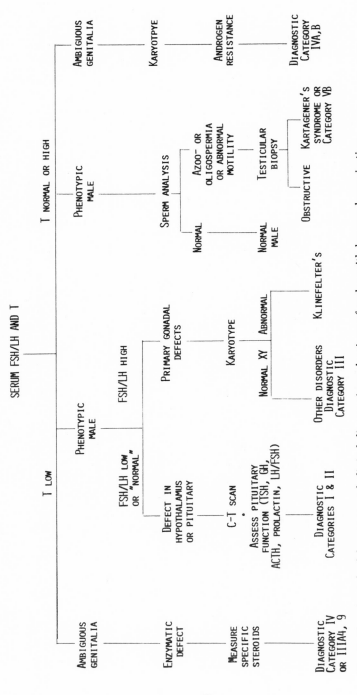

Fig. 8. Flowsheet for laboratory and clinical diagnostic evaluations of males with hypoandrogenization

Diagnostic categories refer to those listed in Table 1. T, testosterone; GH, growth hormone; ACTH, corticotropin; C–T, computerized tomography. Modified from Odell and Swerdloff (34)

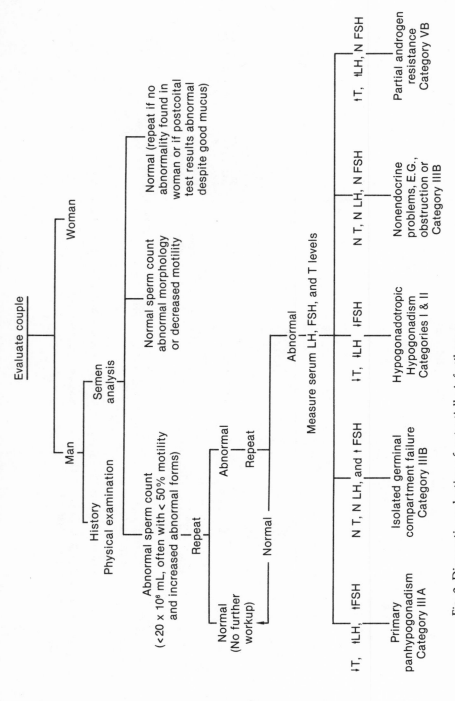

Fig. 9. Diagnostic evaluation of potentially infertile men

Categories refer to those listed in Table 1. N, normal. Modified from Swerdloff and Boyers *(32)*; used with permission

tomography with enhancement, as well as an evaluation of the secretion of the other pituitary hormones, growth hormone, prolactin, thyrotropin, and corticotropin. Patients in categories III, IV, and V should have their karyotype evaluated.

Possible treatment of these disorders is not presented here. Selection of treatment is obviously predicated on obtaining the correct diagnosis.

The second systematic approach to male infertility is exemplified in Figure 9. This approach selects for the male complaining of infertility and begins with a sperm analysis. Using this as a beginning, one then can enter the diagnostic table we have previously discussed in detail. Because this approach does not consider the male with ambiguous genitalia, diagnostic categories IIIA4, IV, and VA are not pertinent.

References

1. Odell WD, Larsen JL. The endocrinology of male infertility. In *Reproduction: The New Frontier in Occupational and Environmental Health Research*, J Lockey, Ed., Alan R. Liss, New York, NY, 1984 (in press).
2. Wiebe JP, Tilbe KS, Buckingham KD. An analysis of the metabolites of progesterone produced by isolated Sertoli cells at the onset of gametogenesis. *Steroids* **35**, 561–577 (1980).
3. Wiebe JP, Tilbe KS. De novo synthesis of steroids (from acetate) by isolated rat Sertoli cells. *Biochem Biophys Res Commun* **89**, 1107–1113 (1979).
4. Lipshultz LI, Murthy L, Tindall DJ. Characterization of human Sertoli cells in vitro. *J Clin Endocrinol Metab* **55**, 228–237 (1982).
5. Means AR, Fakunding JL, Huckins C, et al. Follicle-stimulating hormone, the Sertoli cell, and spermatogenesis. *Recent Prog Horm Res* **32**, 477–527 (1976).
6. Louis BG, Fritz IB. Follicle-stimulating hormone and testosterone independently increase the production of androgen binding protein by Sertoli cells in culture. *Endocrinology* **104**, 454–461 (1979).
7. Franchimont P, Verstraelen-Proyard J, Hazee-Hagelstein MT, et al. Inhibin: From concept to reality. *Vitam Horm* **37**, 243–302 (1979).
8. Baker HWG, Bremner WJ, Burger HG, et al. Testicular control of follicle-stimulating hormone secretion. *Recent Prog Horm Res* **32**, 429–476 (1976).
9. Lumpkin M, Negro-Vilar A, Franchimont P, McCann S. Evidence for a hypothalamic site of action of inhibin to suppress FSH release. *Endocrinology* **108**, 1101–1104 (1981).

10. Odell WD, Swerdloff RS. Etiologies of sexual maturation: A model system based on the sexually maturing rat. *Recent Prog Horm Res* **32**, 245–288 (1976).

11. Nelson WO. Some factors involved in the gameto-genetic and endocrine function of the testes. *Cold Spring Harbor Symp Quant Biol* **5**, 123–135 (1937).

12. Lostroh AJ. Regulation by FSH and ICSH (LH) of reproductive function in the immature male rat. *Endocrinology* **85**, 438–445 (1969).

13. Von Berswordt-Wallrabe R, Mehring M. Fully restored, maintained fertility of hypophysectomized (HE) male rats receiving long-term testosterone proprionate (TP) replacement therapy. *J Steroid Biochem* **5**, 380 (1974). Abstract 352.

14. Ito T, Horton R. The source of plasma dihydrotestosterone in man. *J Clin Invest* **50**, 1621–1627 (1971).

15. Longcope C, Kato T, Horton R. Conversion of blood androgens to estrogens in normal adult men and women. *J Clin Invest* **48**, 2191–2201 (1969).

16. Imperato-McGinley J, Peterson RE. Male pseudohermaphroditism: The complexities of male phenotypic development. *Am J Med* **61**, 251–272 (1976).

17. Odell WD, Swerdloff RS. Feedback control of pituitary gonadotropins. Central actions of estrogenic hormones. *Adv Biosci* **15**, 141–162 (1975).

18. Walsh PC, Swerdloff RS, Odell WD. Feedback regulation of gonadotropin secretion in men. *J Urol* **110**, 84–89 (1973).

19. Patritti Laborde N, Odell WD. Short-loop feedback of luteinizing hormones. Dose response relationships and specificity. *Fertil Steril* **30**, 456–460 (1978).

20. Patritti Laborde N, Wolfsen AR, Heber D, Odell WD. Pituitary gland: Site of shortloop feedback for luteinizing hormone in the rabbit. *J Clin Invest* **64**, 1066–1069 (1979).

21. Patritti Laborde N, Wolfsen AR, Odell WD. Shortloop feedback system for the control of follicle stimulating hormone in the rabbit. *Endocrinology* **108**, 72–75 (1981).

22. Pfeiffer CA. Sexual differences of the hypophyses and their determination by the gonads. *Am J Anat* **58**, 195–226 (1936).

23. Barraclough CA, Gorski RA. Studies on mating behaviour in the androgen-sterilized female rat in relation to the hypothalamic regulation of sexual behaviour. *J Endocrinol* **25**, 175–182 (1962).

24. Barraclough CA. Modifications in the CNS regulation of reproduction after exposure of prepubertal rats to steroid hormones. *Recent Prog Horm Res* **22**, 503–539 (1966).

25. Brown-Grant K, Munch AV, Naftolin F, et al. The effects of adminis-

tration of testosterone and related steroids to female rats during the neonatal period. *Horm Behav* **2**, 173–182 (1971).

26. Dohler KD. Is female sexual differentiation hormone-mediated? *Trends Neurosci* **1**, 138–140 (1978).
27. Dohler KD, Gorski RA. Sexual differentiation of the brain. Past, present and future. *Brain Res Bull* **5**, 5 (1981).
28. Gorski RA. Long term hormonal modulation of neuronal structure and function. In *The Neurosciences —Fourth Study Program*, FO Schmitt, FG Worden, Eds., MIT Press, Cambridge, MA, 1978, pp 969–982.
29. Odell WD, Swerdloff RS. Progestogen-induced luteinizing and follicle-stimulating hormone surge in postmenopausal women: A simulated ovulatory peak. *Proc Natl Acad Sci USA* **61**, 529–536 (1968).
30. Kalra SP, Kalra PS. Neural regulation of luteinizing hormone secretion in the rat. *Endocr Rev* **4**, 311–351 (1983).
31. Slag MF, Morley JE, Elson MK, et al. Impotence in medical clinic outpatients. *J Am Med Assoc* **249**, 1736–1740 (1983).
32. Swerdloff RS, Boyers SP. Evaluation of the male partner of an infertile couple. *J Am Med Assoc* **247**, 2418–2422 (1982).
33. Collins JA, Wrixon W, Janes LB, Wilson EH. Treatment-independent pregnancy among infertile couples. *N Engl J Med* **309**, 1201–1206 (1983).
34. Odell WD, Swerdloff RS. Abnormalities of gonadal function in men. *Clin Endocrinol* **8**, 149–180 (1978).
35. Spencer CA, Challand GS. Interference in a radioimmunoassay for human thyrotropin. *Clin Chem* **23**, 584–588 (1977).
36. Frohman LA, Baron MA, Schneider AB. Plasma immunoreactive TSH: Spurious elevation due to antibodies to bovine TSH which cross-react with human TSH. *Metabolism* **31**, 834–840 (1982).
37. Snyder PJ, Rudenstein RS, Gardner DF, Rothman JG. Repetitive infusion of gonadotropin-releasing hormone distinguishes hypothalamic from pituitary hypogonadism. *J Clin Endocrinol Metab* **48**, 864–868 (1979).
38. Kallman I, Schonfeld WA, Barrera SF. The genetic aspects of primary eunuchoidism. *Am J Ment Defic* **48**, 203–206 (1944).
39. Lieblich JM, Rogol AD, White BJ, Rosen SW. Syndrome of anosmia with hypogonadotropic hypogonadism (Kallmann syndrome). *Am J Med* **73**, 506–519 (1982).
40. Gorlin RJ, Cervenka J, Pruzansky S. Facial clefting and its syndromes. *Birth Defects* **7**, 3–49 (1971).
41. DeMyer W. The median cleft face syndrome. *Neurology* **17**, 961–971 (1967).
42. Prader A, Willi H. Das syndrom von imbezilliatat adipositas, muskelhypotonie, hypogenitalismus, hypogonadismus, and diabetes melli-

tus mit myotonie-anamnese. *Kongr Psych Entu Stor Kindes Alt* **1**, 353–361 (1963).

43. Vasquez SB, Hurst DL, Sotos JF. X-linked hypogonadism, gynecomastia, mental retardation, short stature, and obesity—a new syndrome. *J Pediatr* **94**, 56–60 (1979).

44. Roth AA. Familial hypogonadism—the Laurence–Moon–Biedl syndrome. *J Urol* **57**, 427–445 (1947).

45. Morley JE, Melmed S. Gonadal dysfunction in systemic disorders. *Metabolism* **28**, 1051–1073 (1979).

46. Beitins IZ, Axelrod L, Ostrea T, et al. Hypogonadism in a male with an immunologically active, biologically inactive luteinizing hormone: Characterization of the abnormal hormone. *J Clin Endocrinol Metab* **52**, 1143–1149 (1981).

47. Patritti Laborde N, Odell WD. Effects of short-term hyperprolactinemia on the endocrine reproductive system in male rabbits. *Fertil Steril* (1984) (in press).

48. Odell WD. Prolactin-producing tumors (prolactinomas). In *Pituitary Tumors,* WD Odell, DH Nelson, Eds., Futura Publ. Co., Mount Kisco, NY, 1984, pp 159–179.

49. Benirschke K, Naftolin F, Gittes R, et al. True hermaphroditism and chimerism. *Am J Obstet Gynecol* **113**, 449–458 (1972).

50. Noonan JA, Ehmke DA. Associated noncardiac malformations in children with congenital heart disease. *J Pediatr* **63**, 468–470 (1963).

51. Char F, Rodriquez-Fernandez HL, Scott CI, et al. The Noonan syndrome: A clinical study in 45 cases. *(Proc 4th Conf Clin Delineation of Birth Defects. Part XI. The Cardiovascular System) Birth Defects* **8**, 110–118 (1972).

52. Berthezene F, Forest MG, Grimaud JA, et al. Leydig cell agenesis. A cause of male pseudo-hermaphroditism. *N Engl J Med* **295**, 969–972 (1976).

53. Sagel J, Distiller LA, Morley JE, Isaacs H. Myotonia dystrophica: Studies on gonadal function using luteinizing hormone-releasing hormone (LRH). *J Clin Endocrinol Metab* **40**, 1110–1113 (1975).

54. Lipshultz LI, Caminos-Torres R, Greenspan CS, Snyder PJ. Testicular function after orchiopexy for unilaterally undescended testis. *N Engl J Med* **295**, 15–18 (1976).

55. Benirschke K. Chromosomal errors and reproductive failure. In *Physiology and Genetics of Reproduction,* **1**, EM Coutinho, F Fuchs, Eds., Plenum Publ. Co., New York, NY, 1974, pp 73–90.

56. Jones TM, Amarose AP, Lebowitz M. Testicular chromosomal mosaicism and infertility. *J Clin Endocrinol Metab* **42**, 888–893 (1976).

57. Afzelius BA. A human syndrome caused by immotile cilia. *Science* **193**, 317–319 (1976).

58. Aiman J, Griffin JE, Gazak JM, et al. Androgen insensitivity as a cause of infertility in otherwise normal men. *N Engl J Med* **300**, 223–228 (1979).

59. Wilson JD, Harrod MJ, Goldstein JL, et al. Familial incomplete male pseudohermaphroditism, type 1. *N Engl J Med* **290**, 1097–1103 (1974).

60. Morillo-Cucci G, German J. Males with a uterus and fallopian tube—a rare disorder of sexual development. *Birth Defects* **7**, 229–231 (1971).

61. Brook CGD, Wagner H, Zachmann M, et al. Familial occurrence of persistent Mullerian structures in otherwise normal males. *Br Med J* **i**, 771–773 (1973).

62. Holsclaw DS, Perlmutter AD, Jockin H, Shwachman H. Genital abnormalities in male patients with cystic fibrosis. *J Urol* **106**, 568–574 (1971).

63. Bardwick PA, Zvaifler NJ, Gill GN, et al. Plasma cell dyscrasia with polyneuropathy, organomegaly, endocrinopathy, M protein, and skin changes: The POEMS syndrome. *Medicine* **59**, 311–322 (1980).

64. Driedger H, Pruzanski W. Plasma cell neoplasia with peripheral polyneuropathy: A study of five cases and a review of the literature. *Medicine* **59**, 301–310 (1980).

65. Imawari M, Akatsuka N, Ishibashi M, et al. Syndrome of plasma cell dyscrasia, polyneuropathy, and endocrine disturbances: Report of a case. *Ann Intern Med* **81**, 490–493 (1974).

66. Medical Research Council Working Party Report. Adverse reactions to bendrofluazide and propranolol for the treatment of mild hypertension. *Lancet* **ii**, 539–543 (1981).

67. Levi AJ, Fisher AM, Hughes L, Hendry WF. Male infertility due to sulphasalazine. *Lancet* **i**, 276–278 (1979).

68. Lim VS, Fang VS. Restoration of plasma testosterone levels in uremic men with clomiphene citrate. *J Clin Endocrinol Metab* **43**, 1370–1377 (1976).

69. Antoniou LD, Sudhakar T, Shalhoub RJ, Smith JC Jr. Reversal of uraemic impotence by zinc. *Lancet* **ii**, 895–898 (1977).

70. Strain GW, Zumoff B, Kream J, et al. Mild hypogonadotropic hypogonadism in obese men. *Metabolism* **31**, 871–875 (1982).

Laboratory and Clinical Work-up of the Infertile Couple

Veasy C. Buttram, Jr.

Causes of Infertility and Their Detection

There are three main causes of infertility: inadequate sperm, ovulatory irregularities, and mechanical factors in the female reproductive tract. Although these three kinds of deterrents to conception occur with nearly equal frequency, it is not unusual for several inhibiting factors to co-exist in an infertile couple. In a review of 1421 consecutive infertility cases from 1970 to 1982, I found that there was more than one probable cause for infertility in 31% of patients. The physician's challenge is to determine the cause of infertility as quickly as possible and to inform the couple of the nature of their problem, the modes of therapy available, the risks involved in treatment, and the probability of success. Our role is then to provide up-to-date medical and surgical care.

Sperm-Related Factors

I will not discuss here the numerous male disorders that may reduce the ability of sperm to penetrate the ovum. The gynecologist, however, should order a routine sperm analysis in the initial evaluation and, even if the results are normal, repeat the analysis at three- to six-month intervals. If results are abnormal, or if infertility persists with no obvious cause being detected in the female, the male should be advised to consult a specialist in male infertility.

Post-Coital Test

Although gynecologists today are not expected to be authorities on male fertility, they should be able to perform and interpret a post-coital test when one is indicated. Consequently, I will discuss the test in some detail even though its efficacy may ultimately be questioned.

The post-coital test involves examination of the cervical mucus several hours after intercourse, at approximately the time of ovulation; it is often considered an essential test during the initial workup preceding laparoscopy. Although we perform post-coital tests on almost every couple, its performance before laparoscopy or other indicated tests is not imperative. It is only a crude indicator of the adequacy of coital technique, cervical mucus, and sperm count; moreover, an abnormal result for a post-coital test is inconclusive and difficult to interpret. Results of later post-coital tests frequently are normal even when no treatment has been given. Except in women who are receiving medication or who have undergone cervical surgery, patients with an isolated cervical mucus abnormality that is the sole cause for infertility are rare.

Because of the frequency with which abnormalities of the cervical mucus arise in patients receiving ovulatory stimulants, post-coital tests or examinations of cervical mucus probably should be requested about every three months for patients being treated with clomiphene citrate. Gysler et al. *(1)* reported that post-coital test results were abnormal in 15% of their patients with clomiphene citrate-induced ovulatory cycles. In general, the risk of developing a cervical mucus problem during therapy with clomiphene citrate is dose-related. In addition, because of its long half-life (about five to seven days), clomiphene citrate is more likely to cause inadequate cervical mucus if ovulation occurs on days 13–15 than if it occurs days 16–18, when the clomiphene is given from day 5 through day 9 of the cycle.

For patients who have not had prior cervical surgery, two consecutive normal results for post-coital tests probably are sufficient. If a patient remains unresponsive to treatment of the primary cause of infertility for longer than six months, however, repeating the test is worthwhile even when previous results have been normal.

Technique. Part of the difficulty in interpreting the results of the post-coital test stems from the lack of a generally accepted procedure for performing the test. For example, the suggested interval between intercourse and examination varies from 1 to 16 h; some authors maintain that 6 h is the minimum interval

(2); others routinely use a 2-h maximum interval *(3)*. Proponents of the so-called "fractional post-coital test" believe that the prognostic significance of the test is maximized only when mucus from the internal os is examined *(4)*. Finally, estimates of what constitutes a "normal" result range from a single motile sperm per high-power field (HPF) *(5)* to more than 20 *(6)*.[1] This lack of standardization, making data obtained by different techniques difficult to compare, has limited the usefulness of the test as a research tool. The usefulness of the test to the individual physician depends more upon the consistent application of a well-defined technique than upon the details of the technique chosen. The technique described below has proven over the past 15 years to be both useful and practical; it is by no means the only acceptable way to perform the test, however, nor is it demonstrably better than many others.

The post-coital test should be performed on the expected day of ovulation, as determined by menstrual history or, preferably, from charts of basal body temperature. The couple should abstain from intercourse, douching, and intravaginal medications for 48 h before the test. We generally ask the couple to have intercourse in the morning of the appointed day and to report for examination within 2 h. Limiting examinations to a specific time interval (usually 1–2 h after intercourse) reduces what variability in results may accrue from examining patients at widely divergent intervals.

Cervical mucus is aspirated from the external cervical canal with a sterile glass pipette. No attempt is made to separate mucus from different levels of the canal. As Speroff et al. noted *(7)*, sufficient justification for routine fractional post-coital testing does not exist at present. The mucus is then examined for opacity–viscosity, "ferning," spinnbarkeit, motile sperm, and leukocytes. The test result generally is considered normal if the mucus is abundant, clear, and thin; shows good spinnbarkeit (6 cm or more); and on microscopic examination demonstrates "ferning" (described as 1^+ to 4^+, depending on the degree of arborization) and more than 20 motile sperm per HPF. If the findings meet these criteria, coital technique and cervical mucus are adequate

---

[1] Abbreviations used (not already defined on p. xviii): HPF, high-power field; HPO, hypothalamic–pituitary–ovarian; DHEA-S, dehydroepiandrosterone sulfate; SHBG, sex-hormone-binding globulin; CAT, computerized axial tomography; D & C, dilatation and curettage; HSG, hysterosalpingography.

and the sperm concentration probably exceeds 20 million per milliliter (8).

The most common reason for encountering "inadequate" or suboptimal mucus (thick, opaque, scanty mucus that demonstrates no ferning and poor spinnbarkeit) is an improperly timed test. A body temperature chart should be kept during the months that the test is performed to correlate the timing of the test with the drop in temperature that indicates ovulation. If the chart suggests that the test was performed more than 48 h before the nadir, then the test should be repeated the following month; if the chart shows that the test was timed properly, treatment may be initiated. We begin with 0.625 mg of Premarin (conjugated estrogens) for 10 days, beginning on day 5 of the cycle. This dosage may be increased to 1.25 mg if subsequent tests demonstrate that mucus has remained poor. If the patient is also receiving clomiphene, she is given Premarin for 10 days beginning on day 9. Cervical mucus that contains large numbers of leukocytes should be cultured, and treatment with intravaginal or systemic antibiotics should be initiated as indicated.

Although more than 20 motile sperm per HPF is generally considered normal and no motile sperm per HPF is subnormal, there is less consistent agreement about the significance of finding one to 20 sperm per HPF. Jette and Glass (8) reported no statistically significant difference in pregnancy rates between groups of patients who had from one to 20 motile progressive sperm per HPF, but found that pregnancy rates were significantly higher if more than 20 sperm were present. This is consistent with my own observations and suggests that, although the finding of 21 sperm per HPF should not necessarily be understood as the lower limit of "normal," it is nevertheless a favorable sign.

Other considerations. Despite the fact that more than 20 motile sperm per HPF is almost always associated with a sperm count of more than 20 million/mL, the post-coital test should not be substituted for semen analysis. This association is not invariant, and omission of semen analysis may fail to disclose abnormalities of sperm morphology or inflammatory diseases of the male genital tract. Of particular interest are reports by Soules et al. (9) and others, which suggest that the post-coital test result may be less significant in the evaluation of male infertility than a test of the ability of the sperm to penetrate ova, the so-called sperm penetration assay. In their study, Soules et al. reported that men who had more motile sperm per HPF were more likely to have fertile scores from the sperm penetration assay. In addition, when the latter score was in the fertile range, there was a statistically significant increase in the number of post-coital test results demonstrating five or more motile sperm per HPF. The clinical significance and application of such assays have not yet been fully realized.

The value of a post-coital test has been put in doubt by studies (10–13) examining the frequency with which sperm are found in the peritoneal cavity at pre-ovulatory laparoscopy just after artificial insemination with homologous semen. The data accumulated demonstrate that peritoneal sperm are found as often in patients with a good post-coital test result as in patients with a poor result. These data imply that the post-coital test does not reflect the ability of sperm to migrate to the peritoneal cavity, nor does it indicate adequacy of sperm transport to the uterus and fallopian tubes. The question arises, consequently, of whether a post-coital test is necessary or helpful in evaluating the infertile couple.

Timing of Therapy

Timing is an important consideration in treating the infertile couple. For example, women undergoing conservative surgery for endometriosis are most likely to conceive in the immediate postoperative months. On the other hand, a sperm count reflects the environment of the sperm about three months previously; thus, surgery on the male, e.g., for varicocele repair, should be performed at least three and preferably six months before conservative surgery or completion of medical therapy for the female.

Ovulatory Factors

The basic mechanisms involved in anovulation are many and complex. Not all are clearly identified and understood. Some frequently mentioned causes of anovulation are fairly well established, whereas others are only conjectural. Indeed, anovulation cannot always be explained. In general, however, anovulation can be ascribed to one of the following: (a) immature hypothalamic–pituitary–ovarian (HPO) axis, (b) stress, (c) hyperandrogenism, (d) HPO abnormalities with normal prolactin, (e) HPO abnormalities with excess prolactin, *(f)* use of drugs with normal or excess prolactin, *(g)* metabolic disorders, and *(h)* premature ovarian failure or ovarian dysgenesis.

Immature Hypothalamic–Pituitary–Ovarian Axis

Most females begin menstruating between the ages of 13 and 15 years. At first, a young girl's menstruation is irregular and anovulatory. With time, generally within two years of onset of menarche, she begins to have regular and normal ovulatory menses. One important and unanswered question is why cyclic, ovulatory menses do not occur at the onset. Presumably, the HPO axis must mature before ovulation can occur regularly, and sometimes this maturation process takes much longer than two years. There are other causes of anovulation in the pubertal female, but one of the main causes seems to be slow maturation of the HPO axis. Currently, no laboratory test can document the presence of an immature HPO axis or detail the degree of maturity achieved. Thus the diagnosis is primarily a clinical one.

Stress

Some patients undergoing stress develop anovulation, resulting in dysfunctional uterine bleeding. This stress usually is environmental but may be physiological as well. Response to stress varies with the individual and is difficult to quantify. As with the immature HPO axis, no laboratory markers can either identify stress as a problem or quantify its effect. Again, the diagnosis is a clinical one without laboratory documentation. Gonadotropin concentrations will invariably be reported as normal or low normal. Conceivably, the young girl with an immature HPO axis is even more likely to be affected by stress than one whose HPO axis is mature.

Hyperandrogenism

Current belief is that excess androgen production by the adrenals or ovaries leads to a self-perpetuating cycle of androgen excess (Figure 1). In this condition, excess functional stromal tissue and atretic follicles in the polycystic ovary secrete significant amounts of androgens, principally testosterone. The increased concentrations of androgens (ovarian or adrenal) contribute to the amount of circulating estrogen, as the androgens are converted peripherally to estrone. These augmented concentrations of estro-

173

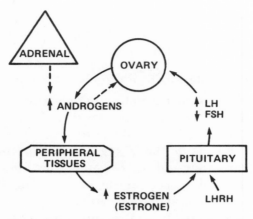

Fig. 1. Hormonal interactions in polycystic ovary syndrome

gen depress the production of follitropin (follicle-stimulating hormone, FSH), while maintaining or increasing the concentrations of lutropin (luteinizing hormone, LH), by increasing the sensitivity of the pituitary to stimulation by luliberin (LH-releasing hormone, LHRH). The result is an increase in the LH/FSH ratio. The chronically (though not totally) depressed concentrations of FSH prevent the normal development of new follicles, so that they undergo premature atresia and become predominantly androgen-producing tissue. Increased production of androgen thereby inhibits future follicular development and perpetuates the anovulatory "steady-state." Current evidence suggests that the high "local" concentrations of androgen contribute to premature atresia of the follicles by counteracting the action of estradiol on the granulosa cells. High concentrations of LH continue to stimulate androgen production. The result is a polycystic ovary with a typical morphological appearance of follicles in all stages of development and atresia within a dense stroma.

The evaluation of hyperandrogenism includes documentation by analysis of peripheral androgen assays. The androgen profile should consist of the following serum tests: testosterone, androstenedione, dihydrotestosterone, dehydroepiandrosterone sulfate (DHEA-S), and sex-hormone-binding globulin (SHBG). Of these, the tests for testosterone and DHEA-S are the most informative.

174

More recently, 3α-androstenediol glucuronide has been added as a possible androgen marker.

In a review of 62 patients with laparoscopically documented polycystic ovaries, we found above-normal values in 66% of the testosterone determinations, 55% of the dihydrotestosterone determinations, 36% of the androstenedione determinations, and 14% of the DHEA-S determinations. A below-normal result for SHBG was found in 15%. All tests were done in the follicular phase of the menstrual cycle. Although one may argue that the "normal" range in this review was too wide, it is more likely that many patients with polycystic ovaries have anovulatory problems not associated with a hyperandrogenic condition.

It is sometimes suggested that patients with polycystic ovaries and a hyperandrogenic condition have an LH/FSH ratio greater than 3. In our 62 patients with polycystic ovaries documented by laparoscopy, 50% had an LH/FSH ratio less than 2; 20% had a ratio between 2 and 3, and 30% had a ratio greater than 3. Not all of our patients had a documented hyperandrogenic condition, but even so, one must not conclude that an LH/FSH ratio greater than 3 is essential for a diagnosis of polycystic ovary syndrome.

Prolactin

Simmond's syndrome is a rare condition that occurs secondary to a thrombotic or embolic infarction of the anterior pituitary gland. Sheehan's syndrome is not so rare, occurring in about 1/2500 deliveries; it is characterized by postpartum hemorrhage or shock resulting in various degrees of hypoxia to the blood vessels supplying the anterior pituitary and the pituitary gland itself. When a normotensive state returns, the anoxic blood vessels allow extravasation of blood into the pituitary gland, producing various degrees of trauma. Both Simmond's and Sheehan's syndromes can result in various forms of pan-hypopituitarism. Typically, though, FSH and LH values remain in the low-normal range. Depending upon the degree of trauma to the pituitary gland, results for other pituitary tests may be normal or abnormal.

Space-occupying lesions of the pituitary gland such as chromophobe adenomas, eosinophilic adenomas, basophilic adenomas, and others can cause pituitary destruction and subsequent anovulation without galactorrhea. Hypothalamic tumors such as cranio-pharyngioma and suprasellar cysts can also result in anovulation by damaging the hypothalamus. Other rare causes of amenorrhea related to intracranial tumors are pineal gland tumors, gliomas, teratomas, and cysts; some of these tumors are associated with precocious puberty.

Approximately 10% of patients with prolonged amenorrhea will have an increased concentration of serum prolactin, as will about 25% of women with isolated, nonpuerperal galactorrhea. When amenorrhea and galactorrhea are both present, prolactin is increased in more than 75% of cases. As Chang has suggested (14), amenorrhea in patients with hyperprolactinemia probably is caused by hypothalamic inhibition of pulsatile secretion of go-nadoliberin (gonadotropin-releasing hormone, GnRH), decreasing the secretion of gonadotropin. However, in these patients, the concentrations of FSH and LH generally are low normal.

Hypothalamic–pituitary pathology (unassociated with drug therapy or hypothyroidism) with excess prolactin production is a relatively uncommon cause of anovulation. Patients with Chiari–Frommel syndrome experience amenorrhea and galactorrhea after delivery, possibly because high concentrations of estrogen and progesterone have hypersuppressed the hypothalamus during ges-tation. In Forbes–Albright syndrome, secretion of prolactin by a pituitary tumor results in galactorrhea and anovulation. There is no known cause of the amenorrhea–galactorrhea in Del Castil-lo's syndrome; in fact, evidence increasingly suggests that such a syndrome does not really exist—rather, about 50% of these patients eventually show radiographic signs of a small pituitary tumor, usually a chromophobe adenoma.

Seldom is there a clinical attempt to categorize hyperprolacti-nemic patients according to any of the afore-mentioned eponyms. More important is ruling out the presence of a prolactinoma (ade-noma). The greater the concentration of prolactin (usually more than 100 ng/mL), the greater the likelihood that an adenoma ex-ists. Macroadenomas can often be detected by coned-down roent-genography of the pituitary gland. Microadenomas are more diffi-cult to demonstrate, requiring computerized axial tomography (CAT scans). A late-morning determination of serum prolactin (at 11:00 hours, after fasting) should be included in the routine screening of the anovulatory woman if her history suggests any of these disorders.

Effect of drugs, with normal or excess prolactin. Many drugs can suppress hypothalamic function, thereby causing anovulation, amenorrhea, and even galactorrhea. The effect is usually dose dependent. Anticholinergic drugs such as the phenothiazines, α-methyldopa, reserpine, and the tricyclic antidepressants initiate galactorrhea by hypothalamic suppression of prolactin-inducing factor. The mechanism of suppression is thought to be mediated through depletion of dopamine or blocking of dopamine receptors.

Investigators still debate whether oral contraceptives (particularly those with high estrogen–progestin concentrations) can cause hypersuppression of the HPO axis. The decreased frequency with which we see "post-pill amenorrhea" or hyperprolactinemia, with or without galactorrhea, in women taking oral contraceptives may be due to the frequent use of "low-dose" pills, which have lower concentrations of estrogen and progestins.

Metabolic Disorders

Although other metabolic conditions may occasionally result in anovulation, the most frequent one is hypothyroidism; less common are hyperthyroidism and Cushing's syndrome. The mechanism by which the anovulatory state is produced by these rarer disorders is not well understood. Possibly, anovulation in the patient with a hypo- or hyperthyroid problem may result from physiological stress. Mild hyperprolactinemia may co-exist with some hypothyroid conditions as a result of decreased hypothalamic dopaminergic activity. Thyroliberin (thyrotropin-releasing hormone, TRH) may have a role in mediating prolactin release by direct action on lactotropes in the anterior pituitary. These patients may have an augmented prolactin release in response to direct stimulation with TRH. Both the basal mild increase of prolactin and its augmented response are normalized when the patient becomes euthyroid. Fortunately, several laboratory tests (for triiodothyronine, thyroxin, thyrotropin, and prolactin) are available to help detect these problems.

Cushing's syndrome, with its excessive production of cortisol, can also be associated with hyperandrogenism. Morning and afternoon measurements of serum cortisol, as well as of serum androgens (androstenedione and DHEA-S), are helpful in evaluating patients suspected of having this condition.

Premature Ovarian Failure or Ovarian Dysgenesis

Premature ovarian failure is a rare cause of anovulation. Its complex etiology has been dichotomized by McDonough et al. *(15)* as follows: chromosomal-incompetent ovarian failure (e.g., XO gonadal dysgenesis and its variants), and chromosomal-competent ovarian failure, which includes 46XY and 46XX forms. The 46XY group includes 46XY gonadal dysgenesis (Swyer's syndrome) and congenital androgen insensitivity syndrome (testicular feminization syndrome). Classified as 46XX are patients with autoimmune disease, 17-hydroxylase deficiency, and gonadotropin-resistant ovary, and those affected by environmental factors such as surgical ablation and irradiation.

Chromosomal-incompetent ovarian dysgenesis usually is associated with primary amenorrhea, but many patients are oligo-amenorrheal. Diagnosis is indicated by persistent occurrence of menopausal-range concentrations of FSH. The serum karyotype is reported as 45XO in 25 to 50% of the patients and as normal 46XX in more than 50%. Not all patients with ovarian dysgenesis and a normal karyotype for peripheral leukocytes will have a normal ovarian tissue karyotype. Because of the impracticality of obtaining ovarian tissue for karyotyping, however, determination of peripheral blood karyotype is indicated in patients with biochemical evidence of premature ovarian failure.

Diagnosis of chromosomal-competent premature ovarian failure, with 46XX karyotype, requires at least two determinations of serum FSH in the menopausal range. In addition, the specific etiology may be investigated, depending on clinical presentation. Women should be informed that the condition may be temporary or permanent: patients have been known to have sudden, transient return of ovulatory function for various periods, with reports of successful pregnancies.

Patients with chromosomal-competent ovarian failure with 46XY karyotype are amenorrheal. Patients with testicular feminization syndrome have a short vagina but no uterus or fallopian tubes. Patients with XY gonadal dysgenesis have a normal vagina associated with a hypoestrogenized uterus. Diagnosis of patients with testicular feminization syndrome is based on a serum karyotype and above-normal concentrations of LH and androgen. In patients with XY gonadal dysgenesis, the concentration of FSH is in the menopausal range. Detection of a mosaic Y chromosome pattern is extremely important. These patients usually require gonadal extirpation to rule out gonadoblastoma.

Assessment of the Anovulatory Female

The work-up of the anovulatory female depends on many factors, including age, degree of oligoamenorrhea, hirsutism, weight, infertility, galactorrhea, acne, and environment. These factors, singly or in combination, generally dictate the type of evaluation. The degree of oligoamenorrhea is particularly important. The longer the duration of amenorrhea, the greater the need for evaluation. Progressive hirsutism obviously dictates a need for assessment. Obesity alone seldom signals a need for extensive endocrine evaluation, but infertility urges the physician to act more quickly. Galactorrhea produces a fear that the patient may have a pituitary tumor. Acne with oligoamenorrhea could possibly be altered by proper hormonal therapy. If there is strong reason to suspect that stress is the problem, a hormonal evaluation may not be necessary.

Method of evaluation. The method of evaluation is not standard. Some physicians think that a progesterone withdrawal test is sufficient if the patient menstruates after injection. They believe that this implies the presence of adequate endogenous estrogen and suggests that no further tests are necessary. Others feel that a "trial of clomiphene citrate" is indicated before laboratory evaluation. Still others are convinced that all anovulatory women need in-depth evaluation.

The components of an in-depth evaluation vary from center to center. Laboratory tests are available for gonadotropins (FSH and LH); androgens (testosterone, androstenedione, dihydrotestosterone, DHEA-S, and SHBG); prolactin; roentgenography (coned-down view of the sella turcica and CAT scans); thyroid hormones; cortisol; and blood or tissue karyotype. However, only those tests that are likely to be informative should be performed.

For example, although evaluations of serum FSH and LH have been recommended for every patient with a history of ovulatory dysfunction, they are helpful only in quite specific and relatively rare circumstances. Because of inherent limitations in sensitivity, neither of these tests is particularly meaningful in hypogonado-

179

tropic patients. Rather, these assays are useful only when the physician suspects, on the basis of preliminary information (especially the history), that a patient is *hypergonadotropic*. Specifically, determination of serum FSH is indicated when ovarian dysgenesis or premature ovarian failure is suspected, in which case the FSH values are increased. Similarly, determination of serum LH should be reserved for patients showing evidence of polycystic ovary syndrome; their LH values are frequently in the high-normal range.

Of the tests available in the androgen profile, determinations of testosterone and DHEA-S are the most helpful. Although researchers do not consistently agree, the concentration of serum testosterone appears at present to be the test of choice for demonstrating hyperandrogenic states of ovarian origin, while DHEA-S may more sensitively indicate increased adrenal production of androgens. Determinations of urinary 17-ketosteroids and 17-hydroxycorticosteroids have been supplanted by these two serum assays.

Unfortunately, determinations of serum estrogen have not been useful in evaluating the anovulatory female. Although serial determinations have been helpful in patients receiving gonadotropin stimulation, folliculograms (ultrasound) seem to be a more sensitive indication of the best time to administer human choriogonadotropin (hCG) with Pergonal (menopausal gonadotropins). Future measurement of estrogen in serum may be limited to evaluation of patients with rare estrogen-producing tumors.

Ovulation Detection

Generally, although not always, if a woman is having regular cyclic menses, she is ovulating properly. The woman with irregular menses probably is not ovulating, particularly if her menses occurs more frequently than every 21 days or less frequently than every 35 days. For less frequent menses, ovulation detection becomes more important.

Detection of ovulation is equally important for evaluating success of treatment when an anovulatory condition has been documented and therapy initiated. Currently there are four methods for assessing ovulation: basal body temperature chart, determination of serum progesterone, endometrial biopsy, and ultrasound.

Basal body temperature. For purposes of documentation, the least expensive, most easily obtained, and most informative and reasonably sensitive indicator of ovulatory activity is the chart of basal body temperature. A midcycle rise of at least 0.5 °F (0.3 °C), sustained for 12 to 16 days in a patient having menses at regular intervals (every 24 to 35 days), is indicative of ovulation. In such instances, additional tests of ovulatory function are seldom indicated unless infertility persists without obvious cause.

To ensure accuracy of this method, the couple are given detailed instructions for the use of the basal thermometer and told of the importance of taking readings immediately upon awakening. For several reasons, they generally are asked to continue recording the woman's temperature throughout the course of evaluation and therapy whether or not she is ovulating regularly. Not only is the basal body temperature the most important guideline for medical ovulation-induction therapy, but also serial temperature charts kept by patients presumed to be ovulating normally aid in detecting individual variations in ovulatory activity as well as stress-associated ovulatory problems. As Morris et al. have pointed out *(16)*, a *single* temperature chart is an inadequate predictor of the day of ovulation during a *given* cycle, because 48 h after the temperature drop, when one can determine that the temperature has changed, the LH surge has already occurred (usually on the same day as the temperature nadir). *Serial* basal body temperature charts, on the other hand, are quite helpful in determining the typical day of ovulation and optimal timing of intercourse. Despite its apparent benefits, however, maintaining a temperature chart may potentially lead to sexual difficulties, particularly in men, because of anxiety associated with sexual performance on demand. The physician should remain vigilant for the development of sexual dysfunction throughout the course of evaluation and therapy.

The significance of the occurrence of a biphasic temperature change (presumed ovulation) before day 10 or after day 21 with a normal (12–14 days) luteal phase is unclear. An obviously monophasic temperature chart is indicative of anovulation. However, improper technique in taking the temperature or a defective thermometer should be considered. The so-called "inadequate luteal phase" is typically associated with either a slow rise in basal temperature at mid-cycle and a luteal phase of 10 days or less, or a sharp rise in basal temperature at mid-cycle followed by a gradual and progressive fall and, again, a shortened luteal phase of 10 to 12 days or less. Clomiphene citrate-induced ovulation usually occurs on day 16 to 18 of the cycle, with menses occurring on day 30 to 32. Finally, a patient who exhibits a sustained rise in basal body temperature for more than 14 days should be presumed to be pregnant.

Serum progesterone. Although a single determination of serum progesterone exceeding 8 ng/mL seven days before menses is indicative of ovulation, this assay is a less practical indicator of ovulation than are the temperature charts. Progesterone concentrations of less than 4 ng/mL are generally considered inconsistent with ovulation, and many clinicians regard concentrations between 4 and 7 ng/mL as marginal or equivocal. False-negative results are not uncommon because of improper timing of the test—too early or too late in the luteal phase. In addition, the significance of an isolated serum progesterone value is questionable because of the fluctuations of its concentration that may occur in any 24-h period. For meaningful data, serial determinations of serum progesterone are needed. Although not very practical, best results are achieved by sampling on days 5, 7, and 9 after supposed ovulation and pooling the blood for testing. If progesterone exceeds 8 ng/mL, one can assume that ovulation, or at least luteinization of the follicle, has taken place.

One of the most frequent rationales for measuring serum progesterone as well as taking an endometrial biopsy is the need to diagnose the so-called "inadequate luteal phase." An endometrial sample that histologically lags more than two days behind the cycle, a serum luteal-phase concentration of progesterone less than 7 ng/mL, or an average of three serum progesterone values of less than 7 ng/mL between 4 and 11 days before menses, have all been said to indicate an inadequate luteal phase. What is meant or understood by this diagnosis is not clear, although the term implies insufficient production of progesterone by the corpus luteum. On this basis, progestins have been administered daily during the luteal phase with reportedly favorable results, although a significant number of pregnancies will occur without treatment. I tend to concur with Strott et al. *(17)* that the inadequate luteal phase occurs as a result of a deficiency in the proliferative phase (perhaps deficient FSH), which leads to poorly stimulated ovaries. We have treated this problem satisfactorily with ovulatory stimulants such as clomiphene citrate. In support of this view, Speroff *(18)* and others postulate that increased FSH is necessary for induction of LH receptors on granulosa cells, which are essential for adequate luteal function. Increasing the FSH also avoids the potential teratogenic risks associated with synthetic progestins. My own experience is that a temperature rise sustained for less than 12 days (as documented by temperature charts) for two successive cycles is an adequate indicator of this problem.

Endometrial biopsy. Many physicians still advocate endometrial biopsy for detection of ovulation, contending that a two-day lag in endometrial maturation is presumptive evidence of inadequate ovulation. However, this test is costly, invasive, and painful and may conceivably disrupt an early pregnancy if performed before onset of menses.

Ultrasound. In ultrasonography, high-frequency sound waves are projected onto an object that is then distinguished by the pattern of "echoes" emanating from its surface. Ultrasound can thus delineate within the body any two neighboring structures that differ sufficiently in their density to absorb or reflect different amounts of sound; e.g., the relatively dense ("echogenic") structures of the developing fetus are easily delineated from the "nonechogenic" fluid surrounding it. In recent years ultrasound has emerged as an invaluable adjunct for the infertility specialist.

In 1979 Hackeloer et al. *(19)* demonstrated that serial ultrasonographic measurements of follicular size correlated with endocrine parameters of ovulation such as serum concentrations of 17β-estradiol and LH. The following year O'Herlighy et al. *(20)* reported a similar correlation between follicular size and volume as predicted by ultrasound and actual follicular size measured at laparoscopy (within the next 12 h).

With this capability for accurate reflection of ovarian function, ultrasound has found numerous clinical applications. Cabau and Bessie *(21)*, among others, have documented the utility of ultrasound in patients undergoing ovulation induction with human gonadotropins. In such patients ultrasound can decrease the incidence of multiple pregnancies by indicating when to withhold hCG (used to initiate ovulation) by noting when multiple follicles are stimulated. Similarly, ultrasound may be of value in decreasing the risk of hyperstimulation syndrome. Hoult et al. *(22)* have demonstrated that combining clomiphene citrate stimulation with ultrasound can lead to a significantly higher recovery rate as well as a significantly improved yield of oocytes for *in vitro* fertilization, as compared with results for spontaneous cycles.

In the recent past, ultrasound has proved valuable in documenting ovulation, whether or not patients were receiving ovulatory stimulants. The initial "folliculogram" usually is best performed on day 8, 9, or 10 of the menstrual cycle; it is repeated every two days until ovulation has been detected. Generally, follicular growth can be documented, and ovulation occurs when the follicle reaches a diameter of 18–26 mm. Occasionally, corpus luteum activity can be recognized when the follicle diameter is less than 18 mm or greater than 26 mm.

Significant findings with ultrasound include the following: *(a)* documentation of inadequate follicular growth without ovulation in some patients who have biphasic basal body temperature charts; *(b)* detection of ovulation as much as three to four days before, and even after, the typical nadir of the basal body temperature; *(c)* demonstration of follicular growth with luteinization of the follicle.

Although data are preliminary, information from folliculograms has been helpful in advising the timing for intercourse, artificial insemination (AID and AIH), and post-coital tests. Documentation of follicular size also has facilitated proper timing for administration of hCG (5000 int. units) when follicle growth reaches 18–20 mm. Administration of hCG before follicular growth is adequate could be detrimental (luteinization without ovulation), and hCG given after corpus luteum formation would be ineffective except for the treatment of documented inadequate luteal phase. Preliminary data indicate that 5 to 10% of natural and clomiphene-stimulated cycles result in luteinization of the follicle; increasing the amount of clomiphene citrate given is generally ineffective, whereas addition of hCG when follicle size is at 18–20 mm effectively abates this problem.

Treatment of Ovulatory Problems

It is rare not to be able to resolve an ovulatory problem with ovulatory stimulants such as clomiphene citrate, cortisone, hCG, menopausal gonadotropins plus hCG, Parlodel (bromocriptine mesylate), or wedge resection of the ovaries. Although space does not allow a comprehensive discussion of each technique, a comment is in order with regard to wedge resection. This surgical procedure is no longer the procedure of choice in women with polycystic ovary syndrome. Between 30 and 50% of patients undergoing wedge resection will develop significant periovarian adhesions, which interfere with conception. The ovary is extremely vulnerable to surgical trauma.

Mechanical Factors

Mechanical problems are currently the greatest problem encountered by the specialist in female infertility, treatment being less often successful than with ovulatory disorders. The mechanical problems encountered most often include pelvic adhesive disease, endometriosis, tubal obstruction (secondary to pelvic inflammatory disease or to tubal ligation), uterine synechia, cervical incompetency, uterine anomalies, and uterine leiomyomata.

Although these anatomical problems may exist alone, they commonly occur concurrently. For example, pelvic adhesive disease frequently is present in patients with moderate or severe endometriosis and should be considered as part of the disease itself. In addition, endometriosis often is seen in patients with leiomyomata and uterine anomalies.

Table 1 indicates the prevalence of each of these mechanical problems as I have encountered them in the past 13 years. These data, to be sure, were gathered in a specialized practice in which endometriosis is the most commonly encountered problem.

Table 1. **Incidence of Mechanical Problems in Female Infertility**

Primary diagnosis	No. (and %) of patients
Endometriosis	566 (58)
Pelvic adhesive disease	232 (24)
Uterine anomaly	60 (6)
Uterine leiomyomata	38 (4)
Bilateral tubal occlusion secondary to bilateral tubal ligation (reversal)	53 (5)
Polycystic ovary syndrome (bilateral wedge resection)	7 (0.7)
Miscellaneous	12 (1)
Total	968 (100)

Whether pelvic adhesive disease is a more common cause of infertility is subject to debate.

Currently there are two primary procedures for evaluating a possible mechanical problem in a female: hysterosalpingography (HSG), and dilatation and curettage (D & C) combined with laparoscopy. Hysteroscopy may be helpful in some conditions.

Hysterosalpingography

HSG involves the injection of radiopaque contrast media through the cervix into the uterine cavity and fallopian tubes, to allow a detailed radiographic examination of the intra-uterine cavity and tubal lumens. It is the noninvasive procedure of choice for demonstrating tubal patency, uterine anomalies, and many abnormalities of the uterine cavity such as endometrial polyps and submucous leiomyomata. In addition, many rare or unsuspected pathologic conditions of the uterus or tubes, such as salpingitis isthmica nodosa, may present with characteristic findings on HSG. The greater sensitivity and specificity of HSG have rendered tubal insufflation obsolete as a test of tubal patency and of the contour of the intra-uterine cavity.

HSG is easily performed and generally quite safe; nevertheless, there is still controversy regarding the contrast medium of choice and possible risks and alleged therapeutic benefits of HSG. At present there is no conclusive evidence favoring either oil- or water-based contrast media for HSG; both have distinct advantages and disadvantages. The increased viscosity and slower dissipation and absorption of the oil-based media provide somewhat more distinct radiographic shadows and allow for delayed films when desired. In addition, oil-based media are generally believed to cause less discomfort and cramping upon injection, although I have not observed this consistently. Water-based media, on the other hand, are generally (although not universally) believed to allow a wider margin of safety. Seven of the nine reported deaths from HSG have occurred with oil-based media (23). The tendency for micelle formation and subsequent blockage of capillaries, as Siegler has described (23), probably causes the risk of intravasation and embolus from oil-based media to exceed that from water-soluble media, although this difference has not been established. The risk may be minimized by halting further injection if circulatory or lymphatic intravasation of contrast media is noted by image-intensifying fluoroscopy. Use of oil-based media also carries a greater risk of granuloma formation, foreign body reaction, and retention cyst formation, findings reported only rarely after HSG with water-soluble media. Finally, though not established by formal study, personal experience suggests that water-based media may produce a lower incidence of false-positive results because they have less tendency to produce tubal spasm.

Most investigators who have stated a preference, however, have selected oil-based contrast media, citing as advantages superior radiographic results, less discomfort, and the ability to take delayed films if desired. They maintain, moreover, that granulomata probably do not form in normal tubes (7).

The contrast medium I prefer is a water-soluble dye (Hypopaque 50; Winthrop). The radiographic results it produces are adequate even for demonstrating details such as endometrial polyps and submucous leiomyomata, and the patient's tolerance is good if the medium is injected slowly. I have not found delayed films to be helpful in reducing the number of false-positive or false-negative results. Furthermore, although granulomata and foreign body reactions probably do not occur in normal tubes, the abnormal tubes in which oil-sequestration and granulomata formation may occur may subsequently be less amenable to correction by tubal plastic procedures. Finally, the rapid dissipation, absorption, and excretion of water-soluble media probably confer upon it a wider margin of safety, and allow the injection of larger amounts of dye into the uterine cavities that may be distorted and enlarged (e.g.) by leiomyomata. Not only does use of oil-based media have the risk of oil embolus, but also injection of larger (> 10 mL) volumes may produce severe peritoneal reaction and pain.

In addition to the problems described above, HSG presents certain other risks, independent of the type of contrast medium used. Because of the rare chance that HSG may disrupt or flush retrograde a concurrent pregnancy, and because of the small radiation hazard, the test should be performed immediately after the cessation of menses. This precaution may also reduce the possibility of circulatory intravasation of dye by involving fewer open blood vessels. In a patient with cervicitis or endometritis, HSG may flush organisms back into the tubes or peritoneal cavity, producing a salpingitis or disseminated peritonitis (19).

Whether the risk of infectious complications would be lessened by use of prophylactic antibiotics before HSG or by delay of laparoscopy or surgery for a month or more after HSG is not known; however, such complications are quite rare in my experience (encountered once in more than 3000 HSGs). Until more substantial evidence suggests otherwise, I doubt that the theoretical benefits of prophylactic antibodies outweigh either the risks and expense of antibiotic administration or the time, stress, and frustration to the couple of delaying laparoscopy or surgery, if indicated.

The risk of complications arising as a result of radiation from HSG has not been quantified. Obviously, however, because the risk of radiation is cumulative and because gonadal tissues are relatively radio-sensitive, radiation should be kept to a minimum. Innovations in fluorographic equipment and technique during the past decade have significantly reduced the HSG-associated radiation hazard to the ovaries. Shirley, for example, in 1971 (24) advocated the use of a "two-film" technique, in which spot films were obtained after the injection of 3 and 10 mL of contrast medium. The average radiation dosage in the posterior fornix was approximately 130 mrad, as compared with approximately 100 mrad with fluoroscopy. By 1978, however, Seppanen et al. (25) reported that the average dosage associated with HSG by 100-mm fluorography with intensification was about 100 to 200 mrad. With current equipment and techniques, therefore, the greater diagnostic accuracy and increased margin of safety (regarding dye intravasation) provided by fluorography are not offset by any significant decrease in radiation dosage simply by using the "two-film" technique alone. In addition, image-intensification fluoroscopy may reduce the total number of films taken. The additional radiation hazard associated with routine delayed films, on the other hand, is not in my experience accompanied by any significant increase in diagnostic accuracy.

Several proponents of hysteroscopy profess that it is better than HSG for evaluation of the uterine cavity. To me, however, it has seemed visually and surgically more limiting than HSG. If the HSG is normal, I do not routinely perform hysteroscopy; if the HSG is equivocal, hysteroscopy is performed.

D & C Laparoscopy

Although some clinicians perform this procedure in the luteal phase of the menstrual cycle, the information obtained (i.e., stigmata of ovulation, as noted by visualization of the ovary, or evidence of secretory activity as detected by a D & C) is not of sufficient significance to warrant the risk of interrupting a pregnancy. Such information is valuable only for that particular menstrual cycle and can be ascertained by noninvasive techniques such as basal body temperature charts, determinations of serum progesterone, and folliculograms.

Before advising major surgery for a woman, the physician should consider several factors:

1. Existence of a mechanical problem such as endometriosis or pelvic adhesive disease does not necessarily mean that the couple is infertile. Many patients with severe pelvic adhesive disease have conceived without surgical intervention. I estimate that one in three patients with endometriosis, particularly those with mild disease, will become pregnant without medical intervention. (This, however, does not disprove the inhibitory effect of the disease on other women.) Couples, particularly those younger than 30 years old, should be encouraged to attempt conception in at least 12 *ovulatory* cycles before considering surgery.
2. In the infertile woman with a mechanical problem that necessitates corrective surgery, documentation of ovulation is not always necessary before surgery. For example, the older infertile woman (older than 30) who has been infertile one or more years, who has a history of regular cyclic menses every 28 to 30 days, and whose partner has a normal semen analysis does not need to be evaluated with basal body temperature charts, serum progesterone determinations, folliculograms, etc. before undergoing surgery. Such testing will be useful after the major problem has been resolved. Similarly, tests such as cervical mucus and post-coital examination need not be performed before surgery, but can be performed in the postoperative follow-up period.
3. One of the major causes of infertility I see is adhesive disease secondary to iatrogenic causes. For example, of 173 patients

who had undergone wedge resection of the ovary for polycystic ovary syndrome, at least 33% developed significant periovarian adhesions postoperatively. The potential consequences of pelvic surgery are particularly significant for the infertile patient.

4. As discussed earlier, if the male cohort has a sperm factor problem, such as varicocele, appropriate therapy should be initiated so that both partners can achieve their fullest fertility potential at the same time.

D & C laparoscopy and possible laparotomy. Major surgery on the day after HSG and on the day of the laparoscopy is acceptable, provided the problem is one such as endometriosis, pelvic adhesive disease, or tubal obstruction secondary to previous ligation. However, when hydrosalpinx exists, conservative surgery is probably best postponed until active infection is not likely to be present. I prefer in all cases to delay conservative surgery so that the condition can be fully explained to the couple, the risks described, and the odds of success discussed before a major decision is made.

D & C laparoscopy after conservative surgery. Currently, many infertility surgeons commonly perform endoscopy one to six weeks after major surgery—both to determine the effectiveness of surgery in terms of formation of postoperative adhesions and to lyse these adhesions (if they exist) before they become more dense or vascular. Patients selected to undergo these procedures have ranged from all patients undergoing conservative surgery in some practices to almost none in others. Although there are theoretical advantages to this follow-up procedure, I have several concerns about its use. No data actually document the effectiveness of this procedure, although recent data indicate that surgical lysis of adhesions via laparoscopy as a primary procedure is effective in selected cases. Hyskon hysteroscopy fluid (dextran in dextrose) can be administered via a secondary puncture site in an attempt to prevent further adhesive formation. The patient in whom no adhesions are found at endoscopy may be consoled with the knowledge that her condition is much improved, and this knowledge may be beneficial in alleviating anxiety. For the patient who has pelvic adhesive disease that is too severe to be corrected laparoscopically, however, the news would be disheartening at a very emotional time. On the other hand, this fact may encourage her to seek adoption earlier than she might have. Although I have performed this procedure on numerous occasions, I am not yet convinced that it is either appropriate or helpful.

References

1. Gysler M, March CM, Mishell DR, Bailey EJ. A decade's experience with an individualized clomiphene treatment regimen including its effect on the post-coital test. *Fertil Steril* **37,** 161–167 (1982).
2. Kistner RW, Patton GW. *Atlas of Infertility Surgery,* Little, Brown & Co., Boston, MA, 1975.
3. Moran J, Davajan V, Nakamura R. Comparison of the fractional post-coital test with the Sims–Huhner post-coital test. *Int J Fertil* **19,** 93–96 (1974).
4. Maathuis JB, Horbach JGM, Van Hall EV. A comparison of the results of hysterosalpingography tube dysfunction. *Fertil Steril* **23,** 428–431 (1972).
5. Grant A. Cervical hostility. *Fertil Steril* **9,** 321–333 (1958).
6. Mastroianni L. Female infertility. In *Current Therapy,* HF Conn, Ed., Saunders, Philadelphia, PA, 1966, pp 731–735.
7. Speroff L, Glass RH, Kase NG. *Clinical Gynecologic Endocrinology and Infertility,* Williams and Wilkins, Baltimore, MD, 1977.
8. Jette NT, Glass RH. Prognostic value of the post-coital test. *Fertil Steril* **23,** 29–32 (1972).
9. Soules MR, Moore DE, Spadoni LR, Stenchever MA. The relationship between the post-coital test and the sperm penetration assay. *Fertil Steril* **38,** 384–387 (1982).
10. Stone SC. Peritoneal recovery of sperm in patients with infertility associated with inadequate cervical mucus. *Fertil Steril* **40,** 802–804 (1983).
11. Asch RH. Laparoscopic recovery of sperm from peritoneal fluid in patients with negative or poor Sims–Huhner test. *Fertil Steril* **27,** 1111–1114 (1976).
12. Asch RH. Sperm recovery in peritoneal aspirate after negative Sims–Huhner test. *Int J Fertil* **23,** 57–60 (1978).
13. Templeton AA, Mortimer D. Laparoscopic sperm recovery in infertile women. *Br J Obstet Gynaecol* **87,** 1128–1131 (1980).
14. Chang RJ. Normal and abnormal prolactin metabolism. Presented at Ovulation Update, Symposium I, San Diego, 1983. Sponsored by Scripps Clinic and Research Foundation.
15. McDonough PR, Byrd J, Phung TT, Mahesh VB. Phenotypic and cytogenetic findings in eighty-two patients with ovarian failure—changing trends. *Fertil Steril* **28,** 638–641 (1977).

16. Morris NM, Underwood LE, Easterling W. Temporal relationship between basal body temperature nadir and LH surge in normal women. *Fertil Steril* **28,** 780–783 (1976).
17. Strott CA, Cosgille CM, Ross GT, Lipsett MD. The short luteal phase. *J Clin Endocrinol Metab* **30,** 246–251 (1970).
18. Speroff L. Mechanism of ovulation. Presented at Ovulation Update (see ref. *14*).
19. Hackeloer BJ, Fleming R, Robinson HP, et al. Correlation of ultrasonic and endocrinologic assessment of human follicular development. *Am J Obstet Gynecol* **135,** 122–128 (1979).
20. O'Herlighy C, DeCrespigny LC, Lopata A, et al. Preovulatory follicular size: A comparison of ultrasound and laparoscopic measurements. *Fertil Steril* **34,** 24–26 (1980).
21. Cabau A, Bessie R. Monitoring of ovulation induction with human menopausal gonadotropin and human chorionic gonadotropin by ultrasound. *Fertil Steril* **36,** 178–182 (1981).
22. Hoult IJ, DeCrespigny LC, O'Herlighy C, et al. Ultrasound control of clomiphene/HCG stimulated cycles for oocyte recovery and in vitro fertilization. *Fertil Steril* **36,** 316–319 (1981).
23. Siegler AM. Dangers of hysterosalpingography. *Obstet Gynecol Survey* **22,** 284–307 (1967).
24. Shirley RL. Ovarian radiation dosage during hysterosalpingography. *Fertil Steril* **22,** 83–85 (1971).
25. Seppanen S, Lehtinen E, Holli H. Radiation dosage in hysterosalpingography: Modern 100 mm fluorography vs full-scale radiography. *Diag Radiol* **127,** 377–380 (1978).

Discussion—Session III

Q: Can one monitor therapy for hirsutism with dexamethasone?

DR. ODELL: This work, largely derived from Richard Horton and Wayne Meikle (e.g., Meikle et al., *J Clin Endocrinol Metab* **48:** 969, 1979, and Horton et al., *J Clin Invest* **69:** 1203, 1982), I think is the most important advance of the last 10 years in understanding hirsutism and androgen action. With their help, we have measured androstanediol glucuronide during treatment with low doses of dexamethasone given at night, as Dr. Lobo has described. Its concentration does change in parallel with the clinical response and with the fall in DHEA-S, for example. We've done this now in perhaps 10 patients.

DR. LOBO: It depends on what type of therapy you're using. With anti-androgen therapy such as spironolactone, the concentrations of 3α-androstanediol glucuronide (3α-diol G) may actually go up—as we will present this year [1984] at the American Fertility Society. These data were a surprise to us, but after thinking about it, we realized we're really looking at a disposal mechanism. Therefore, if you're blocking the androgen receptor, there may be a shunting of androgens towards formation of 3α-diol G. So in somebody undergoing anti-androgen therapy, 3α-diol G may not be the most valuable marker.

Q: Dr. Odell, has GnRH ever been used for therapy of male infertility?

DR. ODELL: Yes; in the patients who lack GnRH it is the physiologically sensible substance to treat with (see Skarin et al., *J Clin Endocrinol Metab* **55:** 723, 1982). Unfortunately, it must be given in a pulsatile fashion, which means the patient must wear a pump, something like an insulin pump, and the pulsations must be given many times daily over many weeks. This treatment is thus time consuming and expensive, but it is theoretically and practically sound and has been done for a few patients.

Q: Dr. Lobo, given our present knowledge, by what mechanism was wedge resection successful for inducing ovulation in the past?

DR. LOBO: We really don't understand why it has been effective, especially since we've tended to abandon it. Generally, after wedge resection, the concentrations of androgen do decrease, at least temporarily, and a lot of patients treated this way have ovulated. We've gone away from it primarily because it often produces pelvic adhesions. Although there's been some resurgence of doing wedge resections because of new microsurgical techniques, we find, at least in our hands, that our protocols for induction of ovulation do as well as the reported wedge resections ever have.

Q: What is a cost-effective practical laboratory approach for evaluation for hirsutism?

DR. LOBO: If the patient has a significant problem, some understanding of all three androgen compartments is necessary. It's probably not absolutely essential for the additional expense to measure free testosterone, but certainly one should measure testosterone for the ovary, DHEA-S for the adrenal, and, if you can, 3α-diol G for the peripheral compartment.

Q: Dr. Goldzieher, what about the use of the new anti-progestin that's recently been tested as a contraceptive?

DR. GOLDZIEHER: The new Roussel compound is probably the most exciting steroidal development in the last 10 to 15 years. This compound is a mild corticoid but also a very powerful anti-progestin. It therefore has great possibilities as a delayed-menses form of oral contraceptive or as a morning-after pill that withdraws the progestational support of an early implantation. If this turns out to be clinically feasible, it will fill one of the biggest gaps in the contraceptive armamentarium.

Q: Dr. Odell, what percentage of impotence in aging men is reversible, and treatable?

DR. ODELL: I'm not aware of any good data for that question. In fact, the occurrence of impotence in aging men is debatable in itself. A large number of publications that show a decrease in testosterone, and sometimes increases in FSH and LH, are from studies with institutionalized men. However, one study by Arman and Tsitouras (*J Clin Endocrinol Metab* **51:** 35, 1980) involved men who were not institutionalized but were still active, working, industrious, fully healthy, and taking no medication; these men showed no change in testosterone up to 70 or so years of age. To answer your question, we need additional studies with normal, active men rather than those in nursing homes and homes for the aged.

Q: Dr. Lobo, is spironolactone safe to use during a cycle in which pregnancy may occur? If not, how can increased testosterone in women be treated during the treatment of infertility secondary to this condition?

DR. LOBO: We generally don't use anti-androgen therapy with patients who are requesting induction of ovulation. In general, I would not recommend spironolactone for those patients; obviously, one should be concerned about giving it to a woman who is going to be pregnant. For a few patients, who are taking only spironolactone, we monitor their cyclicity very carefully, e.g., with basal body temperature charts; if their temperature stays up, we stop the treatment.

COMMENT:[1] We've treated a fairly large number of women with both acne and hirsutism with spironolactone and have been profoundly disappointed in the response. I was surprised when you said 70% were helped.

DR. LOBO: The effects are dose related. I think a lot of women receiving 50 or 100 mg of spironolactone have not been helped. The real benefit comes from about 200 mg. If you look at objective criteria, as Cummings and Yen did (Cummings et al., *J Am Med Assoc* **247**: 1295, 1982)—and there are many ways of doing this— there is real clinical improvement. In addition, in unpublished data, minute biopsies on patients undergoing treatment have actually quantified in vitro that 5α-reductase decreases with treatment and correlates extremely well with patients who have an objective response.

COMMENT: Our regimen has been first to depress the plasma concentration of testosterone as much as possible either with prednisone or with oral contraceptives or both. If there is no clinical response of the acne or the hirsutism after adequate trial of the

---

[1] Unidentified speaker.

195

usual suppressive measures, we then add spironolactone, 10 mg at bedtime, to try to exert an anti-androgenic action on the residual androgens. We have not been too disappointed in the response.

DR. LOBO: Patients who have an adrenal component of androgen excess will not be benefited as much from spironolactone. For some reason, spironolactone affects the adrenal in a different way. Serum DHEA-S is unchanged in patients receiving spironolactone. We are studying this further.

Q: Just as testosterone has been suggested to have an effect on ovarian function, is there evidence of estrogenic effects on testicular function?

DR. ODELL: Some data suggest that estrogens can modify the action of gonadotropins on the rat testes, but I know of no counterpart of that in humans. Although I didn't mention it, obesity and cirrhosis of the liver, for example, which lead to enhanced peripheral aromatization and enhanced estradiol production from testosterone, also lead to a form of hypogonadism with suppressed gonadatropins and sometimes low testosterone and low sperm counts.

COMMENT: There has been some suggestion that prolonged hCG administration would result in subsequent decrease in testosterone formation were this to be an estrogen-receptor mechanism.

Q: Does prolactin have a normal function in men or in nonpregnant women? Should bromocriptine treatment be adjusted to leave some prolactin present?

DR. ODELL: Although prolactin has been extensively investigated in both animal models and humans, to my knowledge there are no widely accepted effects of prolactin on testes function during either prepuberty or adulthood. Several groups have given prolactin to prepubertal female rats and shown precocious vaginal opening. These data suggest a synergism with gonadotropins in female rats prepubertally. Bartke et al. have published several studies suggesting prolactin acts synergistically with LH in male rats (e.g., Bartke et al., *Endocrinology* **101:** 1760, 1977). On the other hand, in studies from our laboratory (Odell and Larsen, in press), partially purified Leydig cells from rats or mice were exposed to a very wide range of prolactin in the presence of LH. Prolactin suppressed LH-stimulated testosterone over a large dose range, but very large doses augmented LH action. However, few data suggest that prolactin is required for testicular function. We've also evaluated very carefully its possible modulation of FSH stimulation of LH-receptor formation and found no effect. But growth hormone enhances the FSH stimulation of LH-receptor formation. In summary, prolactin to date has no well-accepted action in normal men and nonlactating women.

IV

STRATEGIES FOR INDUCING CONCEPTION

And than late her come & she shall conceyue with the grace of god. But she muste drynk that pouder with good wyn; and yf she desire to conceyue a male child, they muste take the marice of an hare & the cunt, and dryen it in the forsaid manere & poudren it & drink the pouder therof with wyne. And yf the woman desire a femel childe, lete her drye the stones of an hare & in the ende of her floures, make pouder thereof and drynk therof to bedde wardes & than go pley with her make. Another medecyn for a woman that may not conceyue: take the stones & the lyuer of a pigge that is deliuered of a sowe allone and make poudre therof, & gyue the woman to drynke with wyne whan she gothe to bedde to her make, & she shall conueyue [sic], witnesse Trotula.

And then let her come and she will conceive with God's grace. But she must drink that powder with good wine; and if she wishes to conceive a male child, the man and woman must take the womb of a hare and its pudendum, dry it in the way previously mentioned, powder it, and drink the powder of it with wine. And if the woman desires a female child, let her dry the testicles of a hare, and at the end of her menstrual period make a powder of it, drink it at bedtime, and then go to play with her mate. Another medicine for a woman unable to conceive: Take the testicles and liver of a pig that has given birth to a single sow, make powder of it, and give the woman it to drink in wine when she goes to her husband in bed, and she will conceive, as Trotula testifies.

—ROWLAND, pp 168–169

New Developments in Ovulation Induction

Gary D. Hodgen and Daniel Kenigsberg

Therapy with ovarian stimulation is notoriously difficult to manage, in part because of the marked individual variability in response to exogenous agents. Over the last 25 years, it has been assumed that the varied underlying pathophysiological conditions necessitating ovulation induction therapy were in great part responsible for the differential responses between patients. However, with the advent of in vitro fertilization, and the wide experience gained with ovarian stimulation in endocrinologically normal women, we now appreciate that there is much inherent variability of response to exogenous gonadotropins, even in these normal women (1–3). Furthermore, the fact that individual response types tend toward a consistent pattern from cycle to cycle (HW Jones and GS Jones, personal communication) suggests a constancy of physiological status, as opposed to a stochastic response.

With this background, we began seeking ways of reducing individual variability of responses to gonadotropin therapy, based on understanding the physiological origin(s) of that variability. Our *first objective* was to identify the source of individual variability in the hypothalamic–pituitary–ovarian axis. We reasoned that by eliminating endogenous pituitary output of gonadotropins, as well as ovarian feedback influencing hypothalamic–pituitary functions, ovarian response to exogenous gonadotropins could be more clearly distinguished. Moreover, if that response was statistically less varied from individual to individual, it would imply that some endogenous supra-ovarian component(s), e.g., the pituitary or hypothalamus, had contributed to the variability observed (Figure 1).

To experimentally eliminate hypothalamic–pituitary contributions, researchers have used three primate models extensively: stalk-sectioned monkeys (4, 5), surgically hypophysectomized animals (6, 7), and radio-frequency or electrically lesioned monkeys

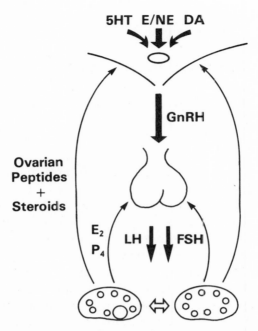

Fig. 1. Hypothalamic–pituitary ovarian axis
and feedback loops

with the medial basal hypothalamus disconnected *(7–9)*. Because
of the unacceptability of direct clinical extrapolations from these
models, we developed a new experimental primate model: the
reversible "medical hypophysectomy," achieved by administration of a gonadotropin-releasing hormone (GnRH) antagonist to
negate endogenous pituitary gonadotropin secretion (Figure 2).

After the elucidation of the structure of GnRH, functional correlates were studied via numerous synthetic analogs of it; some,
with high affinities for the GnRH receptor but no intrinsic biological activity *(10)*, are GnRH antagonists. Here, we used a potent
GnRH antagonist [(Ac-pClPhe^1,pClDPhe^2,DTrp^3,DArg^6,DAla^{10})
GnRH HCl] to diminish pituitary secretion of follitropin (follicle-
stimulating hormone, FSH) and lutropin (luteinizing hormone,
LH), thus producing a hypogonadotropic state approaching "medical hypophysectomy" with respect to the gonadotrope.

For our *second objective*, to assess the validity of our model for
"medical hypophysectomy," it was necessary to determine an ef-

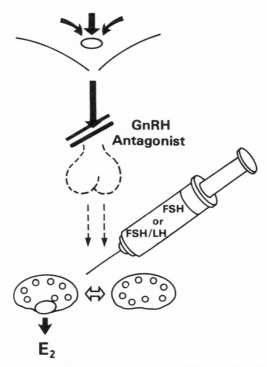

Fig. 2. "Medical hypophysectomy" by a GnRH antagonist

fective dose and regimen of the GnRH antagonist, that is, one able to suppress endogenous hypothalamic–pituitary output and reduce concentrations of circulating gonadotropin to or below the limits of detection in assays. Once a dose–response curve was established in castrates, intact monkeys were given the GnRH antagonist with exogenous gonadotropin. This brought us to the next issue.

A *third objective* was to study the differential actions of FSH treatment alone vs combined FSH/LH therapy in the ovary. Dogma insists that both gonadotropins are required to accommodate their synergistic actions for stimulation of follicular maturation. In brief, the two-cell theory *(11, 12)* of follicular steroidogenesis holds that theca cell production of androgen is a function of LH action and that granulosa cell aromatization of those androgens is a function of FSH action *(13, 14)*. In part because of these concepts, gonadotropin preparations typically used for ovulation induction contain both FSH and LH, often in near equal proportions. Although the efficacy of these preparations is beyond question, the optimal FSH:LH ratios and the relative importance of each component are unresolved.

Although studies on preparations containing different ratios of FSH and LH are not new (15, 16), the GnRH antagonist we used here provides a novel strategy for achieving greater control over ovarian stimulation, through elimination of physiologically important influences of the hypothalamus and pituitary. In addition, the availability of "pure" FSH preparations warranted reexamination of comparisons with more conventional preparations of human menopausal gonadotropin (hMG) having an equal ratio of FSH to LH.

More specifically, these objectives can be reduced to three principal questions:

1. How can individual variation of response to exogenous gonadotropins be reduced; and more fundamentally, what is the endogenous source of this variation?
2. What dose and regimen of GnRH antagonist are required to reduce endogenous secretion of gonadotropin until a state of "medical hypophysectomy" is approached?
3. Is there an optimal FSH:LH ratio that can be used for therapeutic ovarian stimulation; in other words, what is the relative importance of these two gonadotropins in the stimulation of ovarian follicular maturation?

Accordingly, we conducted the following experiments, assigning 50 cycling and eight castrate female cynomolgus monkeys (Macaca fasicularis) to the study. Animal husbandry and blood collection techniques have been previously described (17).

The GnRH antagonist [(Ac-pClPhe^1,pClDPhe^2,DTrp^3,DArg^6, DAla^{10})GnRH HCl] was a generous gift from the Contraceptive Development Branch, CPR, National Institute of Child Health and Human Development (CDB 2085).

Exogenous gonadotropins were either "pure" FSH (Metrodin or Urofollitropin; Serono Laboratories, Inc., Randolph, MA) or hMG (Pergonal; Serono). The "pure" FSH was in vials containing 25 int. units of FSH, with undetectable [<40 int. units/L (Second International Reference Preparation) or <10 ng/mL] LH, by an in vitro bioassay (18, 19), confirming earlier findings (20).

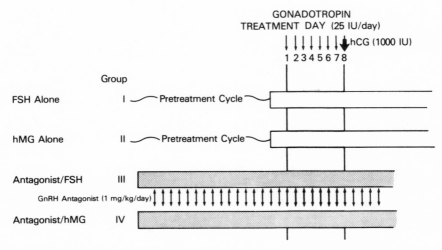

Fig. 3. Protocol for previously normal ovulatory monkeys, groups I–IV

All subjects entered study on cycle day 3. Groups I and II received no pretreatment with GnRH antagonist; therefore, gonadotropin treatment day 1 corresponds to cycle day 3. Groups III and IV received pretreatment and concurrent treatment with the GnRH antagonist beginning on cycle day 3. For an interval of 17 days (cycle days 3–18) pretreatment with GnRH antagonist was give alone. While continuing GnRH antagonist therapy, gonadotropin treatment day 1 corresponds to cycle day 19. In all groups, FSH or hMG (25 int. units per day) was given for seven consecutive days, followed by 1000 int. units of hCG on the eighth day. Thus, days are normalized and referred to as "gonadotropin treatment days 1–8" in all groups

Effects of Gonadotropin Therapy, with and without GnRH Antagonist

Fifty adult ovulatory female monkeys having regular menstrual cycles and no previous exposure to exogenous FSH or LH were assigned to one of four groups (Figure 3). Two variables were studied: (a) no pretreatment vs pretreatment with GnRH antagonist, followed by concurrent administration of the GnRH antagonist and gonadotropin(s) (groups I and II vs III and IV, respectively); and (b) exogenous gonadotropin treatment with "pure" FSH alone vs a combination of FSH plus LH (hMG) (groups I and III vs groups II and IV, respectively). Subjects not receiving the GnRH antagonist were given gonadotropin (FSH or hMG) beginning on cycle day 3. Alternatively, pretreatment with GnRH antagonist alone was begun on cycle day 3 and continued for 17 days before initiating gonadotropin treatment; then, the GnRH antagonist was given in combination with gonadotropin treat-

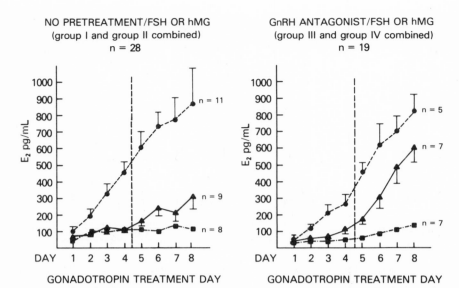

NO PRETREATMENT/FSH OR hMG
(group I and group II combined)
n = 28

GnRH ANTAGONIST/FSH OR hMG
(group III and group IV combined)
n = 19

GONADOTROPIN TREATMENT DAY GONADOTROPIN TREATMENT DAY

Fig. 4. Concentrations of serum estradiol (E_2; $x \pm$ SEM) in the composite of groups I and II vs groups III and IV, i.e., those that did not receive and those that did receive pretreatment and concurrent treatment with the GnRH antagonist, divided into fast (•), slow (▲), and nonresponders (■), on gonadotropin treatment days 1–8

Among responders, for area under the curve (AUC) computations for days 1–4 and days 5–8 (comparing fast and slow responders), analysis of variance and Kramer's modification of Duncan's multiple range test showed a significant difference ($p < 0.05$) between those not treated with GnRH antagonist; however, there was no significant ($p > 0.05$) difference between responses during treatment with the GnRH antagonist. Note n=the number of subjects for AUC analysis, whereas the number of subjects for computing daily mean E_2 values may be greater. CVs among responders for total AUC in groups I–IV were 63.1, 70.5, 43.1, and 28.3%, respectively. In groups I and II vs groups III and IV, the CVs for AUC computations were 69.0 and 47.9%, respectively

ment. All subjects were treated daily with 25 int. units of either FSH or hMG for seven consecutive days, and with 1000 int. units of human choriogonadotropin (hCG) on the eighth day. Hereafter, these days are referred to as *gonadotropin treatment days 1–8* for all groups (normalized, Figure 4). We collected daily 3.5 mL of femoral blood from all monkeys, using aliquots for radioimmunoassays for estradiol, progesterone, FSH, and LH, as described from this laboratory *(21)*. Also, in group III (GnRH antagonist with "pure" FSH), we daily assayed serum for biologically active LH *(18, 19)*.

From previous experiences with ovulation induction protocols in women and monkeys, we anticipated that some subjects would not respond to a set regimen of exogenous gonadotropin therapy, as indicated by serum concentrations of estradiol *(3, 21)*. Consistent with the primary intent of this study, namely, to discover causal factors of variability and the means for constraining differences in individual response patterns, we classified responses as follows: *Responders* had peripheral serum estradiol > 300 pg/mL on or before gonadotropin treatment day 8 (i.e., after seven days of receiving either FSH or hMG). This group was subdivided according to the rapidity of the estradiol increase in serum. *Fast responders* had estradiol > 300 pg/mL by gonadotropin treatment day 5, whereas *slow responders* manifested estradiol > 300 pg/mL later in the treatment regimen, but before or on gonadotropin treatment day 8. Conversely, among *nonresponders,* estradiol concentrations did not reach 300 pg/mL through gonadotropin treatment day 8; that is, based on patterns of estradiol in circulation, ovarian response did not exceed that of the natural cycle; indeed, sometimes it was much less.

The distribution of prospectively assigned and treated subjects by groups is shown in Table 1. We could not determine the area under the curve (AUC) for estradiol in serum for two subjects in groups III and one subject in group IV, because of three missing values; otherwise, the data sets were intact.

Evaluations of the subclasses of responders, i.e., fast responders vs slow responders, were based on AUC values for estradiol in serum. The gonadotropin treatment days 1–8 were divided into AUC days 1–4 and AUC days 5–8 (Figure 4).

The statistical significance of differences in AUC for the estra-

Table 1. **Distribution of Subjects by Response Pattern of Serum Estradiol Production**

Treatment group	Fast responder	Slow responder	Non-responder	Total
I FSH alone	4	2	7	13
II hMG alone	7	7	1	15
III Antagonist + FSH	2[a]	7[a]	4	13
IV Antagonist + hMG	4	2[a]	3	9
Total	17	18	15	50

[a] Denotes that one subject in each of these groups was unavailable for AUC analysis because of a missing estradiol value on gonadotropin treatment day 8. Not all groups are of equal size because subjects were prospectively assigned to groups and random attrition occurred.

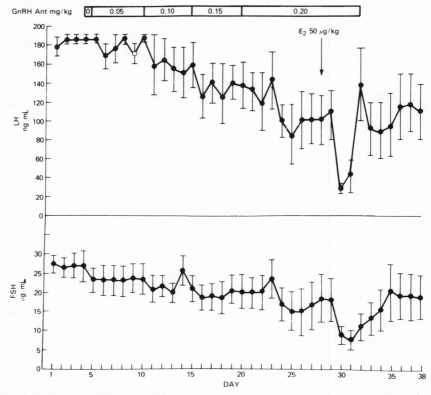

Fig. 5. Plasma LH and FSH values ($x \pm$ SEM) in five long-term castrate female monkeys treated with GnRH antagonist [(Ac-pClDPhe[1],pClDPhe[2],DTrp[3],DArg[6], DAla[10])GnRH HCl] in increasing doses

Estradiol challenge on day 27 provoked an LH surge

diol in serum was assessed by analysis of variance and Kramer's modification of Duncan's Multiple Range Test *(22, 23)*.

Dose determinations with GnRH antagonist. Long-term castrate female cynomolgus monkeys were given increasing doses of the GnRH antagonist in a prospective, two-part protocol. The lower-dose group (n=5) was given daily intramuscular injections of 0.05, 0.10, and 0.15 mg/kg of body weight for five days each, then 0.20 mg/kg for an additional 17 days. In all, therapy lasted 32 days with an estradiol benzoate challenge (50 μg/kg) on day 27 (Figure 5). The higher-dose group (n=3) was given 0.5, 1.0, and 1.5 mg/kg for five days each, then 2.0 mg/kg for an additional 17 days (Figure 6). This protocol allowed comparisons of doses

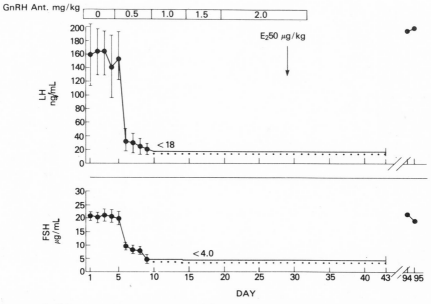

Fig. 6. GnRH antagonist suppresses FSH and LH concentrations in serum to below limits of assay detection

Long-term ovariectomized monkeys did not respond to an estrogen challenge test. Note full recovery of gonadotropin secretion by two months after cessation of treatment

of the GnRH antagonist over a 10-fold range, with the same duration and challenge test of pituitary response to estrogen positive feedback for LH/FSH release (Figure 6).

In the lower-dose group (Figure 5), there was a gradual decrease in mean LH concentrations in circulation and a smaller decrease in mean FSH values over the dose range of GnRH antagonist from 0.05 to 0.20 mg/kg. Notice that the estradiol benzoate challenge (day 27) prompted a biphasic LH response: suppression followed by an LH increase (Figure 5).

In the higher-dose group (Figure 6), after seven days of therapy, mean LH and FSH concentrations in peripheral serum were at or below the minimal detectable limits of the assays. Whereas LH was consistently suppressed to below the detection limits of the assay, FSH values hovered near the threshold for detection. This resulted from the 0.5 to 1.0 mg/kg dose of GnRH antagonist. All higher-dose subjects failed to show any LH or FSH response to the estradiol benzoate challenge on day 27. Reversibility was prompt, however; within two months after treatment, endogenous gonadotropin concentrations were restored to pretreatment, castrate values.

Accordingly, to begin studies in intact females, we selected 1.0 mg/kg per day, intramuscularly, as an effective regimen for achieving a hypogonadotropic state that approached a "medical hypophysectomy."

Table 1 lists the four groups by their estradiol response pattern. All groups contained both responders and nonresponders, as defined above. Because the pre-eminent issue of these studies concerned the variability of the estradiol increase among subjects responsive to gonadotropin therapy, we did not include the nonresponders for AUC analysis. Figure 4 illustrates the estradiol curves for groups I and II (without GnRH antagonist pretreatment) and for groups III and IV (with GnRH antagonist pretreatment), distinguished by response patterns (fast vs slow vs nonresponders).

AUC analysis for gonadotropin treatment days 1–4 and days 5–8 of the fast responders and slow responders showed that there was a significant difference ($p < 0.05$) between them during both intervals, when there was no pretreatment with the GnRH antagonist (groups I and II combined). However, when there was pretreatment with GnRH antagonist followed by treatment with either gonadotropin preparation (groups III and IV combined), the difference between fast and slow responders was absent ($p > 0.05$) (Table 2). There was no difference ($p > 0.05$) in the incidence

---

Table 2. **Comparison of Area-under-Curve Values for Estradiol among Responder Monkeys**

| Treatment group | Response pattern, n | Estradiol, pg/mL, on gonadotropin treatment days | |
		1–4	5–8
No GnRH antagonist	Fast 11	1323.2	2230.2
(Groups I and II)	Slow 9	451.3[a]	723.7[a]
GnRH antagonist	Fast 5	938.2	2075.0
(Groups III and IV)	Slow 7	310.0	1218.9

Notice the significant difference between fast and slow responders in the non-GnRH antagonist groups vs the lack of significant difference between fast and slow responders in the GnRH antagonist-treated groups.

[a] Significant difference by Kramer's modification of Duncan's multiple range test, $p < 0.05$.

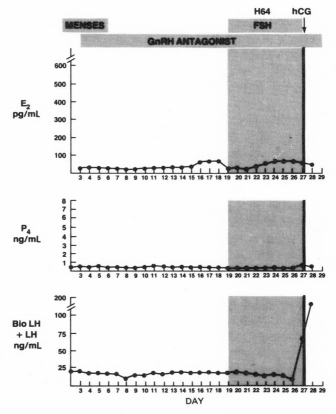

Fig. 7. Representative estradiol (E₂), progesterone (P₄), and LH values (RIA) of a nonresponder from group III

Note lack of prominent E₂ rise, despite treatment with "pure" FSH beginning on day 19. Days 19–27 correspond to gonadotropin treatment days 1–8

of nonresponders either with or without GnRH antagonist pretreatment (Table 1). A representative individual nonresponder hormone profile is shown in Figure 7.

GnRH antagonist induces a hypogonadotropic state. In 21 of 22 previously normal ovulatory females treated with the GnRH antagonist, 1.0 mg/kg (groups III and IV), ovulation was blocked throughout the pretreatment interval of 17 days before administration of exogenous gonadotropin. The responses of the one subject that "broke through" this therapy are depicted in Figure 8. Notice that superimposing exogenous gonadotropin on this pre-

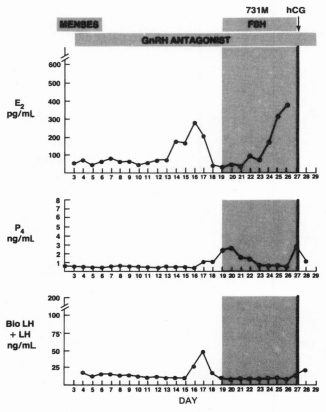

Fig. 8. Estradiol, progesterone, and LH values (RIA) in a subject (group III) pretreated with GnRH antagonist from cycle day 3

Note estradiol increase beginning on day 14, LH increase on day 16, and subsequent progesterone increase on day 17. This is the only monkey (out of 22) in which ovulation was not blocked during the pretreatment interval with the GnRH antagonist. Gonadotropin treatment days and abbreviations as in Fig. 7

sistent ovarian cycle produced an additional ovarian response.

Baseline concentrations of estradiol (gonadotropin treatment day 1) were analyzed by group before the onset of treatment vs that during GnRH antagonist therapy (Figure 9). Clearly, administration of the GnRH antagonist resulted in significant ($p < 0.01$) diminution of serum concentrations of estradiol.

Basal concentrations of serum LH were not perceptibly different

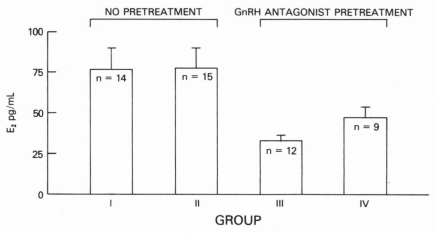

BASELINE (Gonadotropin Treatment Day 1) ESTRADIOL LEVEL

Fig. 9. Baseline concentrations of plasma estradiol ($x \pm$ SEM) on gonadotropin treatment day 1, prior to administration of gonadotropin, in groups I–IV

Comparing non-GnRH antagonist pretreated subjects (groups I and II) with GnRH antagonist-pretreated subjects (groups III and IV) showed a significantly lower mean concentration of plasma estradiol after initiation of GnRH antagonist therapy (Student's t-test, $p < 0.01$); that is, a hypogonadotropic state was created by the analog

between pretreated and nonpretreated groups, in part because many values were near or below assay limits of detection.

Early progesterone increase. We observed that two out of 13 subjects in group III (treated with GnRH antagonist in combination with "pure" FSH) manifested definite increases of progesterone in serum, beginning on gonadotropin treatment day 5 and 7, respectively, and continuing through and beyond gonadotropin treatment day 8, when hCG subsequently was given. That is, there were two to four days of unambiguous increases in progesterone prior to injection of hCG. Moreover, this early progesterone rise occurred in the absence of any increase in endogenous LH, as measured by either bioassay or radioimmunoassay. To illustrate this point, the profiles for one representative individual are shown in Figure 10.

The relative (un)importance of LH vs FSH. Despite ongoing treatment with the GnRH antagonist, nine of 13 monkeys given "pure" FSH (group III) achieved sufficient increases of estradiol in serum

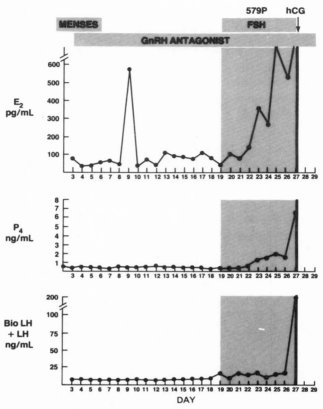

Fig. 10. Representative concentrations of estradiol, progesterone, and LH (by RIA) in a subject from group III in which progesterone serum began to increase on day 23, in the apparent absence of an increase of endogenous LH and without administration of exogenous LH or hCG

The "LH" increase on day 27 is a measurement of exogenous hCG from the previous day. Days 19–27 correspond to gonadotropin treatment days 1–8

to qualify as responders. In other words, in the presence of this induced hypogonadotropic state, as evidenced by sub-tonic serum concentrations of estradiol ($p < 0.01$) and blockade of ovulation in 12 out of 13 subjects, FSH treatment "alone" was capable of stimulating ovarian responses (rising estradiol concentrations) indistinguishable from those during hMG therapy, where exogenous LH was injected. Profiles from a representative individual from group III are shown in Figure 11.

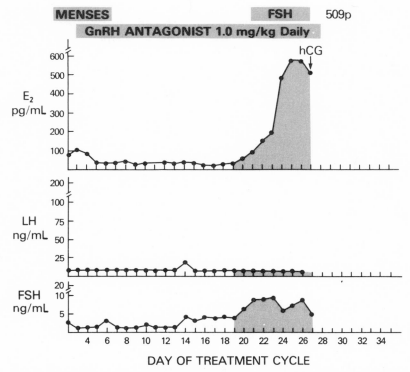

GnRH ANTAGONIST 1.0 mg/kg Daily

hCG

E_2 pg/mL

LH ng/mL

FSH ng/mL

DAY OF TREATMENT CYCLE

Fig. 11. Representative serum estradiol (E_2), LH, and FSH values in a typical group III subject

Plasma E_2 exceeded 300 pg/mL, qualifying this subject as a responder; but because the 300 pg/mL was not reached on or before gonadotropin treatment day 5, this monkey was classified as a slow responder. *Shaded area* corresponds to gonadotropin treatment days 1–8

Additional experiments. These findings were so surprising and anti-dogma (FSH induced prompt ovarian responses in the face of markedly diminished or undetectable concentrations of LH) that we performed additional experiments. In the first, monkeys in group III were mated for 24–48 h after hCG injection; their fallopian tubes were then flushed 72 h later *(24)*. At laparotomy, nine of the 13 subjects had ovulated, as evidenced by the presence of corpora lutea. Importantly, four of these nine had embryos, some of which already contained five cells (Figure 12).

In the final experiment, we attempted ovarian stimulation, as judged by estradiol production and follicular development, in two juvenile female monkeys, ages 16 to 20 months. Small unstimu-

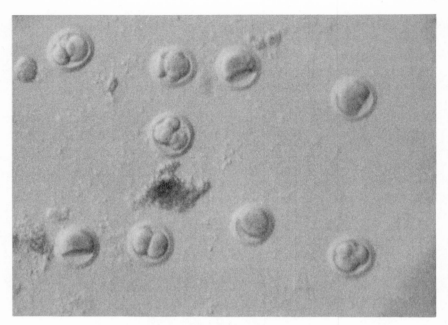

Fig. 12. Nine embryos recovered by tubal flush 48 h after mating and 72 h after hCG injection in a group III monkey

Out of 13 group III monkeys, nine had ovulation sites at subsequent laparotomy; embryos were recovered from four of these females. Some embryos contained as many as five cells

lated ovaries were confirmed at the pretreatment laparoscopy; they had not reached menarche, which would be expected near 30 months of age. They therefore provided a different hypogonadotropic model on which to test FSH. These monkeys, physiologically equivalent to normal girls five to eight years old, were administered "pure" FSH (25 int. units per day). Figure 13 shows the patterns of promptly rising estradiol in serum. When follicular development was confirmed, by laparoscopy or laparotomy (Figure 14), 1000 int. units of hCG was administered. The subsequent increases in progesterone in circulation, as well as menses 12 and 13 days after hCG, are indicative of apparent ovulation.

Discussion

Clinical experience over the last 25 years has shown that it is often easier to manage gonadotropin therapy in severely hypogo-

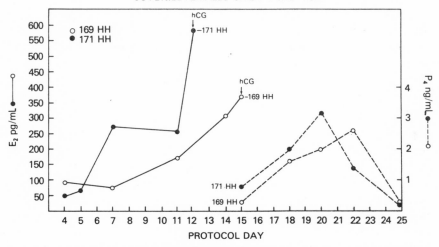

JUVENILE FEMALES GIVEN "PURE" FSH

Fig. 13. Two juvenile (prepubertal) females, 16 to 20 months of age, had unstimulated ovaries at pretreatment laparoscopy

"Pure" FSH (25 int. units per day) was started on protocol day 1 and continued until the day of hCG (1000 int. units) injection. Monkeys were monitored by serial laparoscopies and determinations of serum estradiol (E_2) concentrations. When E_2 exceeded 300 pg/mL and ovarian follicular stimulation was confirmed visually, hCG was administered. The solid lines (*left*) reflect E_2 values and the dashed lines (*right*) represent progesterone (P_4) concentrations in serum. Menses occurred 13 days (171HH) and 12 days (169HH) after hCG injection

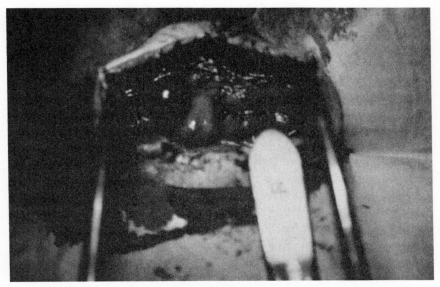

Fig. 14. The stimulated ovaries of 171HH, shown at laparotomy on day 18

217

nadotropic patients than in those presenting with anovulation of other etiologies *(25–28)*. This realization has prompted other attempts at inducing a transient hypogonadotropic state in individuals undergoing induction of ovulation, with the goal of achieving more uniform responses and fewer therapeutic complications for greater ultimate efficacy. Jones et al. *(29)* attempted pretreatment with synthetic steroids to suppress the pituitary over a two-month interval prior to gonadotropin therapy. Fleming et al. *(30)* pretreated patients with a GnRH agonist before administering exogenous gonadotropin. Why have such strategies not been adopted more widely?

The above approaches have notable disadvantages: First, progestins are thought to inhibit folliculogenesis in the primate ovary directly *(31)*; also, exogenous progestins modify the milieu of the uterine endometrium, cervix, and fallopian tubes prematurely, during the proliferative phase. Second, GnRH *agonists* actually enhance gonadotropin and estradiol secretion for the initial 10 to 14 days of treatment, before a state of pituitary suppression is attained *(32, 33)*, whereas in contrast, the GnRH *antagonist* used in the present study only diminishes concentrations of FSH and LH, without concurrent increases in secretion of ovarian steroids. Although GnRH or its analogs may influence the ovaries directly in rodents *(34)*, persuasive evidence obtained in women and monkeys argues against a direct action of these synthetic decapeptides in the primate ovary *(35, 36)*.

Accordingly, we set out to determine whether a GnRH antagonist would reduce individual variation in response to gonadotropin therapy, through diminished functions of the hypothalamus and pituitary.

Gonadotropin Therapy with and without GnRH Antagonist

Pretreatment with the GnRH antagonist increased the homogeneity of ovarian secretion of estradiol during therapy with exogenous gonadotropin, among responsive females, as compared with the responses of non-GnRH antagonist-treated, gonadotropin-responsive subjects. This constraint on individuality of both fast responders and slow responders by the GnRH antagonist suggests that an important part of the source of individual variation in response to gonadotropin therapy is supra-ovarian; that is, hypothalamic-pituitary functions contribute substantially to the variability of ovarian response during gonadotropin treatment.

Further, as Table 1 showed, there was a near even distribution of nonresponder monkeys, irrespective of whether the GnRH antagonist was given. Thus, the source of relative resistance among nonresponders may derive from the ovaries themselves, as opposed to factors contributed by supra-ovarian components that might be influenced by the GnRH antagonist. Whether this relative refractoriness to exogenous stimulation in some females is at the receptor or humoral level remains to be determined.

Unlike the clinical situation, the fixed protocols used here allowed for the nonresponders not to receive more exogenous gonadotropin than others in the study. Conversely, fast responders did not receive less gonadotropin, so that we could compare like-treated individuals in all groups. Probably even greater conformity of subject response could be obtained with daily adjustments of gonadotropin doses. Here, for experimental purposes of precisely evaluating response as an endpoint, the use of a fixed gonadotropin protocol eliminated the confounding effect of having multiple regimens of treatment.

GnRH Antagonist Induction of a Hypogonadotropic State

Hypogonadotropic hypogonadism (Kallmann's syndrome) is a spectrum or degree of disorders presenting with low to undetectable quantities of FSH and LH (37). Often, it is not associated with an agonadotropic state; indeed, such conditions may be analogous to those developed here—a milieu approaching "medical hypophysectomy." That is, the GnRH antagonist was efficacious in blocking the natural ovarian cycle and markedly reducing estradiol in circulation, but did not remove all measurable gonadotropins from the serum of some monkeys. Indeed, one female ovulated in spite of GnRH antagonist treatment. However, all 21 of the remaining monkeys manifested unmistakable evidence of a hypogonadotropic state during GnRH antagonist treatment. This response can be regarded as an internal bioassay, where diminished ovarian secretion of estradiol accompanied suppression of endogenous gonadotropins. The strikingly lower concentrations of estradiol in GnRH antagonist-pretreated animals is further evidence that the regimen did create a hypogonadotropic state, although a total hypophysectomy-like condition, in terms of FSH and LH secretion, was not attained uniformly. Moreover, although we assume that other pituitary glycoprotein hormones were unaffected, these studies remain to be completed.

Whether the rapid and severe diminution of concentrations of endogenous FSH and LH (undetectable) in castrate monkeys (Figure 6) is indicative of a greater sensitivity of castrate females than of intact monkeys, or whether it reflects a response from a higher initial gonadotropin baseline, remains to be elucidated. Clearly, higher doses of the GnRH antagonist would be required to fully suppress pituitary gonadotropin secretion in the primate menstrual cycle.

Early Progesterone Increase

Recent studies (38) have described an increase of plasma progesterone up to 12 h before the start of the LH surge in the normal human menstrual cycle. That this progesterone increase occurs in the absence of perceptible changes in the pulse amplitude or frequency of endogenous LH may implicate an independent intra-ovarian mechanism that begins to shift ovarian steroidogenesis and (or) secretion toward progesterone, even before initiation of the LH surge. Here, we found two monkeys treated with "pure" FSH in the presence of the GnRH antagonist that had undetectable LH in plasma, yet increases in serum progesterone developed as much as four days before treatment with hCG. These observations may fit with a growing body of evidence that steroidogenic shifts to progesterone can be initiated by intra-ovarian events, therein usurping onset of the LH surge. One should appreciate also that this early increase in progesterone occurred without injection of LH.

In the testis, negative feedback of estradiol on 17,20-demolase causes accumulation of precursor steroids, including progesterone (39, 40), although this mechanism has not been fully demonstrated in ovarian tissue of primates. Alternatively, although theca cells of rodents reportedly possess few if any receptors for FSH (41), it has not been definitively shown whether ovarian theca cells in primates have LH receptors that can respond to FSH.

Lastly, none of the above explanations may hold; that is, despite the suppressive influence of the GnRH antagonist on pituitary gonadotropin secretion, even minute quantities of residual endogenous LH or miniscule LH contamination of the "pure" FSH preparation may be present and sufficient, even if below assay detection limits.

The Relative (Un)Importance of LH vs FSH

The two-cell theory of ovarian steroidogenesis has been described at length in several rodent models (11) and to a lesser degree in various higher mammals (12). In brief, it holds that steroidogenic precursors leading to androgens are synthesized in theca cells, which are subject to stimulation by LH; then, precursor androgens are aromatized to estrogens, predominantly estradiol, by granulosa cells under the influence of FSH (13, 14, 42, 43).

Studies in women, involving pituitary FSH preparations for ovulation induction (15, 44, 45), indicated lower estradiol responses when FSH was administered alone than when preparations containing both FSH and LH were given. This could be interpreted as supporting evidence of the two-cell theory, i.e., that LH was deficient; alternatively, the results may have been influenced by the shorter circulatory half-life of pituitary FSH, compared with the longer-acting FSH extracted from postmenopausal urine (46).

Here, we have shown that "pure" FSH of urinary origin is capable of stimulating ovarian secretion of estradiol at a concentration not dissimilar from that obtained with the same dose of a preparation of urinary hMG, containing an equal ratio of FSH to LH. Furthermore, we have demonstrated undiminished ovarian production of estradiol when "pure" FSH was administered in the presence of a GnRH antagonist that maintained a relative hypogonadotropic state (in terms of endogenous gonadotropin secretion).

Results of Additional Experiments

The two additional experiments support an interpretation that "pure" FSH of urinary origin can promptly stimulate ovarian follicular maturation and familiar estradiol production patterns in monkeys, even when concentrations of endogenous LH are vanishingly small during both treatment with GnRH antagonist and juvenile life. Importantly, ovulation of fertilizable oocytes, embryo cleavage, and pregnancy resulted from a combination of GnRH antagonist plus "pure" FSH therapy.

The data presented raise far-reaching questions about the relative importance of FSH vs LH in the primate ovarian cycle. Although these findings do not warrant the discarding of dogma that insists upon the essential nature of an FSH/LH synergism in the promotion of follicular maturation, the data surely bring into question long-held views on the relative importance of LH. Clearly, FSH is the pre-eminent hormone driving folliculogenesis in the primate ovarian cycle. As the above experiments indicate, substantial estrogen biosynthesis and secretion and advanced follicular development are possible with scarcely any LH present.

Conclusion

In summary, we conclude that individual variation in ovarian response to gonadotropin therapy in monkeys is, in large part, supra-ovarian in origin, although failure to respond to gonadotropins was not negated by GnRH antagonist treatment. Furthermore, a milieu approaching "medical hypophysectomy," produced by using a potent GnRH antagonist, deserves consideration as a clinically applicable strategy to reduce variability among responders, thereby improving patient management. Secondly, in our monkey model, the GnRH antagonist promptly produced a relatively hypogonadotropic state that was reversible; these findings have implications for both fertility and anti-fertility research. Finally, the two-cell theory, requiring coordinate action of both FSH and LH to achieve ovarian steroidogenesis culminating in dynamic estrogen production, may need to be re-examined. Indeed, the importance credited to the ratios of these gonadotropins is surely open to question. Although the data presented do not justify denial of an essential role of LH in ovarian follicular maturation, with concurrent estrogen biosynthesis and secretion, FSH is surely of far greater relative significance in the primate ovarian cycle.

Presented in part at the Associate Members Forum, Fortieth Annual Meeting of the American Fertility Society, New Orleans, April 4–7, 1984, and the Thirty-First Annual Meeting of the Society for Gynecologic Investigation, San Francisco, March 21–24, 1984, and the IVF/Andrology International Symposium, Kiawah Island, Charleston, SC, September 13–16, 1984. Supported in part by Ford Foundation Grant no.810–0293. Dr. Kenigsberg is recipient of the National Fellowship in Reproductive Medicine.

References

1. Kenigsberg D, Littman BA, Hodgen GD. Medical hypophysectomy I: Dose-response using a GnRH antagonist. *Fertil Steril* (in press), 1984.
2. Kenigsberg D, Littman BA, Williams RF, Hodgen GD. Medical hypophysectomy II: Variability of ovarian response to gonadotropin therapy. *Fertil Steril* (in press), 1984.
3. Garcia JE, Jones GS, Acosta AA, Wright A. Human menopausal gonadotropin/human chorionic gonadotropin follicular maturation for oocyte aspiration: Phase II, 1981. *Fertil Steril* **39**, 157 (1983).
4. Vaughan L, Carmel PW, Dyrenfurth I, et al. Section of the pituitary stalk in the rhesus monkey. I. Endocrine studies. *Neuroendocrinology* **30**, 75 (1980).
5. Ferin M, Wehrenberg WB, Lam NY, et al. Effect and site of action of morphine on gonadotropin secretion in the female rhesus monkey. *Endocrinology* **111**, 1652 (1982).
6. Knovil E, Greep RO. The physiology of growth hormone and particular reference to its action in the rhesus monkey and the "species specificity" problem. *Recent Prog Horm Res* **15**, 1 (1959).
7. Tullner WW, Gulyas BJ, Hodgen GD. Maternal estrogen and progesterone levels after hypophypsectomy in early pregnancy and in term fetuses or newborn monkeys. *Steroids* **26**, 625 (1975).
8. Norman RL, Resko JA, Spies HG. The anterior hypothalamus: How it affects gonadotropin secretion in the rhesus monkey. *Endocrinology* **99**, 59 (1976).
9. Nakai Y, Plant TM, Hess DL, et al. On the sites of negative and positive feedback actions of estradiol in the control of gonadotropin secretion in the rhesus monkey. *Endocrinology* **102**, 1008 (1978).
10. Schally AV, Arimura A, Coy DH. Recent approaches to fertility control based on derivatives of LH-RH. *Vitam Horm (NY)* **38**, 257–323 (1980).
11. Falck B. Site of production of oestrogen in rat ovary as studied in micro-transplants. *Acta Physiol Scand* **47**, Suppl 163 (1959).
12. Short RV. Steroids in the follicular fluid and the corpus luteum of the mare. A "two-cell type" theory of ovarian steroid synthesis. *J Endocrinol* **24**, 59 (1962).
13. Ryan KJ, Petro Z, Kaiser J. Steroid formation by isolated and recombined ovarian granulosa and theca cells. *J Clin Endocrinol Metab* **28**, 355 (1968).
14. Moon VS, Tsang BK, Simpson C, Armstrong DT. 17β-Estradiol biosynthesis in cultured granulosa and theca cells of human ovarian

follicles: Stimulation by follicle-stimulating hormone. *J Clin Endocrinol Metab* **47,** 263 (1978).

15. Jacobson A, Marshall JR. Ovulatory response rate with human menopausal gonadotropins of varying FSH-LH ratios. *Fertil Steril* **20,** 171 (1969).

16. Kreitman O, Lynch A, Nixon WE, Hodgen GD. Ovum collection, induced luteal dysfunction, in vitro fertilization, embryo development and low tubal ovum transfer in primates. In *In Vitro Fertilization and Embryo Transfer,* ESE Hafez, K Semm, Eds., Alan R. Liss Inc., New York, NY, 1982, pp 303–324.

17. Williams RF, Johnson DK, Hodgen GD. Resumption of estrogen-induced gonadotropin surges in postpartum monkeys. *J Clin Endocrinol Metab* **49,** 422 (1979).

18. Van Damme MP, Robertson DM, Diczfalusy E. An improved in vitro bioassay method for measuring luteinizing hormone (LH) activity using mouse Leydig cell preparations. *Acta Endocrinol* **77,** 672 (1974).

19. Marut EL, Williams RF, Cowan BD, et al. Pulsatile pituitary gonadotropin secretion during maturation of the dominant follicle in monkeys: Estrogen positive feedback enhances the biological activity of LH. *Endocrinology* **109,** 2270 (1981).

20. Goodman AL, Descalzi CD, Johnson DK, Hodgen GD. Composite pattern of circulating LH, FSH, estradiol, and progesterone during the menstrual cycle in cynomolgus monkeys (398 34). *Proc Soc Exp Biol Med* **155,** 479 (1977).

21. Hodgen GD, Werlin LB, Kenigsberg D, et al. Reversible pharmacologic castration of the female: Implications for endometriosis, contraception and ovulation induction. In *LHRH and Its Analogs—Fertility and Antifertility Aspects.* International Workshop, Berliner Gesprache, Berlin, F.R.G., October 10–12, 1983.

22. Kirk RE. *Experimental Design: Procedures for Behavioral Sciences,* Brooks/Cole, Belomont, 1968, pp 69–99.

23. Kramer CY. Extension of multiple range test to group means with unequal numbers of replications. *Biometrics* **12,** 307 (1956).

24. Hodgen GD. Surrogate embryo transfer combined with estrogen–progesterone therapy in monkeys. *J Am Med Assoc,* 2167 (1983).

25. Gemzell CA, Diczfalusy E, Tillinger G. Clinical effects of human pituitary follicle-stimulating hormone (FSH). *J Clin Endocrinol Metab* **18,** 133 (1958).

26. Vande Wiele RL, Bogumil J, Dyrenfurth I, et al. Mechanisms regulating the menstrual cycle in women. *Recent Prog Horm Res* **26,** 63 (1970).

27. Ben-Rafael Z, Dor J, Mashiach S, et al. Abortion rate in pregnancies

following ovulation induced by human menopausal gonadotropin/ human chorionic gonadotropin. *Fertil Steril* **39**, 157 (1983).

28. Wentz AC. *Obstet and Gynecol Survey* **38**, 489–490 (1983).
29. Jones GS, Ruehsen MDM, Johanson AJ, et al. Elucidation of normal ovarian physiology by exogenous gonadotropin stimulation following steroid pituitary suppression. *Fertil Steril* **20**, 14 (1969).
30. Fleming R, Adam AH, Barlow DH, et al. A new systematic treatment for infertile women with abnormal hormone profiles. *Br J Obstet Gynecol* **89**, 80 (1982).
31. diZerega GS, Hodgen GD. Folliculogenesis in the primate ovarian cycle. *Endocr Rev* **2**, 27 (1981).
32. Schmidt-Gollwitzer M, Hardt W, Schmidt-Gollwitzer K, et al. Influence of the LH-RH analog buserelin on cyclic ovarian function and on the endometrium. A new approach to fertility control? *Contraception* **23**, 187 (1981).
33. Werlin LB, Hodgen GD. Gonadotropin-releasing hormone agonist suppresses ovulation, menses, and endometriosis in monkeys: An individualized, intermittent regimen. *J Clin Endocrinol Metab* **56**, 844 (1983).
34. Hseuh AJW, Jones PBC. Extrapituitary actions of gonadotropin-releasing hormone. *Endocr Rev* **2**, 437 (1981).
35. Asch RH, Sickle MV, Rettori V, et al. Absence of LH-RH binding sites in corpora lutea from rhesus monkeys (*Macaca mulatta*). *J Clin Endocrinol Metab* **53**, 215 (1981).
36. Clayton RN, Huhtaniemi IT. Absence of gonadotropin-releasing hormone receptors in human gonadal tissue. *Nature* **299**, 56 (1982).
37. Lieblich JM, Rogol AD, White BJ, Rosen SW. Syndrome of anosmia with hypogonadotrophic hypogonadism (Kallmann syndrome): Clinical and laboratory studies in 23 cases. *Am J Med* **73**, 506 (1982).
38. Hiff JD, Quigley ME, Yen SSC. Hormonal dynamics at midcycle: A reevaluation. *J Clin Endocrinol Metab* **57**, 792 (1983).
39. Kalla N, Nisula B, Menard R, Loriaux DL. The effects of estradiol on testicular testosterone biosynthesis. *Endocrinology* **106**, 35 (1980).
40. Nozu K, Dufau ML, Catt KJ. Estradiol receptor-mediated regulation of steroidogenesis in gonadotropin-desensitized Leydig cells. *J Biol Chem* **256**, 1915 (1981).
41. Richards JS. Maturation of ovarian follicles: Actions and interactions of pituitary and ovarian hormones on follicular cell differentiation. *Physiol Rev* **60**, 51 (1980).
42. Fevold HL. Synergism of the follicular stimulating and luteinizing hormones in producing estrogen secretion. *Endocrinology* **28**, 33 (1941).
43. Chow BF, van Dyke HB, Greep RO, et al. Gonadotropins of the

swine pituitary II. Preparation and biological and physicochemical characterization of a protein apparently identical with metakentrin (ICSH). *Endocrinology* **30,** 650 (1942).

44. Jewelewicz R, Warren M, Dyrenfurth I, Vande Wiele RL. Physiological studies with purified human pituitary-FSH. *J Clin Endocrinol Metab* **32,** 688 (1971).

45. Berger MJ, Taymor ML, Karam K, Nudemberg F. The relative roles of exogenous and endogenous FSH and LH in human follicular maturation and ovulation induction. *Fertil Steril* **23,** 783 (1972).

46. Mancus S, Dell'Acqua S, Donini P, et al. Disappearance rate, urinary excretion and effect on ovarian steroidogenesis of highly purified urinary FSH, administered to a hypophysectomized woman. In *Clinical Application of Human Gonadotropins,* G Bettendorf, V Insler, Eds., Georg Thieme Verlag, Stuttgart, 1970, pp 151–159.

Effects of Ovarian Stimulation on in Vitro Fertilization in Humans

Richard P. Marrs and Joyce M. Vargyas

The first trials of extracorporeal fertilization with humans involved the use of stimulated ovarian cycles to increase the number of oocytes that were collected at the time of laparoscopy *(1)*. After clinical trials with human menopausal gonadotropins and clomiphene citrate failed to produce pregnancy, cycle stimulation was dropped. Thereafter, investigators focused on monitoring the spontaneous ovulatory cycle, trying to collect a single mature oocyte at the time of ovulation for subsequent fertilization in vitro followed by transfer of a single embryo into the uterine cavity. This technique of monitoring oocyte collection resulted in the first human live birth in 1978 *(2)*. Thereafter, the use of the spontaneous, unstimulated ovulatory cycle predominated for the procedure of in vitro fertilization and embryo replacement (IVF-ER)*(3)*. However, in 1981, Trounson et al. *(4)*, reported an increased rate of successful pregnancy with the use of clomiphene-stimulated cycles for multiple oocyte recovery and embryo transfer. Thereafter, centers involved with IVF returned to the use of ovarian stimulation before oocyte retrieval, attempting various regimens of ovarian stimulation with different degrees of success *(5–7)*. Here we will compare the regimens of ovarian stimulation that have been used at our center for performing IVF-ER.

Monitoring of Ovarian Response

Whatever the regimen of ovarian stimulation, a precise method of monitoring response to ovarian stimulus is necessary to obtain oocytes at the appropriate maturational state. Combinations of ultrasound scanning and measurements of estradiol and luteinizing hormone (LH, lutropin) in serum or urine have been utilized in various programs to determine accurately the time for oocyte collection. In our program we use a combination of real-time ovarian scanning and measurements of estradiol and LH in serum *(8)*. In each stimulation regimen, we scan the ovary daily with ultrasound, beginning the sixth day of treatment, and concurrently measure estradiol. Ultrasound is used to monitor the early response to the stimulation regimen, the number of follicles visible on day six of the medication cycle being correlated with the concentrations of estradiol. Moreover, we monitor follicle growth until it reaches the appropriate size, at which time we discontinue the stimulatory agent. Knowledge of the serum concentrations of estradiol are useful in the early part of the cycle to ensure that the cystic spaces seen with ultrasound are functional follicles, as evidenced by their production of estradiol. Moreover, after the stimulatory agent is discontinued, the levelling off of estradiol concentrations is the marker for administering choriogonadotropin (hCG). Serum that is obtained for estradiol measurement is also stored until pre-ovulatory status is determined and a final serum sample is obtained before the injection of 4000 int. units of hCG. LH is measured in all collected samples, to determine the baseline value for LH secretion. If the serum concentration of LH increases significantly before administration of hCG, laparoscopy to harvest oocytes can then be performed 24 to 28 h after the initiation of the LH increase.

Stimulation Methods

In the past two years we have studied various regimens of ovarian stimulation. Initially, we used clomiphene citrate, 150 mg daily for five days, as the primary method for ovarian stimulation. Because studies with primates had indicated that selection of the dominant follicle occurred early in the cycle *(9, 10)*, we tried administering clomiphene citrate at various times (beginning on day 3, 4, 5, or 7 of the menstrual cycle) to determine whether development of multiple follicles would be more successful if the ovaries were stimulated early in the cycle *(11)*. In this group of patients the numbers of follicles generated, oocytes collected and fertilized, and embryos transferred per cycle were optimal when we started clomiphene on day 5 (Figures 1 and 2). This result was somewhat divergent from what we expected from stud-

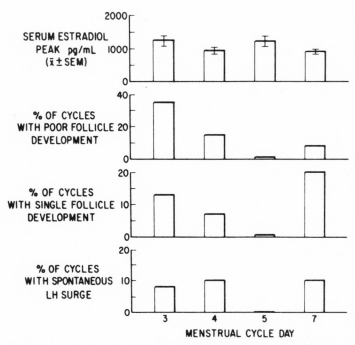

Fig. 1. Comparison of serum estradiol at time of hCG administration *(top panel)*, cycles with poor development *(second panel)*, cycles with single dominant follicle *(third panel)*, and cycles with LH surge *(bottom panel)* after clomiphene citrate, 150 mg for five days

Bars represent mean ± SEM

ies with the primate model; however, when we examined more closely the group receiving clomiphene beginning on day 3, ultra-sound demonstrated multiple follicle development early in the treatment cycle, although most of these follicles did not continue to develop.

We then performed a second study, utilizing combinations of clomiphene citrate and human menopausal gonadotropin, to determine whether a prolonged stimulation cycle might produce larger numbers of multiple follicles in our patients *(12)*. In this study the patients in Group 1 received 150 mg of clomiphene citrate daily from day 3 through 7. The patients in Group 2 received clomiphene citrate (150 mg daily, days 3 through 7), followed by two ampules of Pergonal (human menopausal gonadotropin; Serono Labs) daily thereafter, until two follicles, 18 mm

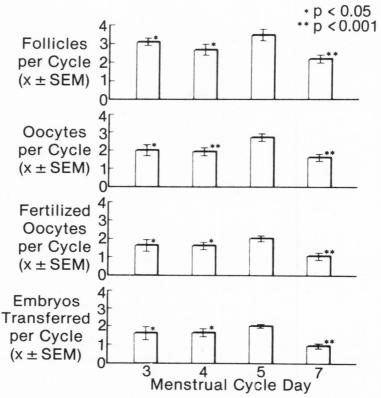

Fig. 2. Comparison of number of follicles aspirated *(top panel)* oocytes recovered *(second panel)* and fertilized *(third panel)*, and embryos transferred *(bottom panel)* after clomiphene citrate, 150 mg for five days

* and ** signify significant difference from results for administration on day 5

or greater, were visible by ultrasound, at which time Pergonal was discontinued. The patients in Group 3 received clomiphene citrate (150 mg daily, days 3 through 7) combined with Pergonal, two ampules a day on days 3, 5, and 7 of the cycle and then continued daily as in Group 2. The fourth group of patients received two ampules of Pergonal daily beginning day 3 of the cycle until two follicles 18 mm or greater were visible; we then monitored concentrations of estradiol until they reached a plateau, at which time we administered hCG. The patients receiving clomiphene citrate followed by or combined with Pergonal had optimal

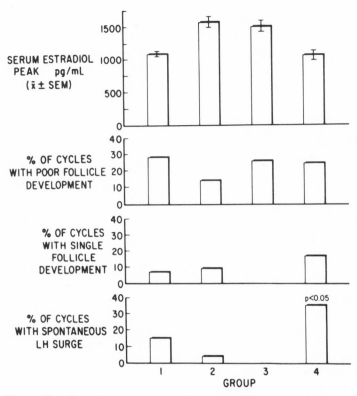

Fig. 3. Results of stimulation with clomiphene citrate, 150 mg daily from day 3 through 7 (Group 1); clomiphene citrate, day 3 through 7, followed by Pergonal, two ampules per day (Group 2); clomiphene citrate, 150 mg per day, day 3 through 7, and Pergonal, two ampules on day 3, 5, 7, and daily thereafter (Group 3); and Pergonal, two ampules daily beginning day 3 (Group 4)

Bars represent mean ± SEM

follicle development and optimal rates of oocyte recovery, fertilization, and embryo transfer (Figures 3 and 4). Group 4, treated with Pergonal only, had a lower oocyte recovery rate and lower embryo transfer rate, presumably because the follicle was overstimulated, making difficult the retrieval of eggs in thick, luteinized follicular fluid. Moreover, postmature ("overripe") oocytes were recovered, which were difficult to fertilize in vitro, and there was a significant increase in spontaneous release of endogenous LH before hCG administration in this group.

Beginning in 1983, we concentrated on two primary regimens

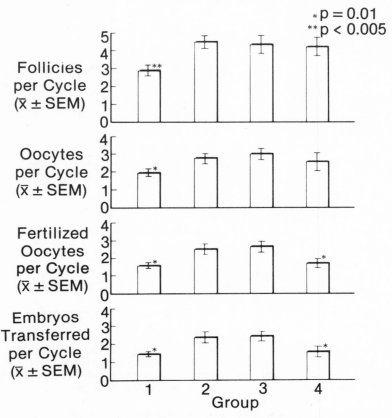

Effect of Various Methods of Ovarian Stimulation
on Folliculogenesis and Embryo Development

Fig. 4. Results of stimulation with clomiphene citrate, 150 mg from day 3 through 7 (Group 1); clomiphene citrate, day 3 through 7, followed by Pergonal, two ampules per day (Group 2); clomiphene citrate, 150 mg per day, day 3 through 7, and Pergonal, two ampules on day 3, 5, 7, and daily thereafter (Group 3); and Pergonal, two ampules daily beginning day 3 (Group 4)

* and ** signify significant difference from results for Group 2 and 3

of ovarian stimulation throughout the year. Clomiphene citrate (150 mg daily) followed by Pergonal, two ampules per day, was administered during 90 treatment cycles. Pergonal was administered until two follicles, 18 mm or greater, were visible; these patients then received hCG when their estradiol concentrations plateaued. For 53 treatment cycles we followed a modified regimen of Pergonal administration. These patients received three ampules of Pergonal, beginning on day 3 of the cycle and continuing until two follicles were visible, at 15 mm or greater; thereafter, when estradiol concentrations plateaued, we administered hCG and performed laparoscopy 36 h later. The number of oocytes collected with Pergonal alone averaged 5.5 ± 0.4 (mean $\pm$ SEM) oocytes per laparoscopy cycle, of which 3.6 ± 0.4 were fertilized and 2.8 ± 0.2 embryos were replaced per cycle. In the group receiving clomiphene followed by Pergonal, 3.3 ± 0.2 oocytes were retrieved per follicle aspiration cycle, of which 2.5 ± 0.2 were fertilized with 2.3 ± 0.2 embryos replaced. The differences between these groups of patients were not statistically significant. In the previous stimulated groups, the patients receiving only clomiphene had fewer oocytes recovered, fertilized, and embryos replaced: 2.7 ± 0.3, 2.0 ± 0.1, and 2.0 ± 0.1, respectively.

We are currently using a modification of the combination therapy. Clomiphene citrate, 100 mg per day, is given on days 3 through 7 concurrently with one ampule of Pergonal daily, which again is continued and extended until two follicles, 18 mm or greater, are seen on ultrasound; hCG is administered when the estradiol concentrations plateau. In these treatment cycles, 4.3 ± 0.3 oocytes have thus far been collected per laparoscopy cycle, of which 3.7 ± 0.3 have been fertilized; 3.1 ± 0.3 embryos have been replaced per cycle.

Pregnancy rates with the various stimulation methods are tending to increase as we fine-tune our approach. Administration of clomiphene citrate alone resulted in pregnancy in 12% of the laparoscopy cycles. The combination of 150 mg of clomiphene citrate followed by Pergonal resulted in 21% of the cases per laparoscopy initiating pregnancy, whereas 20% of the Pergonal-only stimulated cycles that went to laparoscopy resulted in pregnancy. The combination of 100 mg of clomiphene citrate and Pergonal has produced a pregnancy rate of only 15% per laparoscopy, but there are too few cycles yet to make a valid comparison.

Follicular Fluid Profile

Even though the number of oocytes collected and fertilized that result in embryo development is important, one must also pay attention to the follicular fluid environments created by the ovarian-stimulation regimens. With these various regimens of ovarian stimulation, certain changes occur in the steroid concentrations within the follicle, secondary to the type of stimulation utilized. In comparison with concentrations in unstimulated cycles, the use of clomiphene citrate, clomiphene citrate followed by Pergonal, and Pergonal alone significantly increased estrogen concentrations in the follicular fluid, where fertilized oocytes were obtained. However, in analyzing and comparing follicular fluids, we found that progesterone concentrations in follicles that produced oocytes that were capable of being fertilized in vitro showed no significant differences between unstimulated cycles and cycles after stimulation. Moreover, the concentrations of androstenedione in follicular fluid showed no significant pattern of change, whether the follicles were stimulated or unstimulated, nor did testosterone concentrations vary (13). Further studies (14) have demonstrated that protein substances in follicular fluid may be enhanced or diminished, depending upon the type of ovarian stimulation used. Production of inhibin by ovarian follicles does appear to be significantly correlated with the use of Pergonal-stimulation regimens (14). When clomiphene was used as a sole method of ovarian stimulation, inhibin production within the follicular fluid was less than after stimulation with Pergonal but more than in the unstimulated pre-ovulatory follicle. Therefore, the concentrations of various regulatory proteins in follicular fluid appear to depend on the type of stimulation the follicle receives (14).

Summary

The primary advantages of ovarian stimulation for human IVF-ER procedures are the ultimate production of multiple embryos for replacement back into the uterus. In our particular program, successful pregnancy with single embryo replacements occurs in about 11% of cases. Replacing two embryos results in a pregnancy rate of 18%, and replacing three embryos results in a pregnancy 33% of the time. When four embryos have been placed into the uterine cavity, the pregnancy rate decreased to 25%. Therefore, the use of ovarian stimulation to retrieve multiple oocytes is important for increasing successful pregnancies.

However, not all of the effects of ovarian stimulation may be beneficial. The changes in the follicular fluid milieu may adversely affect oocyte quality and ultimately embryo viability. Hyperstimulation and the changes in the endocrine environment may affect endometrial receptivity. Further work in optimizing the type of ovarian stimulation is therefore needed.

The optimal system would be a method of hyperstimulation that would produce multiple oocytes without dramatically changing the endocrine milieu within the follicle compartment or within the reproductive tract. New methods of stimulation that may provide a better mechanism of multiple follicle development include pulsatile administration of gonadotropin-releasing hormone (GnRH; gonadoliberin) and use of pure follicle-stimulating hormone (FSH; follitropin) preparations. Another avenue of approach to avoid the adverse effects of ovarian hyperstimulation is to develop a system for cryopreservation of embryos, whereby multiple oocytes and embryos can be generated by ovarian hyperstimulation, preserved for various periods of time, and replaced during a nonstimulated, natural ovulatory cycle. These approaches may ultimately increase the implantation success rate with human IVF-ER in the future.

References

1. Steptoe PC, Edwards RG. Laparoscopic recovery of preovulatory human oocytes after priming of ovaries with gonadotropins. *Lancet* i, 683–688 (1970).
2. Edwards RG. Test-tube babies. *Nature* **293**, 253–256 (1981).
3. Lopata A, Johnston IW, Hoult IJ, Speirs AL. Pregnancy following intrauterine implantation of an embryo obtained by in vitro fertilization of a preovulatory egg. *Fertil Steril* **33**, 117–120 (1980).
4. Trounson AO, Leeton JF, Wood C, et al. Pregnancies in humans by fertilization in vitro and embryo transfer in the controlled ovulatory cycle. *Science* **212**, 681–682 (1981).
5. Marrs RP, Vargyas JM, Gibbons WE, et al. A modified technique of human in vitro fertilization and embryo transfer. *Am J Obstet Gynecol* **147**, 318–322 (1983).
6. Lopata A. Concepts in human in vitro fertilization and embryo transfer. *Fertil Steril* **40**, 289–301 (1983).
7. Jones HW Jr, Jones GS, Andres MC, et al. The program for in vitro fertilization at Norfolk. *Fertil Steril* **38**, 14–21 (1982).
8. Vargyas JM, Marrs RP, Kletzky OA, Mishell DR Jr. Correlation of ultrasonic measurement of ovarian follicle size and serum estradiol

levels in ovulatory patients using clomiphene citrate for in vitro fertilization. *Am J Obstet Gynecol* **144,** 569–573 (1982).

9. Goodman AL, Nixon WE, Johnson DK, et al. Regulation of folliculogenesis in the cycling rhesus monkey. Selection of the dominant follicle. *Endocrinology* **100,** 155–161 (1977).

10. diZerega GS, Hodgen GD. Folliculogenesis in the primate ovarian cycle. *Endocr Rev* **2,** 27–49 (1981).

11. Marrs RP, Vargyas JM, Shangold GM, Yee B. The effect of the time of initiation of clomiphene citrate on multiple follicle development for human *in vitro* fertilization and embryo replacement procedures. *Fertil Steril* (in press).

12. Vargyas JM, Morente C, Shangold G, Marrs RP. The effect of different methods of ovarian stimulation for human in vitro fertilization and embryo transfer. *Fertil Steril* (in press).

13. Marrs RP, Vargyas JM, Lobo R. Comparison of the intrafollicular hormonal milieu with fertilization of human oocytes *in vitro*. Presented at the Endocrine Society, San Antonio, Texas, June 8–10, 1983.

14. Marrs RP, Lobo R, Campeau JD, et al. Correlation of human follicular fluid inhibin activity with spontaneous and stimulated follicle maturation. *J Clin Endocrinol Metab* **58,** 704–709 (1984).

In Vitro Fertilization, 1981–1983

Howard W. Jones, Jr.

As of December 31, 1983, the program of in vitro fertilization at Norfolk had completed three years of activity, with use of human menopausal gonadotropin (hMG) as a method of recruiting and maturing ovarian follicles. During this period, the successful pregnancy results have improved each year (Table 1). The main purpose of this paper, however, is not to present end results per se, but to emphasize several physiological findings derived during this three years' experience. For this purpose, various subsets of data will be used.

Table 1. **Results of in Vitro Fertilization Program, Norfolk, 1981–1983**

Year	No. of cycles	No. of transfers	No. of pregnancies	Pregnancies per cycle	Pregnancies per transfer
1981	55	31	7	12.7	22.6
1982	207	155	34	16.4	21.9
1983	301	243	64	21.3	26.3
Total	563	429	105	18.7	24.5

Effect of Human Menopausal Gonadotropin Stimulation on the Spontaneous Lutropin Surge

It has been known for many years that an increase in follicular-phase serum estradiol is followed by a surge of lutropin (luteinizing hormone, LH), which is the immediate predecessor of ovulation. However, during stimulation with hMG, serum concentrations of estradiol equal to and higher than those observed in the normal menstrual period failed to stimulate a spontaneous LH surge (Figure 1). For this reason, when using hMG stimulation,

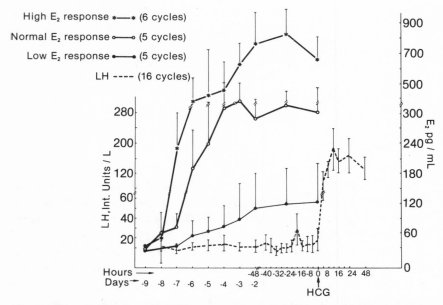

Fig. 1. The relation of serum LH to serum estradiol (E₂) after hMG stimulation in patients with low, normal, and high response to hMG

Note that in spite of peripheral estradiol in excess of 300 pg/mL in the normal and high responders, there is no evidence of an LH increase until hCG is given. *Bars* represent SD of 16 hMG-stimulated cycles

one must also use human choriogonadotropin (hCG) as a surrogate for the spontaneous LH surge.

The inhibition of the LH surge in hMG-stimulated cycles is apparently not absolute, and occasionally an LH surge will occur, presumably when the estradiol concentrations reach extraordinarily high values *(1)*.

Channing et al. *(2)* analyzed follicular fluid from the hMG-stimulated pre-ovulatory follicles and found increased concentrations of an inhibin-like activity, from three- to 10-fold that found in the dominant follicle of a natural cycle. Although porcine follicular fluid "inhibin" preferentially blocks pituitary release of follitropin (FSH), according to Chari et al. *(3)*, it may also inhibit LH if given in sufficient amounts. One may, therefore, postulate that the suppressive effect of hMG on the LH surge is related to the increased amount of inhibin-like protein produced in the hMG-stimulated cycles. Support for this theory is found in the work on the rhesus monkey by Schenken and Hodgen *(4)*.

Patients' Response to hMG

Early in our experience, we determined that, as judged by the concentrations of serum estradiol, individual patients responded differently to the same amount of hMG stimulation. Three patient-response categories were identified—low, intermediate, and high—related to the serum estradiol values. We determined that hMG was best discontinued in the majority of patients when the estradiol concentration peripherally was 300 pg/mL, or above, if the peripheral biological estrogen response had occurred. These patients, characterized as intermediate responders, made up the largest number of patients. In the patients designated high responders, the peripheral estradiol exceeded 600 pg/mL without a peripheral biological response. The low responders were those patients who had had a peripheral estrogen response for three days even though the serum estradiol had not reached 300 pg/mL (5).

We thus determined that in, our program, we would attempt to modulate the stimulation of the patient with hMG rather than give a rigid stimulation pattern, as our initial experience seemed to indicate that patients classified as intermediate produced the best pregnancy results.

The reason for the variation in patients' response to regimens of similar stimulation is not clearly understood. Mantzavinos et al. (6) showed it was not related to the diameter of the largest follicle but was in part related to the number of measurable follicles. It is clearly not related to a higher total hMG dose; early experiences showed that the high responders had received less hMG than the intermediate responders, who had received less than the low responders (5).

The repetitiveness of the response to hMG stimulation with the same amount of hMG in a particular patient has been striking (Figure 2), although a patient's response may be changed by altering the type of stimulation administered. However, low responders, when given more hMG per day, may or may not have an improved response as measured by the estradiol concentration in peripheral serum. Indeed, doses of hMG in excess of two ampules a day can in some cases be counterproductive—the estradiol may begin to fall, even under stimulation, which suggests that follicular response has been muted, perhaps by luteinization by the LH component in the hMG preparation (Figure 3).

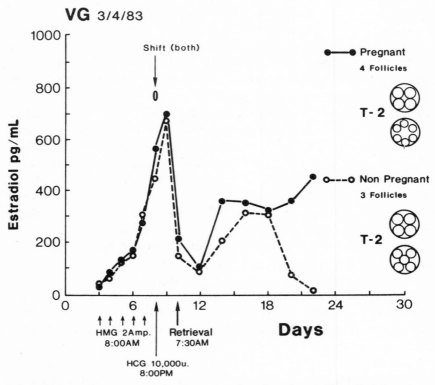

VG 3/4/83

Fig. 2. A patient's response in two menstrual cycles after similar administrations of hMG

Note that her peripheral concentrations of estradiol produced are essentially superimposable. In the second cycle, she became pregnant. Retrieval marks the point of oocyte harvest. T−2= transfer of two concepti (no. of blastomeres indicated by diagram)

The final estradiol response just before and after the discontinuation of the hMG, including the response to the injection of hCG, seems to have an important bearing on the quality of oocytes obtained. The best results, in terms of pregnancy rates, seem to be obtained if the oocytes are harvested from patients whose serum concentrations of estradiol continue to rise, even ever so slightly, after the discontinuation of the hMG and indeed continue to rise after the injection of hCG (Figure 4, pattern *A*). Almost as satisfactory are those patients who exhibit a mild downturn in peripheral concentration of estradiol after the discontinuation of the hMG, provided the estradiol concentration increases after the hCG injection is given (pattern *B*). A very poor pregnancy

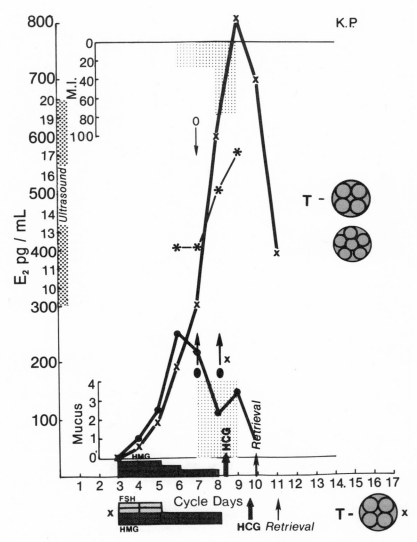

Fig. 3. A variation in estradiol (E₂) response in the same patient, related to the variation in the stimulation pattern

When FSH is added to the stimulation, there is a very high response, but where hMG is used alone, there is a falling estradiol even while the hMG is being given. T, Transfer (no. of blastomeres indicated by diagram). X, FSH-treated cycle; ●, hMG-treated cycle. *Dotted area (upper)*= % maturation index (M.I.); 0 = shift in maturation index in hMG-treated cycle. *Dotted area (lower)*= mucus response (amount): upward arrows indicate adequate mucus in the hMG cycle and the FSH cycle. Ultrasound units in mm

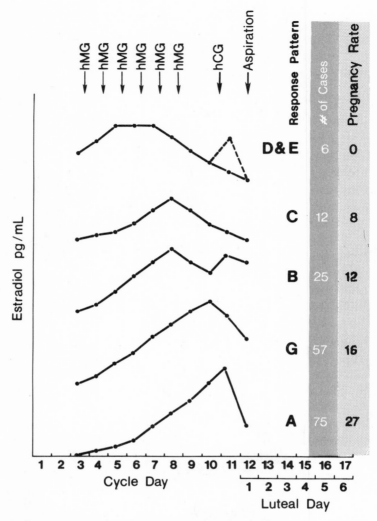

Fig. 4. Diagram of estradiol production patterns in relation to pregnancy rate

See also Fig. 5 and the text for a discussion of the patterns

rate characterizes those patients whose peripheral estradiol decreases after the discontinuation of the hMG and who have no
response to the injection of hCG (patterns *C* and *G*). Even worse
are those patients whose concentration of peripheral estradiol de-

creases in the face of hMG injection (patterns *D* and *E*); indeed, no pregnancy has occurred under this circumstance.

An analysis of the data indicates that these various patterns of peripheral estradiol seem to reflect the quality of the oocytes. This is born out by the fact that the numbers of oocytes obtained per patient, whether for patients with a rising concentration of estradiol or an estradiol that has fallen and yet rises again after hCG, or in those patients who have a falling estradiol after the discontinuation of hMG but who do not respond to hCG, are all about the same. Their oocytes are fertilized at about the same rate, and an equal number of embryos per patient are transferred. However, the pregnancy rate, as mentioned above, progressively declines with various peripheral estradiol patterns. It is difficult to escape the conclusion that the quality of the oocyte, although imperceptible by microscopic examination, deteriorates in some of these estradiol patterns (Figure 5).

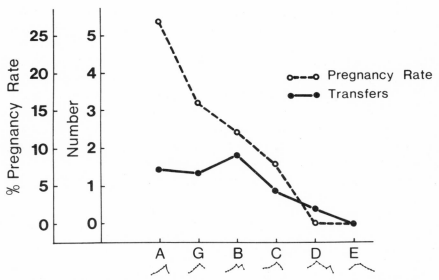

Fig. 5. The number of concepti transferred per cycle in relation to the pattern of estradiol production and the pregnancy rate

The number of transfers per cycle in patterns A, G, and B is essentially the same, but the pregnancy rate varies considerably, suggesting that the quality of the transferred concepti varies. See also Fig. 4

Relation of the Pregnancy Rate to the Number of Transferred Concepti

All programs have observed the fact that the pregnancy rate improves with the number of concepti transferred; however, the optimum number of concepti per transfer is a matter of uncertainty. From an obstetrical point of view, multiple pregnancies (more than twins) cause problems, so that the risk of triplets, quadruplets, and even quintuplets must be considered.

There has been some suggestion that transfers of more than three, or perhaps four, concepti result in a lower pregnancy rate. Our own early data suggested the same thing; however, a careful analysis of pregnancy rates (broken down into very small groups) indicates that, except for the transfer of five concepti, the pregnancy rate seems to increase with the number of transferred concepti (Table 2). Moreover, further analysis of the patients in the five-transfer category indicates that several of the concepti were derived from immature oocytes that had been transferred in the pronuclear stage.

If one assumes that each conceptus has an equal probability of success, one can calculate the theoretical expectation of multiple pregnancies by a simple expansion of the algebraic binomial $(A + B)^2 = 1$ when A equals the probability of a pregnancy, B represents the probability of failure (Table 3). Among our pregnancies, 13 sets of twins and one set of triplets have been identified by ultrasonography early in pregnancy. The use of ultrasonography early in pregnancy has shown that many times one twin will be absorbed and the pregnancy will continue as a singleton. Indeed, this happened to one of the sacs in the triplet pregnancy, which is now continuing as a twin pregnancy; among the 13 twins, this phenomenon has been observed five times.

Table 2. **Pregnancies by Concepti Transferred: Norfolk Series 1–12**

No. of concepti per transfer	Total no. transferred	No. of pregnancies	Pregnancies per transfer, %
1	153	31	20.3
2	147	33	22.4
3	72	21	29.2
4 or more	57	20	35.1
Total	429	105	24.5

Table 3. **Probability of Multiple Pregnancies with Multiple Transfers**

No. of concepti transferred	% probability of						
	Singleton	Twins	Triplets	Quads	Quints	Sextuplets	Total
1	20						20
2	32	4					36
3	38	10	0.8				49
4	41	15	2.6	0.2			59
5	41	20	5.1	0.6	0.03		67
6	39	25	8.2	1.5	0.15	0.006	74

Assumptions: (1) probability of pregnancy from a single transfer = 20%; (2) all concepti have equal chance.

The number of twins encountered is fewer than one would anticipate theoretically from the calculation. This fact, together with the disappearance of some of the twins, suggests that not all concepti are equal, in spite of the inability to determine this by microscopic examination of the concepti at the time of transfer.

Patients' Response to FSH

That the pregnancy rate increases with the number of concepti transferred suggests that the goal would be multiple transfers, the exact number depending on the quality of the concepti; at this moment, the precise number is still a matter of further study. In an attempt to recruit an adequate number of oocytes to assure multiple transfer in all patients, we have tried to recruit a larger number of follicles by the use of FSH alone without any added LH. The theoretical basis for this approach is the concept that FSH is the recruiting hormone for follicles, and that LH may luteinize them too early in the follicular phase if present in undesirable quantities. We have, therefore, had some preliminary experience in the use of FSH alone for follicular recruitment.

One of the astonishing findings in these patients is that many of them, if given the same amount of FSH as they had been given in previous cycles, but in the previous cycles had also had an equal amount of LH added, will in the FSH-only cycles produce the same peripheral estradiol response as in the previous cycles. This seems to be somewhat contrary to the conventional wisdom that estradiol production is a function of LH. Moreover, determinations of FSH and LH in these patients' serum suggest that the native LH is depressed by the use of exogeneous FSH; thus one is forced to conclude either that LH is not at all necessary for production of estradiol in the follicular phase or that very minute amounts of LH are adequate, so minute that they are not measurable by present techniques of radioimmunoassay. Furthermore, the spontaneous LH surge seems to be inhibited in these patients, just as it is when patients are given hMG; therefore, hCG has been used as the surrogate for the spontaneous LH rise. Oocytes obtained 36 h after hCG injection are fertilizable, cleave normally, and when transferred can produce a pregnancy.

This experience brings into question the role of LH in the initiation of the resumption of meiosis. On the basis of our clinical experience with FSH, it would appear that the surrogate surge supplied by hCG is all that is necessary to trigger the resumption of meiosis. Large numbers of oocytes can be collected by this technique.

It is too early to know the exact role of this method of stimulation, because our experience so far has been confined to the use of FSH among those patients who did not respond well to hMG on previous stimulations. It is entirely possible that FSH will be useful as the stimulating agent in patients who have previously been unstimulated, but this remains to be determined.

The Influence of Programs of in Vitro Fertilization on Clinical Gynecology

Although the main thrust of this presentation has been to emphasize astonishing new physiological concepts that have developed by studying follicular and oocyte maturation by stimulation with hMG or FSH, it is perhaps of interest to note that programs of in vitro fertilization are having a substantial impact on the practice of gynecology.

Certain types of tubal surgery, e.g., secondary operations on tubes that have failed a primary surgical attempt, should become very rare indeed. Perhaps in vitro fertilization could even replace the primary operation for tubal obstruction in cases where experience has shown that a very poor outcome is likely, e.g., for thickened tubes obstructed at the distal end and bound down by adhesions along their shaft. Moreover, if the expectation of pregnancy from in vitro fertilization approaches 50%, as it well might, *all* tubal surgery on the peripheral end of the tube might, except in rare circumstances, become a thing of the past.

The last few years have seen a wave of conservatism in the treatment of tubal pregnancies. In view of the fact that the recurrence of ectopic pregnancies in conserved tubes is substantial, it is entirely possible that in the foreseeable future the conservative operation would involve a salpingectomy.

Finally, for many years, it has been accepted practice to remove the uterus whenever it became necessary to remove both fallopian tubes for whatever reason. The theory of this was that the uterus no longer served any useful purpose and indeed was a liability in that malignancies might occur in the future. This practice, however, is no longer tenable, for with programs of in vitro fertilization, pregnancies can occur in the absence of fallopian tubes.

Thus, programs of in vitro fertilization have been extraordinarily productive in allowing us to understand some of the basic mechanisms involved in reproductive biology; equally important, however, has been the influence of the programs on the practice of gynecology. Furthermore, this procedure has offered hope to countless couples who before in vitro fertilization were denied the opportunity for childbearing.

References

1. Ferraretti AF. Superovulation induction with exogenous human gonadotropins. In *Human In Vitro Fertilization and Embryo Development,* G Loverrog, Ed., Bari Congress, Edizini Int., Roma, Italy, 1984, pp 57–70.
2. Channing CP, Tanabe K, Jones GS, et al. Observation of a greater concentration of inhibin activity in follicular fluid of preovulatory follicles of human menopausal gonadotropin-hCG treated women compared to untreated women. Endocrine Society Meeting, San Antonio, TX, June 1983, abstract no. 1224, p 386.
3. Chari S, Hopkinson CRN, Duame E, Sturm G. Purification of "inhibin" from human ovarian follicular fluid. *Acta Endocrinol* **90,** 157–166 (1979).
4. Schenken RS, Hodgen GD. FSH-induced ovarian stimulation in monkeys: Blockade of the LH surge. *J Clin Endocrinol Metab* **57,** 50–55 (1983).

5. Garcia JE, Jones GS, Acosta AA, Wright GL Jr. HMG/hCG follicular maturation for oocyte maturation. Phase II, 1981. *Fertil Steril* **39,** 167–173 (1983).
6. Mantzavinos T, Garcia JE, Jones HW Jr. Ultrasound measurement of ovarian follicles stimulated by human gonadotropins for oocyte recovery and in vitro fertilization. *Fertil Steril* **40,** 461–465 (1983).

Discussion—Session IV

Q: Dr. Jones, when you transfer two concepti, is there any evidence that implantation of one inhibits implantation of the other?

DR. JONES: It's hard to give a dogmatic answer to this. Bob Edwards feels that one helps the other: His data show that when he transfers two, the pregnancy rate is practically double or a little more than that for the transfer of one. The problem is, his pregnancy rate on transferring one is quite low, so I'm not convinced that this is a good procedure. He also thought that the transfer of multiple concepti increased the abortion rate, which we cannot confirm from our data, the miscarriage rate being distributed randomly through our group. At the moment I think all the concepti have an equal environment and my opinion is that the difficulty is inherent within the conceptus.

Q: Is there any evidence that nonaspirated follicles will produce hyperstimulation syndrome?

DR. MARRS: If, for instance, a patient had premature release of endogenous LH before we were performing frequent monitoring and we did not aspirate her oocytes, such a patient would have some ovarian enlargement and tenderness, but we have not seen significant clinical hyperstimulation. It's possible that those patients could, but we think that the endogenous LH that is released and triggers ovulation is different from what you see in a Pergonal-induced cycle with hCG-induced follicle rupture. The LH has a shorter half-life in the system, which may account for the difference in response that we have seen in these patients. Many of the patients will have one inaccessible ovary and may develop multiple follicles on both sides. Again, failure to aspirate follicles from an ovary that's not visualized at laparoscopy has not created any clinical hyperstimulation problems in those patients.

Q: Do you see post-operative adhesions after multiple aspirations?

Dr. Marrs: No, we haven't. In fact, we do a lot of laparoscopic lysis during these follicle aspirations; even those adhesions tend not to reform after the laparoscopy.

Q: Should you give the patient a pregnancy rate statistic based on the number of transfers or based on the number of laparoscopies?

Dr. Marrs: I think it's fairer to give the patient the odds for pregnancy per laparoscopy, that is, for the procedure that's traumatic to her system. Some people have suggested that we correlate our pregnancy rates with the initiation of the treatment cycle, but I don't think that's realistic. I don't think you can tell a patient that the pregnancy rate per stimulated cycle is such and such, because you may give medication for five or six days and drop it for a cycle if she doesn't respond. Patients aren't really too traumatized by that. However, if you put them through a laparoscopy and don't get to transfer a viable embryo, that's more significant—and I think that's a more realistic point from which to judge your rate of success.

In 1983 the vast majority of our patients who underwent laparoscopy had an embryo transfer.

Q: Do you exclude the endometrium, corpus luteum function, etc., in explaining the differences in various rates of successful in vitro fertilization?

Dr. Jones: Yes. We're very concerned about endometrial competence and corpus luteum function. In fact, we treat our patients with progesterone very early. From the results of our studies correlating endometrial biopsy results with the peripheral concentrations of estradiol and testosterone, we believe that pregnancy rates are enhanced when the endometrium is at least 24 h ahead of schedule. Perhaps this ties in with the fact that we transfer the conceptus into the endometrium about 48 or 24 h before it normally would reach there, and at a cell-division stage somewhat earlier than usual.

Q: Is the trigger for the LH surge the estradiol/inhibin ratio, or the rate of change of estradiol concentration, or some other, later, independent factor?

Dr. Jones: If one looks at the estradiol rise in the normal cycle, one is impressed by the fact that this increase has a rather broad base, starting up three or four days before reaching its peak. I'm inclined to believe that the rate of increase may be relevant. In other words, I would expect a broader-base rise to be more effective than an acute rise to 300 pg/mL followed by a quick drop.

Q: What's the rate of fetal anomalies in pregnancy wastage from embryo transfer as compared with that in the general population?

DR. MARRS: To date, no anomalous babies have been delivered, of probably more than 250 babies that have been now delivered by the in vitro program around the world. As regards any abnormalities in the babies, I'm aware of only two, both cardiac defects. One occurred in a twin gestation in one of the Australian deliveries and another here in the United States. These cardiac abnormalities are not thought to be related to any of the manipulations that the oocytes or embryo undergo during the process.

We don't think that there is any increased risk to these children in terms of genetic, developmental, or emotional problems in childhood or adult life. But again, the oldest child is only 5½ years old now. She appears to be completely normal, but we don't know what ultimately will happen. We think everything will be normal in these children.

Pregnancy wastage varies from about 30% to as high as 50% in some programs. These are spontaneous abortions in the first 10 to 12 weeks of pregnancy. The percentage really varies from program to program but is generally more than that expected in the general population of women, which is between 10 and 15%.

Q: Is there a program to follow up these children?

DR. MARRS: Because we have a very active high-risk obstetrical team at our university, we do a little more than some of the other programs. Two of our people, Dr. Larry Platt and Dr. Greg Devore, use ultrasound to examine fully the biophysical characteristics of these children within the first 20 to 24 weeks of pregnancy, including a full cardiac ultrasound evaluation of the fetal cardiac status—primarily because of the two pregnancies that have had cardiac anomalies. These can be picked up very early in pregnancy.

Because many of our patients are over 35, we also strongly recommend amniocentesis to all who become pregnant.

Q: You mention cryopreservation for transfer of frozen embryos. How many have you done?

DR. MARRS: We have not transferred any of these embryos as of yet. We just received approval last week from our research committees and our ethics board to go ahead with it. We do have 12 or 14 embryos that have been stored and we will be utilizing them in the next few months. However, in those patients, we are requiring amniocentesis in early pregnancy, should such pregnancies occur, as we hope.

Only one other team in the work right now is utilizing cryopreserved embryos—Alan Trounson's team in Melbourne, Australia. In our last conversation with them a couple of weeks ago they told us they had two ongoing clinical pregnancies with thawed frozen human embryos. [*Ed. note:* A live birth was reported by this group in April 1984.] They had two other pregnancies that were lost early in pregnancy. I don't know how many transfers they've performed, but it's probably in the range of 20 or 25.

The main problem with cryopreservation is determining the best time to freeze the embryo. In our protocol, we will be freezing eight-cell, 16-cell, and 32-cell embryos, then thawing them and allowing them to approach blastocyst development before transfer. Nobody really knows the optimal stage yet. The Trounson team has been freezing it at the four-cell stage.

Q: Does inhibin act locally to influence oocyte maturation?

Dr. Marrs: We don't think so, but we don't know for sure. Other follicular fluid regulatory proteins are produced within the follicle; oocyte maturation inhibitor is the primary one that we plan to look at in the very near future. That factor does appear to affect oocyte maturation and quality. We don't know whether inhibin does; we know that it has a central effect, but we don't know what type of activity it has within the follicle. Dr. diZerega has looked at some other regulatory proteins that affect granulosa cell production of steroids. Those parameters very definitely are controlled within the follicle by other regulatory proteins that we have identified.

Q: Whether one uses sperm wash capacitation for intra-uterine insemination, or in vitro fertilization, what's the optimal time for sperm incubation?

Dr. Marrs: It's variable. In some males certainly you can separate the semen, wash the spermatozoa, separate the spermatozoa, and add them to the oocyte culture, and fertilization will occur very normally. The capacitation and acrosome reaction occur in the sperm head, not only while the sperm are incubating alone but also while they're co-incubating with the oocyte. In fact the cumulus corona complex may have some effect on the capacitation process in the spermatozoa.

Seminal plasma separation is the first step. How long it takes to fully capacitate human spermatozoa I don't think anybody truly knows. Certainly in different males different times may be required. For instance, in our testing of males in our hamster penetration test, we tried various pre-incubation times in certain males to see if we could improve the penetrating quality of their sperm. Sperm from some males respond to prolonged incubation, others are negatively affected by it, so this is variable. With humans, we started out pre-incubating the sperm for 2 h; now we're using a 6-h pre-incubation. Our fertilization rates per ovum are no different; it's just more convenient in our laboratory system to use a longer sperm pre-incubation interval. We've even used sperm incubated for 24 h with our immature oocytes; again, fertilization appears to be normal if the oocytes have reached maturation.

COMMENT: Some data on hamsters from Larry Lipshultz's lab suggest that an ejaculate contains different populations of sperm so that capacitation may occur in different populations over a period of 16 or 18 h. They feel that at least some of the times where they're seeing increased hamster penetration after prolonged incubation of the sperm at 4 °C a greater percentage of the population of sperm is being totally capacitated by the time they initiate incubation with the hamster eggs. They think this may be important with some of the oligospermic patients.

Q: With the high estradiol concentration during ovarian stimulation, is prolactin increased at the time of ovulation?

DR. MARRS: The early effect may have just been an effect of the anesthetic the patient received, which has been known to increase prolactin, but after 12 to 16 h the prolactin concentrations were not different from those in the nonstimulated patients. Dr. Hodgen showed some data in his primate colony that prolactin tends to be increased in these hyperstimulated models. We have not looked at that specifically. Whether this affects luteal-phase function is another unanswered question. This may again be another effect of the ovarian stimulation regimens that we use. It may possibly interfere with normal implantation and normal pregnancy.

Q: Since hCG is a signal to the corpus luteum, why not use hCG to maintain corpus luteum function?

DR. MARRS: You can argue both sides of this—progesterone vs hCG. My bias is that hCG is fine if you have a functional corpus luteum. But if you have a functional corpus luteum, why do you need hCG supplementation? That's why I feel that supplementation with progesterone is appropriate. If you fear corpus luteum insufficiency, you should supply the hormone that's needed, not something that may drive an already weakened system to produce progesterone.

Q: Dr. Hodgen, has the difference between bioactive LH vs immunoactive LH seen in monkeys at mid-cycle been shown in women as well? Are there any other divergencies between the bioactive and immunoactive LH?

DR. HODGEN: Depending upon the assay systems one uses, one will see either agreement or relative disagreement between results for bioactivity and the radioimmunological activity. One particular assay used for many years to measure lutropin (LH) in the rhesus monkey does not appreciate very well the biological potency of the material.

More recently, a new radioimmunoassay for rhesus monkey LH by Bill Heckem gives results that agree very well with those of the bioassay. In terms of the clinical situation, the results of assays used to evaluate patients again depend largely on the antiserum used. If the antibody is seeing a part of a molecule that relates very well to a biological expression of LH activity, then agreement between the assays will be good. But if many of the antigenic components of the antiserum aren't really related to the expression of biological activity, there will be more disparity. So it simply depends on using an RIA system that gives values that correlate with those of the biological assay.

DR. ODELL: Dr. Hodgen, Harold Papkoff (Greenwald and Papkoff, *Proc Soc Exp Biol Med* **165:** 391, 1980) showed in rats that you could substitute highly purified FSH for LH as an ovulatory hormone. The monkeys you pretreated with highly purified LH/ FSH to develop follicles make a marvelous study tool for trying purified FSH as an ovulatory hormone. Have you done that?

DR. HODGEN: We've not actually done that experiment, but we have given very high doses of pure FSH up to the expected time of ovulation. Those follicles do not luteinize; they do not rupture; the eggs are not released until we give hCG. Furthermore, going to the mid-luteal phase, we have asked whether we could stimulate progesterone production by luteinized granulosa cells, now the luteal cell. Giving high doses of the pure FSH does not measureably increase progesterone secretion. So, at least in our model, we're unable to show an LH-like effect of the highly purified FSH.

Q: How long can you delay the administration of hCG in these hMG-stimulated cycles and still see normal ovulatory response with release of a mature oocyte? In other words, how long after hMG stimulates production of a mature oocyte or a mature follicle can you delay giving hCG?

DR. HODGEN: Remember, a series of follicles are present, typically the most advanced of which are already in need of hCG (the surrogate LH surge) and others are rapidly approaching that stage. So they're only quasi-synchronous in their development. But the ova in these follicles are not going to stay viable for more than about 24 to 36 h. If they don't get the LH-like effect from hCG in that interval, those eggs will fragment and have very poor potential for fertilization.

Q: Do you think there's a role of prolactin in this somewhere? Old studies demonstrate that prolactin may be able to prolong this period of fertilizability. Do you think there's a role for that in normal physiology?

DR. HODGEN: We don't have data that would support or reject that idea. Although prolactin may impair gonadotropin secretion if present in supraphysiological amounts during the development of the pre-ovulatory follicle, it has little or no effect in the luteal phase. If LH is provided, even in the face of very high prolactin concentration, such events as the secretion of progesterone, the length of the menstrual cycle, etc., do not seem to be truncated.

Q: Is pure FSH now available for clinical use?

DR. HODGEN: The material that I first got in 1981 was called Urofollitropin and was used exclusively for animal studies. Dr. Jones presented some very important clinical results with the pure FSH now called Metrodin, which he and his colleagues in Norfolk have used in vitro fertilization protocols. I think it would be fair to represent this as still an experimental drug. It is not ready yet for general distribution, but it is entering clinical trials and the early results are very positive.

Q: Concerning the failure of an estrogen-induced FSH surge, is this not simply the negative-feedback effect of high estrogen concentrations? Was this possibility excluded?

DR. HODGEN: It's excluded only in the sense that one seeing a gradually increasing concentration of estradiol would expect positive feedback when the estrogen reaches 150 to 200 pg/mL. However, the fact that much higher concentrations are reached later still doesn't tell us why those women did not have LH and FSH surges when the estradiol crossed the presumed threshold for positive feedback.

The other point is that the follicle-fluid extracts administered are indeed extracts: more than 99% of all of the free steroid, including estrogen, has been removed. So that material contains nonestrogen activities that are able to prevent estrogen from inducing the LH surge. Further, there is evidence that this material, whatever it is, in the follicle fluid is immunogenic. We therefore have been able to produce antibodies capable of neutralizing the intense effects of follicle fluid in preventing estrogen-induced LH surges. So there's a cascade of answers but the problem is yet to be fully resolved. There appear to be strong data collectively suggesting that it's not simply estrogen preventing the action of estrogen.

Q: Does 5-aminosalicylic acid have the same effect on sulfasalazine?

VOICE: As far as I know it's not been studied. In fact, very many medications haven't yet been evaluated.

Q: Dr. Hodgen, I've always been struck that the castrate rhesus monkey adult male responds so beautifully to an estrogen challenge by positive feedback but the castrate man doesn't, nor does the castrate adult sheep, castrate adult hamster, castrate adult mouse, or the castrate adult rat. Why do you think the rhesus monkey is different?

DR. HODGEN: Considering the number of similarities on other scales, I don't have a good answer because, for many other physiologies and parameters, there's near mimicry among species. This difference is an outstanding one. Drs. Spees and Norman from the Oregon Primate Center presented at the meeting of the Endocrine Society last year elegant experiments that showed how really superficial is the androgenization in the male rhesus monkey. Whereas we looked at the ingrained effect of androgen in causing the hypothalamus to function male-like instead of female-like, they did the following extraordinary experiment. They transplanted ovarian tissue under the skin of male rhesus monkeys, whose hypothalamus and pituitary then, in fact, responded to an ovarian clock. The very experiments Dr. Ross referred to by Dr. Knobil years ago used this as the control mechanism. The male rhesus monkeys, having ovarian tissue, experienced positive feedback to estrogen with an LH/FSH surge, and actually secreted progesterone from the transplanted ovarian tissues. So the male hypothalamus in the rhesus monkey can still function if you just peel back the androgen layer. It's a very shallow degree of maleness.

V

MENOPAUSE

And sume women haue corrupte mater as quyttour passyng away from hem. And otherwhiles suche mater passith from hem in stede of blode; and otherwhiles with the blodes that the blode thei shuld be purged of. And yf they be olde women other women that be bareyn, it nedith nozt to yeue hem no medecyns therof.

And some women have decaying matter when they have a discharge; and sometimes such matter passes from them instead of blood; and sometimes bleeding comes with the blood that they should be purged of. And if they are old women or women that are barren, there is no need to give them medicine.

—ROWLAND, pp 148–149

Normal Physiology during Menopause

Howard L. Judd

According to the 1980 census of the United States, 32 million of the 116 million women in this country were 50 years of age or older. Most of these women have had or shortly will have their last menstrual period, thus becoming postmenopausal. Because, statistically, a 50-year-old woman can expect to live another 28 years, a large minority of our female population are without ovarian function and will live approximately one-third of their lives after their ovaries cease to function. Consequently, physicians caring for women must have an understanding of the hormonal and metabolic changes associated with the menopause.

Etiology and Pathogenesis

Menopause

There are two types of menopause, classified according to cause: physiological and artificial.

Physiological menopause. In the human embryo, oogenesis begins in the ovary around the third week of gestation. Primordial germ cells appear in the yolk sac of the embryo and by the fifth week migrate to the germinal ridge, where they undergo successive mitotic cellular divisions to give rise to oogonia, which eventually give rise to oocytes. The fetal ovaries are estimated to contain about seven million oogonia at 20 weeks' gestation. From then until menopause, the number of germ cells decreases. After seven months' gestation, no new oocytes are formed. At birth, ovaries contain about two million oocytes, which by the time of puberty have been reduced to 300 000 and continue to decrease during the reproductive years. Two general processes are responsible for this: ovulation and atresia. Nearly all oocytes vanish by atresia, with only 400 to 500 actually being ovulated. Very little is known about atresia of oocytes: studies with animals have shown that estrogens prevent whereas androgens enhance the atretic process.

Apparently, menopause in the human female results from two processes. First, oocytes responsive to gonadotropins disappear from the ovary; second, the few remaining oocytes do not respond to gonadotropins. On very careful histologic inspection, isolated oocytes can be found in postmenopausal ovaries, some showing a limited degree of development; but most reveal no sign of development in the presence of excess endogenous gonadotropins.

Various logistic problems have made it difficult to determine the average age at menopause, currently or in the past. There may have been an increase in the age at menopause in the United States and Western Europe, but this is not clear. At this time, we believe the average age at menopause in the U.S. to be 40–50 years. There does not appear to be any consistent relationship between age at menarche and menopause, nor do marriage, childbearing, height, weight, or prolonged use of oral contraceptives seem to influence the age at menopause. Smoking, however, is associated with early menopause.

Spontaneous cessation of menses before age 40 is called *premature menopause* or *premature ovarian failure.* Cessation of menstruation and the development of climacteric symptoms and complaints can occur as early as a few years after menarche. The reasons for premature ovarian failure are unknown.

Some disease processes, especially severe infections or tumors of the reproductive tract, occasionally damage the ovarian follicular structures so severely as to precipitate menopause. Menopause can also be hastened by excessive exposure to ionizing radiation; chemotherapeutic drugs, particularly alkylating agents; and surgical procedures that impair ovarian blood supply.

Artificial menopause. The permanent cessation of ovarian function brought about by surgical removal of the ovaries or by radiation therapy is called an artificial menopause. Irradiation to ablate ovarian function is rarely used today. Artificial menopause is used to treat endometriosis and estrogen-sensitive neoplasms of the breast and endometrium. More frequently, artificial menopause is a side effect of treatment of intra-abdominal disease; e.g., ovaries are removed in premenopausal women because the gonads have been damaged by infection or neoplasia. When laparotomy affords the opportunity, elective bilateral oophorectomy is also used to prevent ovarian cancer. For premenopausal women, this procedure is still highly controversial; for postmenopausal women, it is now generally accepted as good medical practice.

The Premenopausal State

The decades of mature reproductive life are characterized by generally regular menses and a slow, steady decrease in cycle length (1). At age 15 mean cycle length is 35 days, at age 25 it is 30 days, and at age 35 it is 28 days. This decrease in cycle length is due to shortening of the follicular phase of the cycle, with the length of the luteal phase remaining constant. After age 45, altered function of the aging ovary is detectable in regularly menstruating women. The mean cycle length is significantly shorter than in younger women and is attributable, in all cases, to a shortened follicular phase. The luteal phase is of similar length, and concentrations of progesterone are not different from those observed in younger women. Concentrations of estradiol, however, are lower during portions of the cycle, including active follicular maturation, the midcycle peak, and the luteal phase, than in younger women. Concentrations of follitropin (follicle-stimulating hormone, FSH) are strikingly increased during the early follicular phase and fall as estradiol increases during follicular maturation. FSH concentrations at the midcycle peak and late in the luteal phase are also consistently higher than those in younger women and decrease during the midluteal phase. Concentrations of lutropin (luteinizing hormone, LH) are indistinguishable from those observed in younger women. The mechanism responsible for this early increase of FSH, but not of LH, is not defined. It may result from the fewer oocytes still present in the older ovary and probably reflects both the lower concentrations of estradiol in these women and the absence of another ovarian factor, analogous to inhibin in the male, that regulates FSH secretion.

The transition from regular cycle intervals to the permanent amenorrhea of menopause is characterized by a phase of marked menstrual irregularity (2). The duration of this transition varies greatly among women. Those experiencing the menopause at an early age have a relatively short duration of cycle variability before amenorrhea ensues. Those experiencing it at a later age usually have a phase of menstrual irregularity characterized by unusually long and short intermenstrual intervals and an overall increase of mean cycle length and variance.

The hormonal characteristics of this transitional phase are of special interest and importance. The irregular episodes of vaginal bleeding in premenopausal women represent the irregular maturation of ovarian follicles, with or without hormonal evidence of ovulation. The potential for hormone secretion by these remaining follicles is diminished and variable. Menses are sometimes preceded by maturation of a follicle, accompanied by limited secretion of both estradiol and progesterone. Vaginal bleeding also occurs after a rise and fall of estradiol concentrations without a measurable increase in progesterone, as occurs in anovulatory menses. In view of the spectrum of hormonal changes observed during this transitional period, one can postulate that residual follicles are responsible for the limited estradiol secretion that precedes episodes of anovulatory bleeding. Whether ovulation actually occurs during any of these cycles is not known; nevertheless, the potential for conception during this time is minimal.

These findings illustrate clearly that the transitional phase of menstrual irregularity is not one of marked estrogen deficiency. During the menopausal transition, high concentrations of FSH in serum appear to stimulate residual follicles to secrete bursts of estradiol. These outbursts may be followed by formation of a corpus luteum, often with limited secretion of progesterone. Because the episodes of follicular maturation and vaginal bleeding are widely spaced, premenopausal women may be exposed to persistent stimulation of the endometrium by estrogen in the absence of regular cyclic progesterone secretion, which is thought to be related to the irregular uterine bleeding common to this period.

Changes in Hormone Metabolism Associated with Menopause

Following menopause, there are major changes in the secretion of androgen, estrogen, progesterone, and gonadotropin, primarily because of the cessation of ovarian follicular activity. It is not known how soon these changes are established after the last period, but they are definitely present within six months.

Androgens

During reproductive life, the primary ovarian androgen is *androstenedione*, the major secretory product of developing follicles (3, 4). At menopause, the circulating androstenedione decreases to about one-half the concentration found in young women, reflecting the absence of follicular activity. Older women exhibit a circadian variation of androstenedione, with peak concentrations between 08:00 hours and noon, and a nadir between 15:00 and 04:00 hours. This rhythm reflects adrenal activity. The clearance rate of androstenedione is similar in pre- and postmenopausal women, so the concentration of circulating hormone reflects its production. Thus, the average production rate of androstenedione is approximately 1.5 mg/24 h in postmenopausal subjects, or one-half the rate in premenopausal women. The source of most of this circulating androstenedione appears to be the adrenal glands, but the postmenopausal ovary continues to secrete about 20% of the total.

The mean concentration of *testosterone* in postmenopausal women is minimally lower than that in premenopausal women before ovariectomy and is distinctly higher than that observed in ovariectomized young women. There is also a prominent nyctohemeral variation of this androgen, the highest concentrations occurring at 08:00 hours and the lowest at 16:00 hours. There is no difference in the clearance rate of testosterone before and after the menopause. Thus, the production rate in older women is approximately 150 μg/24 h, only one-third lower than the rate in young women.

The source of the circulating testosterone is more complex than that of androstenedione. After menopause, ovariectomy is associated with a nearly 60% decrease of testosterone. Because ovariectomy does not change the metabolic clearance rate of this androgen, the fall in the quantity in circulation reflects alterations of its production rate. Fourteen percent of circulating androstenedione is converted to testosterone. The small simultaneous decrease of androstenedione after ovariectomy can account for only a small portion of the total decrease of testosterone; the remainder presumably represents direct ovarian secretion and exceeds the amount secreted directly by the premenopausal ovary. Large increments of testosterone have been found in the ovarian veins of postmenopausal women, exceeding the concentrations observed in premenopausal women, which supports the hypothesis that the postmenopausal ovary secretes more testosterone directly than does the premenopausal gonad. Hilar cells and luteinized stromal cells (hyperthecosis) are present in postmenopausal ovaries and have been shown to produce testosterone in premenopausal women; presumably, these cells could do the same in postmenopausal subjects. A proposed mechanism for increased ovarian production of testosterone by postmenopausal ovaries is the stimulation of gonadal cells, still capable of androgen production, by excess endogenous gonadotropins, which in turn are increased because of the reduction in estrogen production by the ovaries. This increased ovarian secretion of testosterone, coupled with a decrease of estrogen production, may partly explain the symptoms of defeminization, hirsutism, and even virilism that some older women occasionally develop.

For the adrenal androgens *dehydroepiandrosterone and dehydroepiandrosterone sulfate,* concentrations decrease by 60% and 80%, respectively, with age *(5).* Whether these reductions are related to the menopause or to aging has not been determined. Again, a marked circadian variation of dehydroepiandrosterone has been observed; whether a similar rhythm is present for dehydroepiandrosterone sulfate is not known. As with younger subjects, the primary source of these two androgens is thought to be the adrenal glands, with the ovary contributing less than 25%. Thus, the marked decreases of dehydroepiandrosterone and dehydroepiandrosterone sulfate reflect altered adrenal secretion of androgens, a phenomenon that has been called the "adrenopause." The mechanism responsible for this is unknown.

In summary, there are three major changes in androgen metabolism with the menopause and aging: *(a)* reduction of androgen production, particularly androstenedione by the ovary; *(b)* continuation of ovarian secretion of androgens, particularly testosterone; and *(c)* reduction of adrenal secretion of androgens, particularly dehydroepiandrosterone and dehydroepiandrosterone sulfate.

Estrogens

Most subjects who have passed the menopause show good clinical evidence of decreased endogenous production of estrogens *(3, 4).* In terms of concentrations in circulation the greatest decrease is in *estradiol,* which is distinctly less than that found in young women during any phase of their menstrual cycle and is similar to that in premenopausal women after ovariectomy. There is no apparent nyctohemeral variation of the circulating concentration of estradiol after menopause. The metabolic clearance rate of estradiol is reduced by 30%; its average production rate is 12 μg/24 h.

The source of the small amount of estradiol produced in older women has now been established as primarily the adrenal glands *(6)*; direct ovarian secretion contributes minimally. Investigators who have examined the concentrations of estradiol in adrenal veins have reported only minimal increases, which argues against direct adrenal secretion as a major contributor to the total concentrations. Although both estrone and testosterone are converted in peripheral tissues to estradiol, the conversion of estradiol from estrone accounts for most estradiol in older women.

After menopause, the circulating concentration of *estrone* exceeds that of estradiol and overlaps with values seen in premenopausal women during the early follicular phase of their menstrual cycles. There is a nyctohemeral variation of circulating estrone, with the peak in the morning and the nadir in late afternoon or early evening, but this variation is not as prominent as that observed for the androgens. In postmenopausal women, there is a 20% reduction of estrone clearance, and the average production rate is approximately 55 μg/24 h.

Again, the adrenal gland is the major source of this estrogen, but direct adrenal or ovarian secretion is minimal. Most estrone results from the peripheral aromatization of androstenedione. The average percentage of conversion, double that found in ovulatory women, can account for the total daily production of this estrogen. Aromatization of androstenedione has been demonstrated in fat, muscle, liver, bone marrow, brain, fibroblasts, and hair roots; other tissues may also contribute but have not been evaluated. To what extent each cell type contributes to total conversion has not been determined, but fat cells and muscle may be responsible for only 30 to 40%. Moreover, this conversion correlates with body size, heavy women having higher conversion rates and greater concentrations of circulating estrogen than do slender subjects.

Progesterone

In young women, the major source of progesterone is the ovarian corpus luteum after ovulation. During the follicular phase of the cycle, concentrations of progesterone are low. With ovulation, the concentrations rise greatly, reflecting the secretory activity of the corpus luteum. In postmenopausal women, the concentrations of progesterone are only 30% of those in young women during the follicular phase (5). Because postmenopausal ovaries do not contain functional follicles, ovulation does not occur and progesterone concentrations remain low. The source of the small amount of progesterone in older women is presumed to reflect adrenal secretion, but this matter has not been studied critically.

Gonadotropins

With the menopause, concentrations of both LH and FSH increase substantially. FSH usually exceeds LH, which is thought to reflect the slower clearance of FSH from the circulation. The reason for the marked increase in circulating gonadotropins is the absence of the negative feedback of ovarian steroids, and possibly inhibin, on gonadotropin release. As in young women, the concentrations of both gonadotropins are not steady but show random oscillations, representing pulsatile secretion by the pituitary. In older women, these pulsatile bursts occur every 1 to 2 h, a frequency similar to that seen during the follicular phase of premenopausal subjects. However, the amplitude of the bursts is much greater, secondary to increased release of the hypothalamic hormone gonadotropin-releasing hormone (GnRH) and enhanced responsiveness of the pituitary to GnRH because of the low concentrations of estrogen. Studies with rhesus monkeys suggest that the site governing pulsatile LH release is in the arcuate nucleus of the hypothalamus. The large pulses of gonadotropin in the peripheral circulation are believed to maintain the high concentrations of the hormones found in postmenopausal women.

Climacteric Symptoms

Hot Flashes

The most common and characteristic symptom of the climacteric is an episodic disturbance consisting of sudden flushing and perspiration, referred to as a "hot flush" or "flash." It has been observed in 65 to 76% of menopausal women (7, 8). Varying in severity and frequency, the flashes can occur every 20 min or as infrequently as once or twice per month *(9)*; women with severe flashes have episodes about once an hour. Eighty percent of those having hot flashes will experience intermittent symptoms for longer than a year, whereas 25 to 35% complain of episodes for longer than five years *(7, 10)*.

Measurable changes in physiological function accompany hot flashes, thus supporting the physiological basis of the symptom. Cutaneous vasodilation, perspiration, decreases in core temperature, and increases in pulse rate have been recorded *(9, 11)*; the cutaneous vasodilation is generalized and not limited to the upper trunk and head. No changes of heart rhythm or blood pressure have been observed, however *(11, 12)*.

These alterations in physiological function do not correspond identically to the perception of symptoms. Women first become conscious of symptoms about 1 min after the onset of measurable cutaneous vasodilation, and discomfort persists for an average of 4 min; the physical changes continue for several minutes longer *(9, 13)*.

The exact mechanism responsible for hot flashes is not known. On the basis of physiological and behavioral data, the symptom may result from a defect in central thermoregulatory function. Several observations support this conclusion:

First, the two major physiological changes associated with hot flashes are the result of different peripheral sympathetic functions. Excitation of sweat glands is by sympathetic cholinergic fibers *(14)*, whereas cutaneous vasoconstriction is under the exclusive control of tonic α-adrenergic fibers *(15)*. It is difficult to envision some peripheral event that produces both cholenergic effects on sweat glands and α-adrenergic blockade of cutaneous vessels, but these are well recognized as the two basic mechanisms that are triggered by central thermoregulatory centers to lower the core temperature.

Second, during a hot flash, the central temperature decreases after cutaneous vasodilation and perspiration. If hot flashes were the result of some peripheral event, one would expect the body's regulatory mechanisms to prevent this decrease.

The third indication is the change in behavior associated with the symptom. Women feel warm and have a conscious desire to cool themselves, by throwing off bedcovers, standing by open windows and doors, fanning themselves, etc. These perceptions occur in the presence of a decrease of central temperature.

An analogous dissociation between perception and central temperature is found at the onset of a fever, when the individual feels cold or experiences a "chill" before any change of central temperature. Most investigators working in the field of temperature regulation consider that fever is the result of an increase of the set point of central thermoregulatory centers, particularly those in the rostral hypothalamus (16). Pyrogen elevates the central set point, and the febrile organism actively raises the central body temperature by both physiological (cutaneous vasoconstriction and shivering) and behaviorial mechanisms (curling in a ball, putting on more clothes, drinking hot liquids, etc.) (17).

Analogously, the climacteric hot flash may be triggered by a sudden downward setting of central, hypothalamic thermostats. Mechanisms for heat loss are activated to bring the core temperature in line with the new set point, thus causing the core temperature to fall.

Because hot flashes occur after ovarian function has ceased, the underlying mechanism is presumed to be endocrinological, and has something to do with either enhanced secretion of gonadotropins or reduced ovarian secretion of estrogens. Studies have now correlated the occurrence of the symptoms with the pulsatile release of LH from the pituitary (18, 19). This close temporal relationship suggests that LH or the factors that initiate pulsatile LH release are involved with the triggering of these thermoregulatory events. LH or increased pituitary activity is not responsible, because hot flashes have been described in patients after surgical hypophysectomy, persons who have low concentrations of gonadotropin and no pulsatile release (20, 21).

Most probably, a suprapituitary mechanism initiates hot flashes and is somehow influenced by the hypothalamic factors responsible for pulsatile LH release. In monkeys the hypothalamic site governing pulsatile release of LH from the pituitary is the arcuate nucleus, through the pulsatile release of gonadoliberin (gonadotropin-releasing hormone, GnRH) (22). Secretion of GnRH is governed by neurotransmitter input, including factors such as norepinepherine, dopamine, endorphins, and prostaglandins (23, 24). Thus, GnRH or the neurotransmitters that influence its release may somehow alter the set point of the thermoregulatory centers to trigger hot flashes.

This symptom complex is a greater disturbance than most physicians have recognized. Patients experiencing flashes frequently complain of "night sweats" and insomnia, there being a close temporal relationship between the occurrence of hot flashes and waking episodes (25). In women with frequent flashes, the average occurrence rate of flashes and waking episodes is hourly, resulting in a profound sleep disturbance.

Because of the subjective nature of the complaint, it is not surprising that numerous agents have been used in an attempt to relieve the symptom, and that many are said to be effective. Adding to the confusion are observations of several investigative teams, who have found marked effects with placebo (26, 27). Studies showing a placebo action have usually quantified the occurrence of flashes by subjective criteria. The use of objective measurements of flashes, however, has largely eliminated this apparent placebo effect (28, 29).

The principal medications used to relieve hot flashes are estrogens. Good randomized, prospective, double-blind, cross-over studies show beneficial effects of this treatment (21). Estrogens block both the subjective sensation and the physiological changes (3, 20, 21). Daily doses of 625 μg of conjugated estrogens or its equivalent are frequently effective, but higher doses may be required. Progestins are also effective (22), daily doses such as 10–20 mg of medroxyprogesterone acetate being recommended. Clonidine, an α-adrenergic agonist, is partly effective but at doses (200–400 μg) that result in frequent side effects (23). Propranolol, an α-adrenergic antagonist, is not more effective than placebo. Vitamins E and K, mineral supplements, belladonna alkaloids in combination with mild sedatives, tranquillizers, sedatives, and antidepressants have all been used, but their efficacies have not been critically evaluated.

Osteoporosis

Osteoporosis is the single most important health hazard associated with menopause. An estimated 700 000 new fractures associated with osteoporosis occur annually in America, and acute care of these fractures costs more than $1 billion each year (30, 31).

The breaking strength of bone is linearly related to its mineral content; when bone mass falls below a critical threshold level, the bone can fracture without a precipitating traumatic cause. On the basis of epidemiological data and roentgenographic appearances of bone, the "fracture threshold" can be identified as bone mass values that are one standard deviation (1 SD) below the mean for young normal women in respect to fractures of the distal forearm and 2.5 SD below the mean for young normal women for fractures of the neck of the femur (32). The increased incidence of fractures that are age- and sex-related can be attributed to the progressive increase in the proportion of the population whose dimensions fall below these thresholds with advancing age.

Bone mass is determined by two factors—the amount of bone mass at skeletal maturity and the rate of bone loss with age. Variance of initial bone density explains some of the racial and sexual differences in the occurrence of osteoporotic fractures, with white women having the lightest skeletons and black men the heaviest; white men and black women are intermediate in skeletal structure (33). Because most individuals achieve satisfactory bone mass in young adult life, bone loss with aging must be the main determinant of osteoporosis.

Age-related bone loss is two- to threefold greater in women than in men (34), and is accentuated by the cessation of ovarian function, which is a particular problem in women who have been castrated at an early age or have gonadal dysgenesis. Thus, women are more likely to sustain fractures from osteoporosis. Cross-sectional studies show that one-third of the white women in the northern United States will sustain a hip fracture by the ninth decade of life (35). There is a 10-fold increase of Colles' fractures (just above the wrist) in women from age 35 to 65 years, but no similar increase is seen in men (36). More than 150 000 women in the United States sustain hip fractures annually (37), of whom 12% will die from these fractures in the four to five months following the injury. Hip fractures are the number one cause of accidental deaths in women over the age of 75, and falls are the tenth leading cause of death of all women in this country (38).

The mechanisms responsible for the increase in bone loss at menopause have not been completely defined. At first, it was thought to be due to decreased bone formation (39); today, controversy continues on whether osteoporosis results from an absolute increase in bone resorption or an absolute decrease in bone formation. Discrepant results probably can be explained by differences in and limitations of methods for assessing bone turnover and also the heterogeneity of the disease. Nevertheless, all studies, regardless of the methods used, show that bone resorption exceeds formation in osteoporotic patients.

The onset of bone loss is associated with slight increases in the concentrations of calcium, phosphate, and alkaline phosphatase in plasma as well as of calcium and hydroxyproline in urine (40). The transient increase of serum calcium decreases the secretion of parathyrin (PTH, parathyroid hormone). Both the decrease in PTH and the resulting increase in phosphate in serum lower the rate of production of 1,25-dihydroxycholecalciferol and thus reduce the absorption of calcium from the gut (41). Low serum concentrations of PTH also reduce renal tubal reabsorption of calcium. Decreased calcium absorption from the gut and increased calcium loss through the kidney normalize the serum concentration of calcium. Thus, in elderly women this concentration is maintained more by bone loss than by absorbed dietary calcium.

PTH, the principal hormone that stimulates bone resorption, plays a central role in the genesis of osteoporosis: in animal and human studies, osteoporosis does not develop in its absence (42). Concentrations of PTH in most patients with osteoporotic fractures are normal or low (43). This suggests that bone may become more sensitive to concentrations of PTH after the menopause.

Reduction of ovarian production of estrogen also plays a key role, as shown by the increase in bone loss with discontinuation of ovarian function and the reductions in measures of bone resorption with estrogen replacement. Researchers currently hypothesize that estrogen decreases the sensitivity of bone to PTH, and the decrease of estrogen at the menopause thus accelerates bone loss. The mechanisms by which estrogen accomplishes this are not clear. In vivo animal studies have shown that estrogens do indeed decrease the effect of PTH on bone (38), but in vitro data are not as convincing (45). These latter observations are supported by the inability of investigators to document the presence of estrogen receptors in bone (46).

If estrogen receptors are not present, then estrogen must exert its action on bone resorption indirectly. A likely possibility for this action is through its effect on the secretion of calcitonin, a potent inhibitor of bone resorption. The concentrations of calcitonin and the rates of its secretion are lower in women than men, and decrease with age in both sexes *(47)*. After age 50, the response of calcitonin secretion to calcium challenge is negligible.

Estrogen enhances calcitonin secretion in both animals and humans *(48)*; thus the increased secretion of calcitonin could inhibit calcium loss from bone and possibly prevent the development of osteoporosis. Several studies indicate low-dose estrogen therapy can arrest or retard bone loss if begun shortly after the menopause. This effect continues for at least 10 years *(49)*. The lowest dosage that is effective in most older women is 625 μg of conjugated estrogens or its equivalent *(50)*. Estrogen therapy also apparently reduces the incidence of fracture.

Calcium supplements also inhibit bone loss *(51)* and should be given (1000–1500 mg/day) in combination with vitamin D in patients with malabsorption. Administration of vitamin D or its metabolites alone is not successful, possibly because of the bone-resorbing action of these agents. Progestins also appear to have a beneficial effect, but need more thorough evaluation *(52)*. Small doses of calcitonin combined with calcium have increased the total body content of calcium during the first 24 months of therapy but not thereafter *(53)*. To date, histological studies of bone have failed to confirm this increase, however *(54)*. Sodium fluoride increases trabecular bone volume, and in high doses may reduce the vertebral fracture rate *(55)*. It has generally been used in combination with large doses of vitamin D and calcium, which makes the beneficial effects of fluoride alone difficult to assess. Moreover, at the doses studied, fluoride has toxic side effects. Anabolic steroids have been widely used, and may also be effective, but are associated with severe androgenic symptoms in some patients.

In summary, a growing list of publications indicates that the menopause and the associated reduction of endogenous estrogens play major roles in the development of osteoporosis in older women. The mechanisms by which estrogens exert this action have not been completely defined. Osteoporosis remains the most serious complication accompanying the loss of ovarian function and represents the major reason to contemplate replacement therapy.

Cardiovascular Symptoms

In general, the incidence of death from coronary heart disease increases with age in all populations and both sexes. In the United States, cardiovascular disease is the leading cause of death in men and women (56). Cardiovascular disease is less prevalent in women than men before the age of 55, with a man's chance of dying of a heart attack being five- to 10-fold greater than a woman's before this age (57). The ratio falls off dramatically somewhere between the ages of 55 and 65, and reaches unity in the ninth decade. A closer look at the statistics reveals that the data for cardiovascular mortalities among women, when plotted against age, produce a curve of essentially constant slope, not changing as it passes through the age of the menopause; rather, it is the change in slope of the male curve at this age that eventually results in both curves coinciding.

Two types of studies have been used to determine whether cessation of ovarian function is associated with an increased incidence of heart disease. The first type involves an examination of the relationship between the menopause and carefully defined cardiovascular disease within the context of an entire population. In Sweden, systematic samples from cohorts of women were examined and classified on the basis of past history of myocardial infarction, angina pectoris, and electrocardiographic evidence of ischemic heart disease (58). The women with cardiovascular disease were found to have undergone menopause earlier than their cohorts. The Framingham study reported the results of 24 years of biennial exams of nearly 3000 women (59) and showed that, indeed, the increased incidence of heart disease in women after menopause was not just age related. The impact of the menopause was substantial and relatively abrupt, with the incidence of heart disease afterwards increasing only slowly, if at all. Heart disease in premenopausal women was unusual and, when present, was usually mild, being just angina pectoris. Other investigators assessed the risk of nonfatal myocardial infarction among groups of American nurses (60): risks were inversely related to age of natural menopause and especially to age of surgical menopause; the risk to women who underwent oophorectomy before the age of 35 was greater than sevenfold that of nurses with intact ovaries.

275

The second type of study has been case-control studies, in which the degree of coronary heart disease or the incidence of myocardial infarction in women who have undergone early castration is compared with that in age-matched controls who still had ovarian function (61). Some of these studies found an increased risk of cardiovascular disease in the castrated subjects. Most of these reports, however, have been criticized for inadequate numbers of study subjects, imprecise methods for assessing heart disease, or bias in patient selection, particularly the controls.

Skin Changes

With aging, noticeable changes of the skin occur: gradual thinning and atrophy, which are more pronounced in areas exposed to light, and wrinkling, which is attributed to degeneration of elastic and collogenous fibers by exposure to solar radiation (62). The epidermis thins in old age and the basal layer becomes even. Dehydration and vascular sclerosis are also present to various degrees. Sudoriferous and sebaceous glands atrophy and decrease activity. According to some investigators, these changes begin by age 30, and intensify between 40 and 50 years of age.

Very few studies have been performed to isolate the effect of menopause from that of aging on human skin. Several investigators have shown decreased uptake of radiolabeled thymidine (a marker of mitosis) and decreased thickness of the skin after oophorectomy, but appropriate surgical controls were not evaluated (62, 63). More work is clearly needed in this area.

Estrogen does affect skin. Using skin from animal and human models, investigators have shown that the hormone increases the thickness of skin, its hyaluronic acid and water content, vascularization, uptake of tritiated thymidine, and synthesis, maturation, and turnover of collagen (64). Estrogen also reduces the size and activity of sebaceous glands and the rate of hair growth. Some studies, however, have not confirmed all of these biological actions.

These effects are probably the result of direct actions of the hormone on skin elements. Estrogen receptors have been identified in skin of humans and laboratory animals. In mice, the receptors are localized to specific elements of skin, including fibroblasts in the dermis and nuclei of basal cell layers of perineal skin, but not in skin from other areas of the body (65). In humans, high-affinity, low-capacity, estrogen-specific binding has been identified (66). The amount of receptor is highest in facial skin, followed by breast and thigh skins. The number of receptors per cell is considerably lower than in other hormone-responsive tissues, probably because of localization of receptors in only a few elements of skin, as observed with laboratory animals, but further studies are awaited to define this.

A few investigators have examined the effects of estrogen on skin in vivo (62, 64, 67). Most of these studies have been troubled by inadequate controls, nonspecific changes, or inconsistent results. Thus, no compelling body of data exists to show a beneficial effect of estrogen on the integument.

Psychological Effects

Several studies have shown an increase in psychological complaints at the time of the menopause (68, 69) and an associated increase in consultations for emotional problems and use of psychotropic drugs (70). The frequency of psychological symptoms tends to be maximal just preceding the menopause, then declines during the year or so after the cessation of menses. This increase of symptoms does not appear to be associated with an increase in the occurrence of severe psychiatric illness (71).

Two physiological alterations related to the menopause affect psychological function and could explain, in part, the increase of psychological complaints at the climacteric. As mentioned previously, hot flashes during the night are closely related with waking episodes, resulting in a chronic sleep disturbance (25). Such a disturbance can lead to alterations of psychological function, including both cognitive and affective elements. The impact of this on the rate of psychological complaints in perimenopausal women needs to be determined.

Vaginal atrophy can also affect psychological function. At the time of menopause, a majority of women experience an apparent decrease in sexual interest (72). This decline is not seen in all women, and some report increased interest, at least temporarily. However, vaginal atrophy can affect sexual interest by influencing vaginal dryness and dyspareunia. With more prolonged estrogen deficiency, the vaginal epithelium becomes atrophic, the vaginal canal narrows and shortens, and the thinned epithelium is susceptible to trauma. These all lead to complaints of dyspareunia, resulting in a decline in sexual enjoyment and interest and affecting psychological function.

Whether the menopause alters psychological function by mechanisms other than those related to hot flashes and vaginal atrophy is not clear. Future investigators seeking to answer this question will need to control carefully for the confounding effects of these two variables.

Also, the influence of estrogen replacement on psychological symptoms is not established, and again is influenced by the confounding variables of hot flashes and vaginal atrophy. Estrogen replacement clearly diminishes the occurrence of hot flashes and improves certain aspects of sleep in comparison with placebo (25, 27): its beneficial effects include decreases in insomnia, sleep latency, and the number and duration of episodes of wakefulness; and increases in length of sleep and the amount of rapid-eye-movement (REM) sleep (73). These actions are different from those observed with most hypnotic agents, which reduce both sleep latency and the time of REM sleep (74). Improvements of sleep presumably explain the measurable improvements of memory and the decreases of anxiety and irritability that follow estrogen administration in women with severe flashes (27). Estrogen replacement also diminishes the symptoms of vaginal atrophy, leading to improved sexual enjoyment and interest. Whether estrogen influences other aspects of female sexuality is far less clear. Controlled studies of estrogen treatment of perimenopausal women have not found an effect on sexuality other than improved vaginal lubrication (27). Two studies of oophorectomized women have produced conflicting results: one showed no effect on "libido," whereas in the other, estrogens enhanced the women's sexual interest and enjoyment (75, 76).

Does estrogen have mood-elevating effects, other than those exerted by reducing hot flashes or improving vaginal lubrication? Carefully controlled studies will be necessary to answer this question. If it does, it may affect cerebral function through actions on metabolism of indoleamines. Given that reduced concentrations of 5-hydroxytryptamine, 5-hydroxyindoleacetic acid, and serotonin in the brain may lead to depression (77), it may be important that estrogen displaces tryptophan from binding sites on albumin, which could increase availability of this amino acid to the brain *(78)*. Indirect evidence *(79)* indicates that the rate-limiting step in the synthesis of brain 5-hydroxytryptamine is the concentration of L-tryptophan, which is not readily available to the brain because it is bound to plasma albumin *(80)*. Increased availability of tryptophan to the brain could conceivably influence brain function, but this biochemical hypothesis is quite speculative.

References

1. Vollman RF. *The Menstrual Cycle*, W. B. Saunders, Philadelphia, PA, 1977, p. 193.
2. Sherman BM, Korenman SG. Hormonal characteristics of the human menstrual cycle throughout reproductive life. *J Clin Invest* **55**, 669 (1975).
3. Judd HL. Hormonal dynamics associated with the menopause. *Clin Obstet Gynecol* **19**, 775 (1976).
4. Vermeulen A. The hormonal activity of the postmenopausal ovary. *J Clin Endocrinol Metab* **42**, 247 (1976).
5. Abraham GE, Maroulis GB. Effect of exogenous estrogen on serum pregnenolone, cortisol, and androgens in postmenopausal women. *Obstet Gynecol* **45**, 271 (1975).
6. Siiteri PK, MacDonald PC. Role of extraglandular estrogen in human endocrinology. In *Handbook of Physiology, Sect 7, Endocrinology*, vol **2**, pt. 1, RO Greep, E Astwood, Eds., Williams & Wilkins, Baltimore, MD, 1973, pp 615–629.
7. Jaszmann L, Van Lith ND, Zaat JCA. The perimenopausal symptoms. *Med Gynaecol Androl Sociol* **4**, 268–276 (1969).
8. McKinlay S, Jefferys M. The menopausal syndrome. *Br J Prev Soc Med* **28**, 108–115 (1974).
9. Tataryn IV, Lomax P, Meldrum DR, et al. Objective techniques for the assessment of postmenopausal hot flashes. *Obstet Gynecol* **57**, 340–344 (1981).
10. Thompson B, Hart SA, Durno D. Menopausal age and symptomatology in general practice. *J Biol Sci* **5**, 71–82 (1973).
11. Molnar GW. Investigation of hot flashes by ambulatory monitoring. *Am J Physiol* **237**, R306–310 (1979).
12. Sturdee DW, Wilson KA, Pipili E, Crocker AD. Physiological aspects of menopausal hot flush. *Br Med J* **ii**, 79–80 (1978).
13. Ginsberg J, Swinhoe J, O'Reilly B. Cardiovascular responses during menopausal hot flush. *Br J Obstet Gynaecol* **88**, 925–930 (1981).

14. Venables R. *Methods in Psychophysiology.* CC Brown, Ed., Williams & Wilkins, Baltimore, MD, 1967, pp 1–26.
15. Greenfield AD. The circulation through the skin. *Handb Physiol, Sect* 2, vol **2**, 1325–1351 (1963).
16. Kluger MJ. The evolution and adaptive value of fever. *Ann Sci* **66**, 38–43 (1978).
17. Reynolds WW, Casterlin ME, Covert JB. Behavioral fever in teleost fishes. *Nature* **259**, 41–42 (1974).
18. Tataryn IV, Meldrum DR, Lu KH, et al. LH, FSH, and skin temperature during the menopausal hot flash. *J Clin Endocrinol Metab* **49**, 152–154 (1979).
19. Casper RF, Yen SSC, Wilkes MM. Menopausal flushes: A neuroendocrine link with pulsatile luteinizing hormone secretion. *Science* **205**, 823–825 (1979).
20. Mulley G, Mitchell JRA, Tattersall RB. Hot flushes after hypophysectomy. *Br Med J* **ii**, 1062 (1977).
21. Meldrum DR, Erlik Y, Lu JHK, Judd HL. Objectively recorded hot flashes in patients with pituitary insufficiency. *J Clin Endocrinol Metab* **52**, 684–687 (1981).
22. Plant TM, Krey LC, Moossy J, et al. The arcuate nucleus and the control of gonadotropin and prolactin secretion in the female rhesus monkey. *Endocrinology* **102**, 52–62 (1978).
23. Leblanc H, Lachelin GCL, Abu-Fadil S, Yen SSC. Effects of dopamine agonists on LH release in women. *J Clin Endocrinol Metab* **44**, 728–732 (1976).
24. Pang CN, Zimmerman E, Sawyer CH. Morphine inhibition of the preovulatory surges of plasma luteinizing hormone and follicle stimulating hormone in the rat. *Endocrinology* **101**, 1726–1732 (1977).
25. Erlik Y, Tataryn IV, Meldrum DR, et al. Association of waking episodes with menopausal hot flushes. *J Am Med Assoc* **245**, 1741–1744 (1981).
26. Coope J. Double-blind cross-over study of estrogen replacement therapy. In *The Management of the Menopause and Postmenopausal Years.* S Campbell, Ed., University Park Press, Baltimore, MD, 1978, pp 159–168.
27. Campbell S, Whitehead M. Estrogen therapy and the postmenopausal syndrome. *Clin Obstet Gynecol* **4**, 31 47 (1977).
28. Erlik Y, Meldrum DR, Lagasse LD, Judd HL. Effect of megestrol acetate on flushing and bone metabolism in postmenopausal women. *Maturitas* **3**, 167–172 (1981).
29. Laufer LR, Erlik Y, Meldrum DR, Judd HL. Effect of clonidine on hot flashes in postmenopausal women. *Obstet Gynecol* **60**, 583–586 (1982).

30. Owens RA, Melton LJ III, Gallagher JC, Riggs BL. National cost of acute case of hip fractures associated with osteoporosis. *Clin Orthop* **150**, 172–176 (1980).
31. Melton LJ III, Riggs BL. Epidemiology of age-related fractures. In *Osteoporotic Syndrome: Detection and Prevention*, LV Avioli, Ed., in press.
32. Newton-John HF, Morgan DB. Osteoporosis—disease or senescence? *Lancet* **i**, 232–233 (1968).
33. Trotter M, Broman GE, Peterson RR. Densities of bones of white and negro skeletons. *J Bone Jt Surg* **42A**, 50–58 (1960).
34. Riggs BL, Wahner HW, Seeman E, et al. Changes in bone mineral density of the proximal femur and spine with aging: Differences between the postmenopausal and senile osteoporosis syndrome. *J Clin Invest* **70**, 716–723 (1982).
35. Gallager JC, Melton LJ, Riggs BL, Bergstralh E. Epidemiology of fractures of the proximal femur. *Clin Orthop* **150**, 163–171 (1980).
36. Knowelden J, Buhr AJ, Dunbar O. Incidence of fractures in persons over 35 years of age. *Br J Prev Soc Med* **18**, 130–141 (1964).
37. Gordan GS, Vaughan C. Sex steroids in the clinical management of osteoporosis. *Curr Prob Obstet Gynecol* **5**, 6–45 (1982).
38. *Accident Facts. 1982.* National Safety Council, Chicago, IL, 1982.
39. Albright F, Smith PH, Richardson AM. Postmenopausal osteoporosis. *J Am Med Assoc* **116**, 2465–2474 (1941).
40. Crilly RG, Francis RM, Nordin BEC. Ageing, steroid hormones and bone. *Clin Endocrinol Metab* **10**, 115–139 (1981).
41. Gallagher JC, Riggs BL, Eisman J, et al. Intestinal calcium absorption and serum vitamin D metabolites in normal subjects and osteoporotic patients: Effective age and dietary calcium. *J Clin Invest* **64**, 729–736 (1979).
42. Houssain M, Smith DA, Nordin BEC. Parathyroid activity and postmenopausal osteoporosis. *Lancet* **i**, 809–811 (1970).
43. Gallagher JC, Riggs BL, Jerpbak CM, Arnaud CD. The effect of age on serum immunoreactive parathyroid hormone in normal and osteoporotic women. *J Lab Clin Med* **95**, 373–385 (1980).
44. Gallagher JC, Williamson R. Effect of ethinyl estradiol on calcium and phosphorus metabolism in postmenopausal women with primary hyperparathyroidism. *Clin Sci Mol Med* **45**, 785–802 (1973).
45. Atkins D, Zanelli JM, Peacock M, Nordin BEC. The effect of oestrogens on the response of bone to parathyroid hormone in vitro. *J Endocrinol* **54**, 107–117 (1972).
46. Chen TL, Feldman D. Distinction between alpha-fetoprotein and intracellular estrogen receptors: Evidence against the presence of estradiol receptors in bone. *Endocrinology* **102**, 236–242 (1978).
47. Deftos LJ, Weisman MH, Williams GW, et al. Influence of age and

sex on plasma calcitonin in human beings. *N Engl J Med* **302**, 1351–1353 (1980).

48. Morimoto S, Tsuji M, Okada Y, et al. The effect of oestrogens on human calcitonin secretion after calcium infusion in elderly female subjects. *Clin Endocrinol* **13**, 135–143 (1980).

49. Lindsay R, Hart DM, Forrest C, Baird C. Prevention of spinal osteoporosis in oophorectomized women. *Lancet* **ii**, 1151–1154 (1980).

50. Genant HK, Cann C, Ettinger B, Gordan GS. Quantitative computed tomography of vertebral spongiosa: A sensitive method for detecting early bone loss after oophorectomy. *Ann Intern Med* **97**, 699–705 (1982).

51. Recker RR, Saville PD, Heaney RP. Effect of estrogens and calcium carbonate on bone loss in postmenopausal women. *Ann Intern Med* **87**, 649–655 (1977).

52. Lindsay R, Hart DM, Purdie D, et al. Comparative effects of oestrogen and a progestogen on bone loss in postmenopausal women. *Clin Sci Mol Med* **54**, 193–195 (1978).

53. Jowsey J, Riggs BL, Kelly PJ, Hoffman DL. Calcium and salmon calcitonin in treatment of osteoporosis. *J Clin Endocrinol Metab* **47**, 633–639 (1978).

54. Milhaud G, Talbot JN, Coutris G. Calcitonin treatment of postmenopausal osteoporosis: Evaluation of efficacy by principal components analysis. *Biomedicine* **22**, 223–232 (1975).

55. Riggs BL, Seeman E, Hodgson SF, et al. Effect of fluoride/calcium regimen on vertebral fracture occurrence in postmenopausal osteoporosis. *N Engl J Med* **306**, 446–450 (1982).

56. World Health Organization. Sixth report on the world health situation. Part I. Global analysis. Geneva, Switzerland 1980.

57. Furman RH. Coronary heart disease and the menopause: Menopause and aging. In *Menopause and Aging* (summary report and selected papers from a research conference on menopause and aging), KJ Ryan, DC Gibson, Eds., DHEW Publ. No. (NIH) 73–319, U.S. Government Printing Office, Washington, DC, 1973, pp 39–55.

58. Bengtsson C. Ischemic heart disease in women. *Acta Med Scand* **549** (Suppl), 75–81 (1973).

59. Gordon T, Kannel WB, Hjortland MC, McNamara PM. Menopause and coronary heart disease: The Framingham Study. *Ann Intern Med* **89**, 157–161 (1978).

60. Rosenberg L, Hennekens CH, Rosner B, et al. Early menopause and the risk of myocardial infarction. *Am J Obstet Gynecol* **139**, 47–51 (1981).

61. Roberts WC, Giraldo AA. Bilateral oophorectomy in menstruating

women and accelerated coronary atherosclerosis: An unproved connection. *Am J Med* **67**, 363–365 (1979).

62. Punnoven R. Effect of castration and peroral estrogen therapy on the skin. *Acta Obstet Gynecol Scand* **5** (Suppl 21), 1–44 (1972).

63. Rauramo L. Effect of castration and peroral estradiol valerate and estriol succinate therapy on the epidermis. In *The Management of the Menopause and Postmenopausal Years,* S Campbell, Ed., MTP Press, Lancaster, 1976, pp 253–262.

64. Shahrad P, Marks R. The effects of estrogens on the skin. *Ibid.,* pp 243–251.

65. Stumpf WE, Sar M, Joshi SG. Estrogens target cells in the skin. *Experientia* **30**, 196–198 (1974).

66. Hasselquist MG, Goldberg N, Schroeter A, Spelsberg TC. Isolation and characterization of the estrogen receptor in human skin. *J Clin Endocrinol Metab* **50**, 76–82 (1980).

67. Goldzieher J. The direct effect of steroids on the senile human skin. *J Gerontol* **1**, 104–112 (1946).

68. Ballinger CB. Psychiatric morbidity and the menopause: Screening of a general population sample. *Br Med J* **iii**, 344–346 (1975).

69. Bungay GT, Vessey MP, McPherson CK. Study of symptoms in the middle life with special reference to the menopause. *Br Med J* **281**, 181–183 (1980).

70. Skegg DC, Doll R, Perry J. Use of medicine in general practice. *Br Med J* **i**, 1561–1563 (1977).

71. Weissman MM, Klerman GL. Sex differences and the epidemiology of depression. *Arch Gen Psychiatry* **34**, 98–111 (1977).

72. Hallstrom T. *Mental Disorder and Sexuality in the Climacteric.* Scandinavian Univ. Books, Esselte Studium, Stockholm, 1973.

73. Schiff I, Regestein Q, Tulchinsky D, Ryan KJ. Effects of estrogens on sleep and psychological state of hypogonadal women. *J Am Med Assoc* **242**, 2405–2407 (1979).

74. Kales A, Kales JD, Bixler EO, Scharf MB. Effectiveness of hypnotic drugs with prolonged use: Flurazepam and pentobarbital. *Clin Pharmacol Ther* **18**, 356–363 (1975).

75. Utian WH. The true clinical features of postmenopausal and oophorectomy, and their response to estrogen therapy. *S Afr Med J* **46**, 732–737 (1972)

76. Dennerstein L, Burrows GD, Wood C, Hyman G. Hormones and sexuality: The effects of estrogen and progestogen. *Obstet Gynecol* **56**, 316–322 (1981).

77. Ridges AP. Biochemistry of depression: A review. *J Int Med Res* **3** (Suppl 2), 42–54 (1975).

78. Aylward M. Estrogens, plasma tryptophan levels in perimenopausal patients. In ref. *63*, pp 135–140.
79. Jequier E, Robinson DS, Levenberg W, Sjverdsma A. Tryptophan-5-hydroxylase activity and brain tryptophan metabolism. *Biochem Pharmacol* **18**, 1071–1081 (1969).
80. McMenamy RH, Oncley JL. Specific binding of ʟ-tryptophan to serum albumin. *J Biol Chem* **233**, 1436–1447 (1958).

Menopause: Hormone Therapy and the Effects on Estrogen/Progesterone Receptors

William E. Gibbons

Introduction

Administration of exogenous estrogen has been used in the therapy of the estrogen-deficient, postmenopausal woman for many years. The acute beneficial effects of reducing vasomotor flushing (hot flashes) and reversing the thinning of urogenital tissues have led to widespread acceptance of estrogen therapy in this country. Only more recently has there been sufficient documentation of the benefits of estrogen therapy for women with osteoporosis. The difficulty in demonstrating these benefits stemmed from the slow nature of the onset of osteoporosis, the multiple factors (e.g., exercise) that affect changes in bone mass, the necessary technology for monitoring changes, and the duration of estrogen therapy required to demonstrate benefit.

Before the osteoporosis issue could be resolved, the course of estrogen replacement therapy in the United States was irreversibly altered with the observation that use of exogenous estrogen was associated with adenocarcinoma of the endometrium (1, 2). As a result, the use of estrogens during menopause began to decline. Subsequently, however, the relationship of estrogen administration and the progressive development of abnormal endometrial histology has been shown by Paterson et al. (3) to depend on both dose and duration of treatment. By following endometrial biopsies at six-month intervals, Paterson et al. noted that increasing the concentration and potency of the estrogen stimulus increased the incidence of abnormal endometrial pathology, but these changes could be antagonized by administering a progestin. Further, if the progestin was administered for at least 10 days, no abnormalities of the endometrial histology were noted. This suggested a duration-related effect of the progestin use as well.

Even though progestins antagonize the effects of estrogens on endometrial growth, they do not antagonize the benefits of estrogen therapy. Schiff *(4)* has shown that progestins themselves can reduce vasomotor flushing. Mandel et al. *(5)* have also shown that oral medroxyprogesterone acetate can reduce calcium loss through urine. The data of Christiansen et al. *(6)* suggest a synergistic effect between estrogen and progestin that may even increase bone mineral content, an effect only seen by very high doses of estrogen *(7)*.

Whitehead et al. *(8)* have shown that the 19-nortestosterone progestins effectively antagonize the biochemical effects of nuclear accumulation of estrogen receptor, a measure of estrogen activity, and thymidine labeling, an index of cellular mitotic activity. However, the 19-nortestosterones appear to lower the serum concentrations of high-density lipoproteins (HDL), which potentially might increase the risk of arteriosclerotic heart disease *(9)*. Because this adverse affect is not noted with medroxyprogesterone acetate, my colleagues and I eveluted the effects of different concentrations of medroxyprogesterone acetate on endometrial histology and estrogen receptor concentrations in postmenopausal women receiving different dosages of conjugated equine estrogens *(10)*.

Study

In these studies, three groups of postmenopausal women (five women per group) were administered 0.3, 0.625, or 1.25 mg of conjugated equine estrogens, respectively, for 25 days every other month. After an initial month of estrogen alone, the women in each group received in successive treatment-cycles 2.5 mg, then 5.0 mg, then 10 mg of medroxyprogesterone acetate on the last 11 days of the estrogen therapy (cycle days 15 to 25). From endometrial biopsies obtained on the twenty-fifth day of estrogen therapy, we evaluated the concentrations of cytosolic and nuclear estrogen receptors and cell histology. Data from the different dosages of estrogen with and without progestin, as well as from the different concentrations of administered progestin, were compared with baseline histology findings and estrogen receptor concentrations.

Receptor measurement. Figure 1 illustrates the difference between

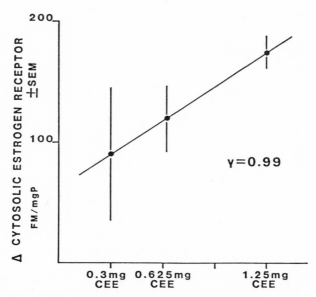

Fig. 1. The relationship between the dosage of conjugated equine estrogens (CEE) and the amount of increase in estrogen receptor (femtomoles per milligram of protein) measured in the cytosol as compared with pretreatment values

the baseline, pretreatment concentrations of cytosolic estrogen receptors and the concentrations after stimulation with estrogen only, for each subject-matched pair of samples. The concentration of estrogen receptor in the cytosol varied linearly with the amount of estrogen administered, with a correlation coefficient of 0.99.

The addition of 2.5 mg of medroxyprogesterone acetate to the estrogen-treatment cycles suppressed the concentrations of cytosolic estrogen receptors to pretreatment values for women receiving 0.3 and 0.625 mg of conjugated estrogens, but not for those receiving 1.25 mg per day (Figure 2, *left*). Addition of 5 or 10 mg of the progestin suppressed cytosolic estrogen receptor content to baseline values in all estrogen-treatment groups. In the cell nuclei, estrogen receptor accumulation was antagonized by all dosages of medroxyprogesterone (Figure 2, *right*).

Histology. Each endometrial biopsy specimen was evaluated for gland epithelial height, gland diameter, percentage of glands

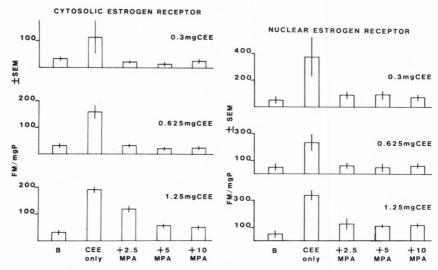

Fig 2. Concentrations of endometrial cytosolic *(left)* and endometrial nuclear *(right)* estrogen receptors from postmenopausal women receiving various doses of conjugated equine estrogen (CEE) to which increasing doses of medroxyprogesterone acetate (MPA) were added

B, baseline values; estrogen receptor concentrations in femtomoles per milligram of protein

showing secretion, quality of secretion, pseudodecidual stroma, and percentages of subnuclear vacuoles. Before treatment, all the biopsy specimens revealed an atrophic endometrium, as did all specimens from biopsies performed four weeks after the last treatment cycle. There was only minimal estrogenic change in the 0.3-mg estrogen group, whereas marked estrogenic stimulation occurred with the 0.625-mg and 1.25-mg estrogen-only specimens.

When medroxyprogesterone acetate was added to the estrogen therapy, the morphological effects varied with the dose. None of the endometrial biopsies from women receiving 2.5 mg of medroxyprogesterone acetate daily demonstrated a progestational response. Because of their biochemical similarity, we compared the responses to the 5-mg and 10-mg medroxyprogesterone acetate treatments. Three women in the 0.625-mg estrogen group and four in the 1.25-mg estrogen group supplied sufficient material for evaluting all of the morphologic parameters (Table 1). In both of these groups the progestagenic response to 10 mg of medroxyprogesterone acetate always exceeded the response to 5 mg. Fur-

Table 1. Comparison of Histologic Effects of Medroxyprogesterone Acetate (MPA) in Postmenopausal Women Receiving Conjugated Equine Estrogens (CEE)

	0.625 mg of CEE daily (n = 3)			1.25 mg of CEE daily (n = 4)		
	MPA dose, mg/day			MPA dose, mg/day		
	5	10	p	5	10	p
Gland epithelial height, μm	17.33 ± 4.04	23.33 ± 7.64	<0.2	23.5 ± 4.43	35.75 ± 9.95	<0.05
Gland diameter, μm	63.33 ± 20.8	105 ± 35	<0.1	91.25 ± 27.5	127.5 ± 35.71	<0.1
Glands showing secretion, %	6.67 ± 5.77	50 ± 14.14	<0.05	42.5 ± 27.2	88.75 ± 9.46	<0.01
Quality of secretion (+)	0.5 ± 0.5	2.16 ± 1.76	<0.1	2 ± 1.08	3.5 ± 0.58	<0.025
Pseudodecidual stroma (+)	0 ± 0	1.13 ± 1.15	<0.1	0.875 ± 1.44	2.5 ± 1.0	<0.1
Subnuclear vacuoles, %	5 ± 7.07	1 ± 1.41		13.75 ± 7.50	3.75 ± 1.50	<0.1

ther, the 10-mg dose of medroxyprogesterone acetate promoted a more homogeneous secretory change in the stroma and glands than the more focal change noted with the 5-mg dose.

Discussion

From a risk/benefit point of view, the most defensible reason for administering estrogens to a postmenopausal woman on a long-term basis is the prevention of osteoporosis. Epidemiologic evidence suggests that those who are at high risk for osteoporotic bone fractures include: fair-skinned or slender persons, smokers, heavy drinkers, those with early menopause, etc. (11). Negative associations for hip fracture include: estrogen-replacement therapy, intact ovaries, and increased weight (12). Hip-fracture patients appear to have lower ideal body weights and higher concentrations of sex-hormone-binding globulin in their serum, which results in lower concentrations of biologically available estradiol and testosterone (13). Subsequently, it has been shown that exogenous estrogens can prevent loss of bone mineral content (14); further, 0.625 mg of conjugated equine estrogens every day orally appears to return urinary calcium/creatinine ratios to their premenopausal range (15). Lindsay et al. (16) have recently reported that conjugated equine estrogens in doses of 0.625 and 1.25 mg per day were equally effective in reducing bone loss, as evaluated by single-photon absorptiometry, but that doses less than 0.625 mg were ineffective.

The route of the estrogen administration may be oral, subcuticular, transdermal, or vaginal. The subcuticular implants appear to produce the highest levels of continuous estrogen stimulation of the endometrium (3) and breast (17), and may pose the highest risk of neoplastic change. A transdermal route such as in an estradiol-containing gel offers several apparent advantages over oral administration: there is less conversion to the less-active estrone and, metabolically, there is less stimulation of estrogen-sensitive proteins (18); however, long-term efficacy in reducing calcium loss still requires clarification (19). The vaginal route similarly can deliver effective local estrogenic stimulation and adequate systemic stimulation but, at least for the conjugated estrogens, requires a higher dose per weight than the oral form for the same effect (20).

The widespread use of estrogen-replacement therapy in post-menopausal women has led to the observation of its relationship to the development of carcinoma of the endometrium *(2)*. This risk has been shown by Gambrell *(21)* and others to be effectively minimized by the concurrent use of a progestin; indeed, Gambrell reports that the addition of a progestin to estrogen replacement can reduce the risk to less than that expected for women on no estrogen replacement. Perhaps of even greater significance, Gambrell et al. *(22)* have reported that the use of progestin postmenopausally may markedly reduce the incidence of breast cancer. The protective effect on the endometrium appears dose-related, with greater benefits when the duration of progestin use each cycle exceeds 10 days. This mirrors the above-mentioned short-term results of Paterson et al. for endometrial histology after estrogen stimulation *(3)*.

The choice of progestin is still controversial. The 19-nortestosterone compounds such as norethindrone are effective in antagonizing the estrogenic stimulation of the endometrium *(8)*, but appear to decrease high-density-lipoprotein concentrations, which might thus increase the risk for ischemic heart disease *(23)*. Such does not seem to happen with natural progesterone or medroxyprogesterone acetate.

In our study we found a disparity between the biochemical and morphological results. Even though 5 and 10 mg of medroxyprogesterone acetate behaved identically in antagonizing increases in cytosolic estrogen receptor, 10 mg was superior by morphological criteria. Further, the progestational change seen with the 10-mg dose resulted in a more pervasive (homogeneous) change, whereas the effect of 5 mg of medroxyprogesterone acetate daily was more focal in nature. Data on abnormal endometrial histology including adenocarcinoma after long-term administration of 5 mg of medroxyprogesterone acetate daily are lacking, but a focal, nonhomogeneous antagonism of estrogen effect would not seem optimal.

This dissociation of the biochemical and endometrial events has been hinted at in the past. For example, Whitehead et al. *(8)* demonstrated a plateauing of effects of treatment after six days of administration. The epidemiological data, on the other hand, suggest that seven days of therapy alone is insufficient to completely block abnormal histological changes *(3, 21)*.

Recommendations

What, then, would be the current recommendation for therapy? If administered orally, and cyclically, 0.625 mg of conjugated equine estrogens currently appears to be the minimal dose for preventing osteoporosis. A progestin should be added to all women on estrogen replacement. The benefits of reduced neoplasia of breast and uterus along with synergistic effects on bone mineral content and vasomotor instability outweigh the inconvenience of withdrawal bleeding. A progestin should be administered for 10 or more days per estrogen cycle. If medroxyprogesterone acetate is used, then 10 mg daily is the lowest recommended dosage.

In our study, 0.3 mg of conjugated equine estrogen provided minimum stimulation of the endometrium. The effects of progestins on endometrial histology is biphasic. In an initial "acute" response, the endometrium converts to a secretory pattern; more chronic exposure results in atrophic change. The synergistic effect of estrogen/progestin on bone loss may allow a further decrease of the "minimum" requirements for each. A combined administration of estrogen/progestin throughout a cycle may result in minimal stimulation of endometrial growth, and the atropic effect of chronic progestin administration may eliminate breakthrough bleeding. Preliminary trials of combination therapy are currently underway.

Who should be treated? Therapy could be limited to symptomatic subjects or those at high risk for osteoporosis. However, because of the suggestion that progestin therapy may reduce breast cancer risk, and until there is an practical, objective method for determining which women don't need hormonal replacement, I recommend that all those without contraindications to therapy should receive estrogen/progestin therapy.

How long should therapy continue? Indefinitely. The limitations or duration of therapy are not defined. The potential for benefits continues throughout the lifespan. Patient compliance or changes in medical status will affect management. Because the understanding and rationale for postmenopausal hormonal replacement is still evolving, one can expect that treatment recommendations will continue to be modified. It is important now that we recognize the benefits of estrogen therapy, comprehend the risks rationally, and add a progestin to all who receive estrogen-replacement therapy.

References

1. Gray LA, Christopherson WM, Hoover RN. Estrogens and endometrial carcinoma. *Obstet Gynecol* **49**, 385–389 (1977).
2. Mack T, Pike M, Henderson, B, et al. Estrogens and endometrial cancer in a retirement community. *N Engl J Med* **294**, 1262–1267 (1976).
3. Paterson ME, Wade-Evans T, Sturdee DW, et al. Endometrial disease after treatment with oestrogens and progestins in the climacteric. *Br Med J* **282**, 822–824 (1980).
4. Schiff I. The effects of progestins on vasomotor flushes. *J Reprod Med* **27**, 498–502 (1982).
5. Mandel FP, Davidson BJ, Erlik Y, et al. Effects of progestins on bone metabolism in postmenopausal women. *J Reprod Med* **27**, 511–514 (1982).
6. Christiansen C, Christensen MS, Transbol I. Bone mass in postmenopausal women after withdrawal of oestrogen/gestagen replacement therapy. *Lancet* **i**, 459–461 (1981).
7. Horsman A, Jones M, Francis R, et al. The effect of estrogen dose on postmenopausal bone loss. *N Engl J Med* **309**, 1405–1407 (1981).
8. Whitehead MI, Townsend PT, Pryse-Davies J, et al. Effects of estrogens and progestins on the biochemistry and morphology of the postmenopausal endometrium. *N Engl J Med* **305**, 1599–1605 (1981).
9. Hirvonen E, Malkonen M, Manninen V. Effects of different progestins on lipoproteins during postmenopausal replacement therapy. *N Engl J Med* **304**, 560–563 (1981).
10. Gibbons WE, Moyer D, Roy S, et al. Biochemical and histological effects of combined estrogen/progestin therapy on the endometrium of postmenopausal women. *Obstet Gynecol* (in press).
11. Saville PD. Postmenopausal osteoporosis and estrogens. Who should be treated and why? *Postgrad Med* **75**, 135–138 (1984).
12. Kreiger N, Kelsey JL, Holford TR, et al. An epidemiologic study of hip fractures in postmenopausal women. *Am J Epidemiol* **116**, 141–148 (1982).
13. Davidson BJ, Ross RK, Paganini-Hill A, et al. Total and free estrogens and androgens in postmenopausal women with hip fractures. *J Clin Endocrinol Metab* **54**, 115–120 (1982).
14. Lindsay R, Hart DM, Aitken JM, et al. Long-term prevention of postmenopausal osteoporosis by oestrogen. Evidence of an increased

bone mass after delayed onset of oestrogen treatment. *Lancet* **i,** 1038–1041 (1976).

15. Geola FL, Frumar AM, Tataryn IV, et al. Biological effects of various doses of conjugated equine estrogens in postmenopausal women. *J Clin Endocrinol Metab* **51,** 620–625 (1980).

16. Lindsay R, Hart DM, Clark DM. The minimum effective dose of estrogen for prevention of postmenopausal bone loss. *Obstet Gynecol* **63,** 759 (1984).

17. Hulka BS, Chambless LE, Deubner DC, et al. Breast cancer and estrogen replacement therapy. *Am J Obstet Gynecol* **143,** 638–644 (1982).

18. Holst J. Percutaneous estrogen therapy. Endometrial response and metabolic effects. *Acta Obstet Gynecol Scand (Suppl)* **115,** 1–30 (1983).

19. Laufer LR, DeFazio JL, Lu JK, et al. Estrogen replacement by transdermal estradiol administration. *Am J Obstet Gynecol* **146,** 533–540 (1983).

20. Mandel FP, Geola FL, Meldrum DR, et al. Biological effects of various doses of vaginally administered conjugated equine estrogens in postmenopausal women. *J Clin Endocrinol Metab* **57,** 133–139 (1983).

21. Gambrell RD Jr. The menopause: Benefits and risks of estrogen–progestin replacement therapy. *Fertil Steril* **37,** 457 (1982).

22. Gambrell RD Jr, Maier RC, Sanders BI. Decreased incidence of breast cancer in postmenopausal estrogen–progestin users. *Obstet Gynecol* **62,** 435–443 (1983).

23. Fahraeus L, Larsson-Cohn U, Wallentin L. L-Norgestrel and progesterone have different influences on plasma lipoproteins. *Eur J Clin Invest* **13,** 447–453 (1983).

Discussion—Session V

Q: Please comment on nonsteroidal treatments of vasal motor symptoms in patients in whom steroids are contraindicated.

DR. JUDD: Our current understanding of this very important issue is as follows. As Dr. Gibbons showed, the use of progestational agents is unequivocally effective in treating hot flashes. The agents that have been examined include Depo-Provera, 150 mg every six weeks to three months; proveritan, 30 mg daily; megestrol acetate, 20 to 80 mg daily; and norethindrone acetate.

For most contraindications of estrogen replacement, the use of progesterone is probably acceptable. Such conditions would include endrometrial cancer, at least in my opinion, and breast cancer; a tendency for clot formation should also probably be included, but this is not clear-cut.

Concerning the use of nonsteroidal preparations, the only one that has been critically evaluated is clonidine (Catapres). In some studies, involving subjective measurements, this has been said to be effective, but not in other studies. I believe we're the only group that has used objective criteria in looking at this drug: we saw a significant decrease in the occurrence of hot flashes at daily doses of 0.4 mg, but all of our patients without exception became symptomatic and all wanted to discontinue the agent. At smaller doses the patients were not symptomatic but we did not see a significant decrease in the number of hot flashes.

Q: What is the current projected duration of estrogen–progesterone therapy? Is post-menopausal therapy to last a lifetime?

DR. GIBBONS: What we have stated as a general qualifier is the fact that by administering the estrogen–progesterone for potentially 10 or 15 years we can place that woman high enough on the curve for loss of bone mass that whenever she finally discontinues estrogen—and some women become intolerant of estrogen therapy as they grow older, which is an individual response—her bone mass will be sufficient that her rate of calcium loss will not reach the point at which she would enter a greatest risk until past her predicted life expectancy. However, we don't have sufficient data to give a specific answer to that.

Secondly, what makes the question difficult is that I really don't believe that the current medications are going to continue to be utilized. That is, it may be found possible to decrease the concentrations of both estrogen and progesterone, especially if they are truly synergistic as some studies suggest, so that we would potentially get fewer side effects from the combinations, so that the patients will tolerate them better. I would be interested in Dr. Judd's comments on this.

There is also some suggestion that women who utilize progestins have a decreased incidence of breast carcinoma. These data are not solid but if such is the case, then we will have something certainly more important than even concern about the risk of osteoporosis.

DR. JUDD: I think the issue of how estrogens—or estrogens plus progesterone—are ultimately given is clearly going to change. The regimes you've been presented today, however, are probably the best regimes currently available.

Q: What are the common complications of osteoporosis that lead to untimely death?

DR. JUDD: This issue is directly related to fracture, particularly fracture of the hip. Then, placing the elderly in bed for extended periods means that the problems of pulmonary embolus and pneumonia become acute.

Q: Is calcium therapy before menopause effective in preventing postmenopausal decrease in bone density?

DR. JUDD: I am not aware of any data that either support or deny that.

Q: Please comment on recent reports that calcitrol, a vitamin D metabolite, can reverse the process of osteoporosis.

DR. JUDD: The problem of aging and bone loss is not just osteoporosis alone; it is a combination of osteoporosis and osteopenia, bone loss. Many postmenopausal women are vitamin D deficient. If you are going to administer calcium to these individuals as therapy for their osteomalacia or even in attempting to prevent osteoporosis, your results will be very limited unless you provide them with vitamin D. There are two ways to approach this. One is to determine whether a patient is or is not vitamin D deficient; the other is to administer vitamin D to all patients

296

you are giving calcium. I have chosen the latter approach. Calcium is an alternative form of therapy in treatment or prevention of osteoporosis. Whether it will be as effective as estrogen replacement we do not yet know. There is no question that calcitrol, the active metabolite of vitamin D, is highly effective in reversing vitamin D deficiency. However, because it is so potent, it can generate problems of vitamin D toxicosis and hypercalcemia.

Q: How do you recommend managing anovulatory or oligoovulatory premenopausal women to avoid problems of estrogen excess later?

DR. JUDD: You don't need to worry about estrogen excess later; rather, you need to worry about unopposed estrogen stimulation of the endometrium in premenopausal women. All patients with reasonable concentrations of estrogen who are not ovulating should be considered for progestational substitution.

Q: If FSH and LH increases are secondary to GnRH release, why is the pattern of FSH not parallel to that of LH?

DR. JUDD: A very perceptive question. We have been unable to show an association between the occurrence of hot flashes and pulsatile FSH release, although Dr. Yen has showed a limited association. The problem is that the clearance rate of FSH is much lower than that of LH. The LH pulse is very sharp and distinct, but the FSH pulse is much more blunted, making it more difficult to show that association. Dr. Elkind-Hirsch showed an association not only between LH and the occurrence of hot flashes, but also between the pulsatile release of GnRH and the occurrence of hot flashes.

Q: Should all postmenopausal women be treated, or only those who are symptomatic? That is, should we expect that bone loss is present in all of these women so that diagnostic lab tests be done for all of them? What are the side effects of treatment?

DR. GIBBONS: From some of the data shown by Dr. Judd, one can generalize that women who are more obese are going to have a greater peripheral conversion of testosterone to estrogen and therefore may have higher circulating concentrations of estrone; certainly, obese women are less prone to be symptomatic. However, women who are overweight have an increased risk for developing endocarcinoma of the endometrium. Overweight women tend to carry a slightly greater bone mass, so they may be at less risk from osteoporosis. However, the concern about the increased risk of endocarcinoma still dictates the need for these women to receive, at some interval, some type of progesterone challenge to antagonize that effect of estrogen.

Thinner women, whether symptomatic or not, should receive estrogen and progesterone. Obese women and women who refuse the progesterone, which is often accompanied by withdrawal bleeding, should have endometrial sampling at some interval, maybe every one or two years to determine that they are not developing a hyperplastic endometrium or worse.

The side effects of treatment vary. There's some concern about weight gain or problems with depression, but I have not found these to be a consistent effect. Some of my patients ask to stay on the progesterone the entire month because that's the only time they don't feel depressed. The weight gain may occur in some patients but this may be slightly antagonized by the progesterone use.

Q: Is treatment different for a patient who's had a hysterectomy than for a postmenopausal patient, since the former has no endometrium?

DR. GIBBONS: The questions can be interpreted in two ways. The woman who loses ovarian function in her thirties is at high risk for experiencing hot flashes and for developing osteoporosis in later years. Whether or not someone who has had a hysterectomy needs a progestin since they do not have the chance of developing endocarcinoma will be answered when we have better data on whether progestins can reduce the incidence of breast cancer. At present I'm recommending that every woman should be receiving progestin to prevent breast cancer.

DR. JUDD: Some very preliminary studies with very limited numbers of patients suggest that progesterone may potentially be protective. But even the best of these, the Nachtigall study, is not conclusive, and it's hard for me to recommend at this time that all postmenopausal women who do not have a uterus go on estrogen plus progesterone.

Concerning which women should or should not receive estrogen replacement, as I see it, the issues of estrogen replacement have to do with alleviating symptoms—hot flashes, vaginal atrophy. The other issues really concern prophylaxis. The two major reasons to consider estrogen replacement for prophylaxis is to prevent osteoporosis in a woman who is entirely asymptomatic and to prevent heart disease in a woman who is entirely asymptomatic. We have scarcely addressed the issue that the menopause appears to be potentially associated with an increase of heart disease. If that proves to be the case, then you can reduce the incidence of deaths from heart attacks in women between the ages of 40 and 60 by two-thirds—which would overwhelm the risk/benefit ratio entirely in favor of therapy. Without any question, this is the most important issue currently being addressed in regard to estrogen replacement.

DR. COOPER: Dr. Judd, I'm really glad you mentioned the cardiovascular aspect. The Lipid Research Clinics have just finished publishing their data, which are of great concern. For instance, at age 50 or so, the cholesterol data for women are much higher than for men. From the values for high-density lipoprotein cholesterol and also its ratio with low-density lipoprotein cholesterol, we are concerned that certain women have a greater chance for heart disease.

Index

Abortion
 repeated (habitual), 51–62, 91, 92, 113
  abnormal karyotypes in, 51–54
  diethylstilbestrol (DES) related, 55–57
  HLA incompatibilities, 59–60
  incompetent cervix, 55–58
  infection, 60
  psychosocial management of, 60–61
  systemic lupus erythematosus, 58–59, 61
  uterine factors, 54–58, 60–61
 saline-induced, 68, 70
 spontaneous, 51–53, 83, 90, 91, 93, 249, 251
Acetylcholinesterase, marker for neural tube defect, 77
Acne, 119–120, 131, 179, 195
Acrosin, 115
Acrosomal hyaluronidase, 115
ACTH, *see* Corticotropin
Adrenal
 hyperplasia, 127, 130
 hypoplasia, 66–68, 79
 production of androgen, 121–122, 124, 128–130, 133, 173, 180, 194, 196, 266
 production of estrogens, 267
AFP, *see* α-Fetoprotein
Ambiguous genitalia, *see* Genitalia
Amenorrhea, 41, 119, 176, 177, 179, 263–264
Amniocentesis, 60, 79, 251
Amnion, avascular, 69–70

Androgen-binding protein (ABP), 125, 138–140
Androgen excess
 associated conditions
  acne, 119–120, 131, 179, 195
  amenorrhea, 119
  anovulation, 119–121, 131, 177–175
  hirsutism, 119–121, 124, 126–131, 193–195
  luteal dysfunction, 119, 120
  obesity, 120
  polycystic ovary syndrome (PCO), 120–121, 123–125, 129–132, 173–175, 180, 185, 190
 causes of, 126–130
  adrenal hyperplasia, 127, 130
  Cushing's syndrome, 130, 177–178
  enzymic defects, 127–128
  hyperstimulation with gonado-liberin (GnRH), 130
  ovarian hyperandrogenism, 126
 markers for
  3α-androstanediol glucuronide (3α-diol G), 123–125, 130–133
  dehydroepiandrosterone sulfate (DHEA-S), 121–122, 124, 130–133
  sex-hormone-binding globulin (SHBG), 125–127, 132–133
  testosterone, salivary, 125
 treatment of, 129, 132–133
Androgen profile in infertile women, 174
Androgen-receptor blocking, 132–133, 193

Androgen-resistance syndromes, 155–157

Androgens, 10–15, 25, 67, 76, 119–133, 139–147, 151–152, 154–162, 173–175, 177, 179, 180, 194, 195, 203, 221, 257, 262, 264–267
  sources of production of, 121–124, 126–127, 129–133, 173, 174, 180

"Androgen sterilization," 142–143

3α-Androstanediol glucuronide (3α-diol G), 123–125, 130–133, 175, 193, 194

Δ^5-Androstenediol, 128, 129

Androstenedione, 178, 179, 234, 265–267

Anencephaly, 67

Anovulation, 119–121, 131, 172–175

Anterior pituitary, 66–67, 111, 175
  neurohumoral control of, 19–30
  See also Hypothalamic–pituitary

Antibodies to zona pellucida, in infertile women, 115–117

Antinuclear antibodies and habitual abortion, 58–59, 61

Anti-Rh₀D, 110

Antisperm antibodies, 109, 114–115

Antral fluid contents, 3, 6–16, 76, 78
  and follicular size, 11, 15, 78
  androgens, 10, 13
  estrogens, 8–15
  progesterone, 8–15, 76, 78

Arachidonic acid and parturition, 69–73, 79

Arcuate nuclei, 22, 31–33, 36, 37, 41, 268, 270

Aromatase activity in developing follicles, 12–15

Ascorbic acid depletion, ovarian, 31, 85

Autoimmune disease, 110, 114, 178

Autosomal trisomy, 51–52

Azoospermia, 154, 159

Breast cancer, *see* Cancers

Bromocriptine, 184, 196

Calcitonin, 273–274

Calcitrol, 296–297

Calcium, 72, 73, 273–274, 296–297

Cancers, sex-related, x–xi, xvi, 83, 88, 94, 130–132, 262–263, 285, 291, 292, 295–297

Cardiovascular disease, *see* Menopause

Cerclage treatment, 55–58

Cervix, incompetent, 55–58, 185

Chiari–Frommel syndrome, 176

Chorioamnionitis, 58, 60

Choriocarcinoma, 88, 94

Choriogonadotropin
  amino-acid sequence homology with other hormones, 83–84, 111
  human (hCG), x, 6, 10, 42, 79, 83–94, 110–114, 117, 150, 152, 159, 180, 183–184, 196, 206–222, 228–233, 238, 240, 242–243, 246, 249, 254–255
    beta subunit, 42, 83–84, 87–94, 111–114
  in nonpregnancy clinical tests, 94
  in other species, 112–114
  in pregnancy tests, 83–93
  standardization of reference material for, 88–89

Chorion laeve, 69–72

Chromophobe adenomas, 175, 176

Chromosomal abnormalities, 51–54, 145–146, 152–157, 178–179

Cimetidine, 133

Climacteric, *see* Menopause

Clomiphene citrate (Clomid), 15, 40, 78–79, 92, 120, 169, 171, 179, 182–184, 227–234
  use in males, 142, 159

Clonidine, 271, 295

Congenital abnormalities, diethylstilbestrol-related, 55–57

Congenital adrenal hyperplasia, *see* Adrenal

Estrogens (*continued*)
  treatment in menopause, 273–274, 276, 278, 285–293, 295–299
Estrone, 4, 5, 7, 12–14, 22, 173, 174, 267, 297

Fallopian tubes, 6, 12, 16, 109, 114, 157, 172, 178, 185–188, 190, 218
  surgery on, 91, 92, 185, 246–247
Female infertility, *see* Infertility
Fertility regulation, *see* Contraception
Fetal
  adrenal hypoplasia, 66–68
  cortisol production, 66, 68
  initiation of parturition, 66–73
  prolactin, 76
  studies (sheep), 84
  testosterone, 84
  urine and synthesis of prostaglandins, 72–73
α-Fetoprotein, 77
Fetus, anencephalic, 67–68
Fibroids, *see* Leiomyomata
Fluoroimmunoassay pregnancy test, 89, 90
Follicles (ovarian), 3–16, 142, 183–184, 245, 249, 252, 254, 255
  atretic, 3, 7, 12, 15, 120, 173, 174, 261–262, 268
  corpus luteum, 3–6, 29, 84, 93, 182, 184, 215, 250, 254, 264, 267–268
  dominant, 3–6, 228
  estradiol content in luteal phase, 3–6, 29, 228
  follitropin (FSH) in, 12, 13, 15, 245–246
  maturation of, 203, 215, 218, 222, 227–229, 232, 235, 237, 240, 264
  nonovulatory, 7, 9, 13, 263–264
  nonsteroidal markers of maturation, 16
  preovulatory, 4, 6–8, 10, 13, 15, 29
  production of inhibin, 234
  size in relation to hormone concentration in stimulated ovulation, 42, 78, 183–184

Follicular fluid, 231, 233–235, 238, 252, 256
Follitropin (follicle-stimulating hormone, FSH), 10, 12, 13, 15, 20–26, 28, 29, 37–42, 83, 92, 111, 130–132, 137–145, 147, 149–152, 154, 155, 157–162, 174–176, 178–180, 182–183, 194, 197, 202–209, 213–222, 235, 238, 241, 245–246, 254–257, 263–264, 268, 297
  half-life, 38, 221
Forbes–Albright syndrome, 176
FSH, *see* Follitropin

Galactorrhea, 176–177, 179
Gene therapy/counseling, 16, 60, 62, 78, 79
Genetic disorders, *see* Chromosomal abnormalities
Genitalia, ambiguous, 146–147, 153, 157
Glycerophospholipids, amnion and chorion laeve, 70–72, 79
GnRH, *see* Gonadoliberin
Gonadal failure, primary, 40
Gonadoliberin (gonadotropin-releasing hormone, GnRH), 4, 20, 130, 144, 151, 154, 158, 193, 201, 235, 268, 270, 297
  agonist, 121, 123, 218
  antagonist, 202–216
  antigonadotropic contraceptive, 108
  inhibition of, 176
  pulsatile secretion of, 4, 144, 151, 193, 270, 297
  therapy in male infertility, 144, 193
  See also Luliberin (LHRH)
Gonadotrophs, 25–26, 28, 37, 38, 144, 152, 202
Gonadotropins, 4, 15, 22, 26–30, 36–40, 43, 120, 130, 173, 196, 201–207, 209–222, 255, 262, 264, 266, 270
  See also Choriogonadotropin, Lutropin, Follitropin

Granulosa cells, 7, 8, 10, 12–15, 174, 183, 203, 221, 252
ovarian cell cultures of, 12–13
Gynecomastia, 137, 147, 151, 158

Habitual abortion, see Abortion
HAI, see Hemagglutination-inhibition
hCG, see Choriogonadotropin
Hemagglutination-inhibition (HAI) tests for pregnancy, 85–86
Hermaphroditism, 153
High-density lipoprotein (HDL) cholesterol, 286, 299
Hirsutism, 119–121, 124, 126, 131, 193–195, 266
hMG, see Menopausal gonadotropins
Hormone receptors, cell membrane, 87
See also specific hormones
Hyaluronidase, acrosomal, 115
Hybridoma antibodies, 110
17α-Hydroxyprogesterone, 67, 127–130
15-Hydroxyprostaglandin dehydrogenase (PGDH), role in prostaglandin inactivation, 70
Hypergonadotropic patients, 179–180
Hyperprolactinemia, 147, 152, 158, 176–177
Hypertelorism (Noonan's syndrome), 153
Hypertension (pre-elampsia), 52, 58
Hyperthecosis, 266
Hyperthyroidism, 144, 177
Hypogonadism, 38, 43, 140–141, 143–144, 147–155, 158–160, 162, 196, 202, 214, 216, 218–222
Hypophyseal portal circulation, 19–21
Hypophysectomy
"medical" (chemical), 202–204, 210, 219, 222
surgical, 201, 270
Hypothalamic
anenorrhea, 41
mediobasal, see Medial hypothalamus

Hypothalamic (continued)
–pituitary function, 4, 19–25, 28–29, 138, 160, 204, 218, 270
–pituitary–ovarian (HPO) axis, 120, 172, 173, 177, 201–203, 256
Hypothalamus, 19–23, 27, 28, 35, 66, 141–146, 151, 158, 159, 176, 257, 268, 270
Hypothyroidism, 59, 147, 152, 177
Hysterosalpingography (HSG), 60, 186–188

Immunization, active vs passive, 110–111, 116, 117
See also Contraception
Immunoglobulin allotypes, 58, 110
IgG half-life, 110
Immunology of pregnancy, x, 59–60
Impotence, 147, 158–159, 194–195
drug-caused, 158
Infertile couple, evaluation of, 148, 168–191
coordination of surgical treatment of, 172
post-coital test, 169–172, 184, 189
Infertility, female
associated conditions
amenorrhea, 119
hirsutism, 119–121, 124, 126–131, 193–195
luteal dysfunction, 119, 120
obesity, 120
polycystic ovary syndrome (PCO), 120–121, 123–125, 129–132, 173–175, 180, 185, 190
testicular feminization syndrome, 178–179
causes of
androgen excess (hyperandrogenism), 119–132, 172–175
anovulation, 119–121, 131, 172–175
hyperstimulation with luliberin (LHRH), 174
immature hypothalamic-pituitary-ovarian axis, 172, 173
"inadequate luteal phase," 181, 182

In vitro fertilization and embryo replacement (IVF-ER) (continued)
lutropin (LH), 245–246
menopausal gonadotropins (hMG, Pergonal), 227, 229–234, 237–243, 246, 249
pregnancy wastage, 251
sperm capacitation, 252–253
ultrasound monitoring
of developing fetus, 244, 251
of ripening follicle, 227–228, 233

Kallman's syndrome, 41, 43, 151, 219
Kartagener's syndrome, 155
Karyotypes, abnormal, 51–55
Klinefelter's syndrome, 152, 155

Labor, onset of, 66–70, 78
premature, 56–58, 68, 70, 73
See also Parturition
Lactate dehydrogenase (LDH) in sperm, 115
LAI, see Latex-agglutination inhibition
Laparoscopy, 169, 172, 175, 183, 186, 188, 190, 216, 227, 228, 233, 249–250
Latex-agglutination inhibition (LAI) pregnancy tests, 85–86
Laurence–Moon–Biedl syndrome, 151
Leiomyomata, 55–56, 185, 187
Leriche syndrome, with impotence, 159
Leydig cells, 84, 137, 139, 140, 146, 153, 154, 196
LH, see Lutropin
LHRH, see Luliberin
Luliberin (luteinizing-hormone-releasing hormone, LHRH), 20, 22–43, 131, 174
activity separate from FSH-RH, 20, 24
agonists, 28
analog, 27–28, 41
axons, 34

Luliberin (continued)
biosynthesis, 26–27
deficiency, 40
degradation, 26, 27, 36
during ovulation, 4
dynamic testing with, 38–40
effect of calcium on release of, 27
in central nervous system cells, 31–35
in cerebrospinal fluid, 31, 35
injections, 40
in urine, 33
nasal spray administration, 41, 76–77
negative feedback, 28–29
neurons, 33–35
pulsatile release of, 36–38, 40–41
pulsatile treatment with, 78
receptors, 20, 26, 37
structure of, 24
transport of, 27, 35
See also Gonadoliberin
Lupus erythematosus, systemic, 58–59, 61
Lutropin (luteinizing hormone, LH)
bioactivity vs immunoreactivity, 130–132, 152, 254
cross reactivity with tests for other hormones, 83–84, 86–88, 110–116
deficiencies of, 151–152
drug-induced increase, 86
effect on follicular maturation, 29, 245–246
endocrine reproductive system, 137–140
half-life of, 249
inhibition of, 22, 25, 28, 37, 141, 196, 202, 218, 237–238, 246
in hyperprolactinemia, 176, 196
in hypogonadism, 150–152, 154, 155, 157–162, 194, 219–220
in menopause, 268
in polycystic ovary syndrome (PCO), 130–132, 174–175, 179–180
in studies of ovulation induction, 203–204, 206, 208–209, 211–212,